Pocket Paediatrics

To
Amanda, Lucy, Susan and Bethany

For Churchill Livingstone:

Publisher: Georgina Bentliff
Project Editor: Elif Fincanci-Smith
Production Controller: Nancy Henry
Design: Design Resources Unit
Sales Promotion Executive: Hilary Brown

Pocket Paediatrics

Christopher O'Callaghan

B Med Sci BM BS MRCP

Senior Lecturer in Child Health,
University of Leicester;
Honorary Consultant,
Leicester Royal Infirmary,
Leicester

Terence Stephenson

BSc BM BCh MRCP

Senior Lecturer in Child Health,
University of Nottingham;
Honorary Consultant,
Queen's Medical Centre,
Nottingham

CHURCHILL LIVINGSTONE
EDINBURGH LONDON MADRID MELBOURNE NEW YORK
AND TOKYO 1992

CHURCHILL LIVINGSTONE
Medical Division of Longman Group Limited

Distributed in the United States of America by
Churchill Livingstone Inc., 650 Avenue of the Americas,
New York, N.Y. 10011, and by associated companies,
branches and representatives throughout the world.

First published 1992
  Reprinted 1993
  Reprinted 1995

ISBN 0-443-04360-4

British Library Cataloguing in Publication Data
A catalogue record for this book is available from the British Library.

Library of Congress Cataloging in Publication Data
O'Callaghan, Christopher.
    Pocket pediatrics / Chris O'Callaghan, Terence Stephenson.
       p.   cm.
    Includes index.
    ISBN 0-443-04360-4
    1. Pediatrics—Handbooks, manuals, etc.   I. Stephenson, Terence.
    II. Title.
    [DNLM: 1. Pediatrics—handbooks.   WS 39 015p]
RJ48.027 1992
618.92—dc20
DNLM/DLC
for Library of Congress   91–33878
                                                              CIP

Printed in Hong Kong
LYP/03

Preface

Although there are many 'pocket books' dealing with common paediatric problems, none of them is actually pocket-size, particularly as paediatrics is one of the few hospital specialties in which doctors do not wear white coats. As a result of seeing other junior doctors share our own experience of having a pocket stuffed full of aides-memoire and photocopies of relevant charts, we decided to write a truly pocket-sized book that would encapsulate this information. We have not confined ourselves to paediatric emergencies, as it is important to have information to hand in clinic for dealing with problems which are common though not emergencies.

We have written this book with senior house officers and registrars particularly in mind. It will also be useful for community paediatricians in training, general practitioners and, indeed, anyone who encounters children and their problems in the course of their work.

We wish to acknowledge all the help we have had from our many teachers over the years and continue to welcome any suggestions or corrections which would improve the text or format. We have modified our 'in house' protocols in the light of published articles and other textbooks but, in a small book of this size, we have had to be didactic. For many conditions there will be several ways of treating the problem and the solution in any one hospital will sometimes be a matter for style and local experience.

We have made great efforts to check for any mistakes in the text and drug doses, and are grateful to those who have helped to check the manuscript, but any mistakes are our own. If you are in any doubt about a treatment or drug dose, always check this with another formulary or experienced colleague.

Finally, we apologise for the many abbreviations used throughout the text but again this was essential if the size of the book was to conform to the size of modern pockets.

Leicester and   C.O'C.
Nottingham   T.S.
1992

Contents

List of abbreviations ix

1. Introduction 1
2. Resuscitation 2
3. Fluids, electrolytes and acid–base balance 16
4. Nutrition 32
5. Growth 45
6. Development 62
7. Cardiology 79
8. Respiratory medicine 101
9. Gastroenterology 122
10. Renal and urogenital problems 148
11. Endocrine and metabolic problems 168
12. Neurology 185
13. Infectious diseases 208
14. Haematology and oncology 230
15. Poisoning 258
16. Ear, nose and throat problems 269
17. Ophthalmology 281
18. The skin 288
19. Neonatology 299

20.	Child abuse	318
21.	Death	323
22.	Orthopaedics and trauma	329
23.	Burns and heat related problems	338
24.	Surgical problems	344
Appendices		349
	Drug doses	349
	Normal values	362
	Clinical chemistry	362
	Haematology	363
	Blood pressure charts	364
	Surface area nomogram	367
Index		368

List of abbreviations

ACTH	adrenocorticotrophic hormone
ADH	antidiuretic hormone
AFB	acid fast bacilli
ALL	acute lymphoblastic leukaemia
ANA	antinuclear antibodies
ANF	antinuclear factor
ARF	acute renal failure
AS	aortic stenosis
ASD	atrial septal defect
ASOT	antistreptolysin O titre
AST	aspartate glutamine transferase
ATP	alloimmune thrombocytopenic purpura
AV	atrioventricular
AXR	abdominal X-ray
BMstix	rapid blood glucose estimation
BP	blood pressure
BPD	bronchopulmonary dysplasia
CDH	congenital dislocation of the hip
CF	cystic fibrosis
CHD	congenital heart disease
CMV	cytomegalovirus
CNS	central nervous system
CP	cerebral palsy
CPAP	continuous positive airway pressure
CRF	chronic renal failure
CRP	C-reactive protein
CSF	cerebrospinal fluid
CVP	central venous pressure
CXR	chest X-ray
DCT	direct Coombs' test
1,25-DHCC	1,25-dihydroxycholecalciferol
DDAVP	desamino-D-arginine vasopressin
DIC	disseminated intravascular coagulation
DMSA	dimercaptosuccinic acid technetium isotope
2,3-DPG	2,3-diphosphoglycerate
DTPA	diethylene triamine penta acetic acid technetium isotope
EBM	expressed breast milk

ECF	extracellular fluid
ECG	electrocardiogram
ECM	external cardiac massage
EDD	expected date of delivery
EEG	electroencephalogram
ERG	electroretinogram
ESR	erythrocyte sedimentation rate
ETT	endotracheal tube
FBC	full blood count
FDPs	fibrin degradation products
FFA	free fatty acids
FFP	fresh frozen plasma
FiO_2	fractional inspired oxygen concentration
FSH	follicle stimulating hormone
FTT	failure to thrive
GA	general anaesthetic
GBS	group B streptococcal infection
GCS	Glasgow coma scale
GFR	glomerular filtration rate
GH	growth hormone
GI	gastrointestinal
GOR	gastro-oesophageal reflux
G6PD	glucose-6-phosphate dehydrogenase
GVHD	graft versus host disease
Hb	haemoglobin concentration
HbA	adult haemoglobin
HbF	fetal haemoglobin
HbS	haemoglobin found in sickle cell disease
HBsAg	hepatitis B surface antigen
25-HCC	25-hydroxycholecalciferol
HDU	high dependency unit
HIE	hypoxic ischaemic encephalopathy
HIV	human immunodeficiency virus
HOCM	hypertrophic occlusive cardiomyopathy
HSE	herpes simplex encephalitis
HSP	Henoch Schönlein purpura
HUS	haemolytic–uraemic syndrome
HVA	homovanillic acid
ICP	intracranial pressure
ICU	intensive care unit
i.m.	intramuscularly
i.n.	intranasally
INR	International normalised ratio
IPPV	intermittent positive pressure ventilation
IRBBB	incomplete right bundle branch block
ITP	idiopathic thrombocytopenic purpura
IUGR	intrauterine growth retardation
i.v.	intravenously
IVU	intravenous urogram

JCA	juvenile chronic arthritis
JRA	juvenile rheumatoid arthritis
LA	left atrium
LAH	left atrial hypertrophy
LBW	low birthweight (< 2.5 kg)
LFT	liver function tests
LH	luteinising hormone
LHRH	luteinising hormone releasing hormone
LP	lumbar puncture
LSE	left sternal edge
LV	left ventricle
LVH	left ventricular hypertrophy
MAS	meconium aspiration syndrome
M, C & S	microscopy, culture and sensitivity
MCUG	micturating cysto-urethrogram
MCT	medium chain triglycerides
MCV	mean corpuscular volume
MSU	midstream urine
NEC	necrotising enterocolitis
NG	nasogastric
NGT	nasogastric tube
NNU	neonatal unit
NPA	nasopharyngeal aspirate
OFC	occipital–frontal circumference
PA	pulmonary artery
$PaCO_2$	partial pressure of carbon dioxide in arterial blood
PaO_2	partial pressure of oxygen in arterial blood
PDA	patent ductus arteriosus
PEEP	positive end expiratory pressure
PFC	persistent fetal circulation
PGE	prostaglandin E
PGI_2	prostacyclin I
PIE	pulmonary interstitial emphysema
PMN	polymorphonuclear leukocytes (neutrophils)
p.o.	orally
POP	plaster of Paris
PPF	plasma protein fraction
PPT	partial prothrombin time
p.r.	rectally
Preterm	< 37 completed weeks' gestation
PROM	prolonged rupture of membranes (>24 hours)
PS	pulmonary stenosis
PT	prothrombin time
PTH	parathyroid hormone
PTT	partial thromboplastin time
PUJ	pelviureteric junction
PUO	pyrexia of unknown origin
PVH	periventricular haemorrhage
RAD	right axis deviation

RAH	right atrial hypertrophy
RBBB	right bundle branch block
RBC	red blood cell count
RDS	respiratory distress syndrome
RHD	rhesus haemolytic disease
RSV	respiratory syncytial virus
RTA	renal tubular acidosis
RVH	right ventricular hypertrophy
SBE	subacute bacterial endocarditis
SBR	serum bilirubin
SG	specific gravity
SGA	small for gestational age (birthweight < 10th centile)
SCG	sodium chromoglycate
SIADH	syndrome of inappropriate antidiuretic hormone secretion
SIDS	sudden infant death syndrome
s.l.	sublingually
SLE	systemic lupus erythematosus
SPA	suprapubic aspiration of urine
SR	sinus rhythm
SVC	superior vena cava
SVT	supraventricular tachycardia
SXR	skull X-ray
T_3	tri-iodothyronine
T_4	thyroxine
TAPVD	total anomalous pulmonary venous drainage
TB	tuberculosis
$TcPO_2$	transcutaneous oxygen tension
TGA	transposition of the great arteries
TORCH	toxoplasmosis, rubella, cytomegalovirus, herpes & hepatitis B
TRH	thyrotrophin releasing hormone
TSH	thyroid stimulating hormone
TPN	total parenteral nutrition
TT	thrombin time
TTN	transient tachypnoea of the newborn
UAC	umbilical arterial catheter
U & E	urea and electrolytes
URTI	upper respiratory tract infection
USS	ultrasound scan
UTI	urinary tract infection
UVC	umbilical vein catheter
VLBW	very low birthweight (< 1.5 kg)
VMA	vanillyl mandelic acid
VP	ventriculo-peritoneal
VSD	ventricular septal defect
VUJ	vesicoureteric junction
VUR	vesicoureteric reflux
WBC	white blood cell count
WPWS	Wolff Parkinson White syndrome

1

Introduction

The first rule of this book is if in doubt, ask. This book is effectively 'get you by in paediatrics' until you can consult a more senior colleague. Because of the constraints on space available, we have tended to be didactic. We would not wish to suggest that the management recommended in this book for a problem represents the only or perfect way to treat that condition but simply this is one way of doing it which is tried and tested. Every hospital is different and the management strategies recommended in this small book should not be followed slavishly if your own local practice dictates otherwise or if the clinical condition is atypical compared with that described in the text. The management strategies recommended are based on protocols which have been drafted for use in the Nottingham hospitals and have continually been up-dated to incorporate changing fashions and new drugs.

If you encounter a problem which is not covered, you should not forget the simple rubric of taking history, examining the child, forming a differential diagnosis and performing the simple investigations first. If you are still unclear as to the nature of the problem, advice should be sought from a senior colleague after this initial assessment.

In an emergency, it is very easy to lose sight of the parents, so try to think of them as well as the child.

Again, because of the constraints of space, the text referring to less urgent or common problems has been reduced to a small font size. Finally, all drug doses have been given in an appendix and also in the text where the information may be needed urgently.

Resuscitation

1. Respiratory arrest is common.
2. Cardiac arrest is often secondary to respiratory arrest.
3. Commonest of all is the child who has not yet arrested but is clearly moribund with shallow, irregular breathing, feeble pulse and decreased conscious level. In all three situations (Table 2.1) the initial management is identical (see Ch. 8 for the management of severe upper airway obstruction).

Initial assessment and management

1. Note the time.
2. Keep the child warm: hypothermia is detrimental to resuscitation.

A. AIRWAY

1. Clear the child's mouth and pharynx using a wide-bore catheter ('Yankauer' paediatric size, suction pressure of 20–30 kPa). Aspirate the nasal passages.

Table 2.1 Common causes of cardiorespiratory arrest

Respiratory	Choking on foreign body or secretions
	Inhalation of vomit
	Croup or epiglottitis
	'Near miss' SIDS
	Asthma
	Following general anaesthesia
	Drowning
Neurological	Meningitis
	Serious head injury
	Seizures
	Muscle weakness
Cardiac	Arrhythmias during or after cardiac surgery or catheterisation
	Electrolyte imbalance
Other	Septicaemia
	Poisoning

2. If breathing remains obstructed despite this, inspect the oropharynx directly, using Magill's forceps to remove any foreign body (neonatal straight-blade laryngoscope for any child < 1 year, larger curved blade for an older child). If there is a definite history of aspiration of a foreign body, and this is not obvious on direct inspection, invert a small child and smack him on the back, or apply the Heimlich manoeuvre (a brisk 'bear hug') to an older child.

3. If the child is breathing but unconscious and unable to protect his airway, insert an oropharyngeal airway (Table 2.2).

4. If the child is not breathing and you are confident and have intubated a child before, insert an ETT (see below). If not, make do with an oropharyngeal airway and commence mask ventilation (see below).

5. If breathing remains critically obstructed despite the above measures, and you are unable to insert an ETT, an emergency tracheostomy is necessary. The safest emergency access is through the cricothyroid membrane, the transverse rut immediately below the Adam's apple. A scalpel should be inserted at this relatively avascular site and rotated and then a neonatal ETT inserted. Alternatively, insert one or more large-bore intravenous cannulae or a minitracheostomy tube at this site.

B. BREATHING

1. Give O_2 by mask (6 l/min) as soon as the airway has been cleared.

2. If cyanosis persists despite O_2 and clearing of the airway, there are three options:

a. Mouth-to-mouth breathing
This should only be used until the facilities for (b) or (c) (below) are available.

b. Mask ventilation (Table 2.3)
For both (a) and (b) the principles are the same:
(i) Insert an oropharyngeal airway.
(ii) Slightly extend the child's neck and hold the angle of the jaw forward with your left hand.

Table 2.2 Guedel airway sizes

Age	Size
Newborn to 6 months	000
6–18 months	00
18 months to 3 years	0
3–9 years	1
> 9 years	2

Table 2.3 Laerdal mask sizes

Age	Laerdal mask size
Premature infant	00
Term infant to 2 years	0/1
3–8 years	0/2

(iii) Either by using your own exhalation or by squeezing the 'ambubag', inflate the child's lungs at 30 breaths/min.

If the child does not become pink within 1 min of commencing either of these techniques, ensure that:
— The airway is definitely not obstructed.
— There is a good seal between your mouth or mask and the child's mouth. Pinch the child's nose or, in a younger child, cover the mouth and nose with your mouth or mask.
— The child's chest rises 1–2 cm with each inflation. This is the best evidence that an adequate tidal volume (10 ml/kg) is being given.

If an O_2 supply is available, this is connected to the inlet port of the 'ambubag' at 4 l/min.

c. Intubation and IPPV (Table 2.4)

(i) Clear the mouth and pharynx with suction.
(ii) Slightly extend the child's neck.
(iii) Holding the laryngoscope with your left hand, slide the blade down the right side of the mouth until the tip of the blade is in the groove between tongue and epiglottis.
(iv) Lift the blade to push the tongue away from you. This may require more effort than you anticipate as muscle relaxants should only be given by an anaesthetist.
(v) Only insert the ETT if the vocal cords have been visualised. The commonest error is to insert the laryngoscope blade too far so that the tip is beyond the epiglottis and you are looking at the oesophagus.

Table 2.4 Endotracheal tube sizes

Age (years)	Tube diameter (mm)	Length* (cm)	Appropriate suction catheter (French gauge)
Newborn	3	12	6
1	4	13	8
3	4.5	14.5	8
6	5	17	10
8	6	19	10
10	7	20	12
14	8	22	12

*The length recommended is from the lips to the midtrachea.

(vi) Insert the tip of the ETT 2 cm beyond the cords, connect the 'ambubag' to the ETT and inflate the chest at 30 breaths/min. Do not let go of the ETT at any time.

(vii) The vocal cords must be visualised. It is better to revert to mask ventilation than to attempt a blind intubation.

(viii) If breath sounds are louder on the right side, the ETT may be too far down. However, louder breath sounds on the right may also occur with
— foreign body in the left main bronchus
— left pneumothorax
— left-sided pneumonia

Consider these before withdrawing the ETT too far and, if the child becomes pink anyway, wait for more experienced help.

(ix) If the chest does not rise with inflation, aspirate the ETT. If the chest still does not move, remove the ETT and revert to mask ventilation as the ETT is probably in the oesophagus. Auscultating over the chest and stomach is not a reliable indicator of ETT position; chest inflation is.

C. CIRCULATION

Shock equals pallor, tachycardia (Table 2.5) and a feeble peripheral pulse, irrespective of cause. The central BP may be normal or low (see Figs A.1–A.3, pp 364–366).

As a rough guide: term infant = 75/40

after 1 year of life, systolic = 90 + age (in years)
diastolic = 55 + age (in years)

The normal range of readings is approximately ± 20% from the above mean values.

Shock may be due to inadequate vascular tone, inadequate intravascular volume or inadequate cardiac output.

1. Septicaemia is the commonest cause of shock in a child previously thought to have a normal heart and with no history to suggest excessive volume losses. Anaphylaxis is another possibility.

2. Intravascular volume may be inadequate because of:
   a. haemorrhage
   b. GI loss

Table 2.5 Normal resting heart rates

Age	Heart rate (beats/min)
1 week	100–190
1 month	70–170
1 year	80–160
6 years	75–115
12 years	65–110
16 years	55–100

    c. renal losses, including diabetic ketoacidosis
    d. hypoadrenalism
    e. severe burns
3. The cardiac output may be inadequate because of:
    a. heart failure
    b. arrhythmia
    c. outflow obstruction (including pericardial tamponade and
        tension pneumothorax)

The latter three are most likely in a child with CHD or one who
has recently had cardiac surgery. They are rare in previously
healthy children, in whom the cause is more likely to be hypovolaemia or infection.

Assessment and immediate management
1. Provided the child has not previously had cardiac catheterisa-
    tion, the best site for palpating the pulse is the right brachial
    artery (the femoral pulses will be absent in undiagnosed
    coarctation).
2. The presence of heart sounds on auscultation is irrelevant if the
    pulses are not palpable.
3. The initial resuscitation of the shocked child is the same irre-
    spective of the underlying cause. If the brachial pulse is absent,
    slow (see Table 2.5) or feeble, start ECM.

Cardiac massage. Lie the child supine on a hard surface and, for
an older child, use the heel of your hand to compress the lower
sternum towards the spine by 2 cm at the rate of 80/min. In a
toddler or baby, place both hands under the child's back and
use both thumbs to compress the sternum. Adequacy of cardiac
massage is gauged by the presence of a palpable brachial pulse.

Venous access.
a. Insert a cannula and start to infuse 15 ml/kg plasma (4%

Table 2.6 Approximate weight and surface area (50th centile)

Age	Weight* (kg)	Surface area* (m²)
Newborn	3	0.2
6 months	7	0.35
1 year	10	0.4
3 years	15	0.6
6 years	20	0.8
8 years	25	0.9
10 years	30	1.0
13 years	40	1.4
14 years	50	1.5

* These figures have been rounded to reduce the likelihood of errors in
calculating drug doses.

human albumin solution) over 15–30 min or, if this is not available, 0.9% saline. If the shock is severe and obviously due to haemorrhage, give O negative uncrossmatched blood 15 ml/kg. (See Table 2.6 for approximate body weights at different ages.) A large-bore cannula is preferable but a 24G cannula in a baby is better than none at all.

b. If a second cannula can be inserted, give 1 mmol/kg (1 ml/kg 8.4% solution) NaHCO$_3$ i.v. to all children receiving ECM.

c. If peripheral venous access cannot be obtained, and you are reluctant to attempt central venous catheterisation (the easiest site for the inexperienced is the femoral vein which is immediately medial to the femoral pulse), then:

   (i) Hypovolaemia can be ameliorated by giving 10 ml/kg 0.9% saline into the peritoneal cavity (insert a 19G cannula through the abdominal wall of the right lower quadrant and remove the stylet) or via the marrowspace of the tibia (use a large-bore spinal needle).

   (ii) Arrhythmias can be treated (see Tables 2.6 and 2.7) by giving atropine, adrenaline or lignocaine down the ETT (but not Ca^{2+} or HCO$_3^-$). Endotracheal administration is safer than intracardiac administration which may cause pneumothorax or pericardial tamponade.

Electrocardiogram (ECG). Attach ECG leads to the right upper chest, left upper chest and left abdomen, or monitor the ECG from the defibrillator paddles. ECM may have to be stopped briefly to observe the ECG.

a. If there is *sinus rhythm but no palpable pulse* (electrome-chanical dissociation) and the child has no cardiac history, the problem is usually hypovolaemia.

b. If there is *sinus rhythm but the child has a cardiac anomaly* or recent thoracotomy, the problem may be:
   (i) heart failure
   (ii) pericardial tamponade
   If the child was receiving IPPV prior to the arrest, consider:
   (iii) pneumothorax or pneumopericardium

c. *Sinus bradycardia.* Give atropine (0.02 mg/kg = 0.03 ml/kg of a 0.6 mg/ml solution) i.v. (paediatric resuscitation drug doses are small volumes and need to be followed by a saline flush to ensure the whole dose is given) or via the ETT.

d. *Asystole.* Check that the electrodes are attached to the child and that the leads are attached to the monitor.
   Give adrenaline (0.01 mg/kg = 0.1 ml/kg of 1 : 10 000 solution) i.v. or via ETT and calcium gluconate (0.2 ml/kg of 10% calcium gluconate) i.v. These doses can be repeated at 2-min intervals until either sinus rhythm or ventricular fibril-lation occurs. Fibrillation is then managed as below.

e. *Ventricular fibrillation* (Table 2.8). Exclude electrical or mechanical interference as the cause of the irregular trace.

Table 2.7 Emergency drug doses

Drug	Usual concentration	Route	Dose
1 : 10 000 Adrenaline	0.1 mg/ml	i.v./ETT*	0.01 mg/kg = 0.1 ml/kg (minimum total dose 0.5 ml)
1 : 1000 Adrenaline	1.0 mg/ml	i.v./ETT*	0.01 mg/kg = 0.01 ml/kg
Aminophylline	25 mg/ml	i.v.	5 mg kg = 0.2 ml/kg over 20 min, assuming no theophylline in last 24 hours
Adenosine		i.v.	0.05–0.3 mg/kg (see text)
Atropine	0.6 mg/ml	i.v./i.m./ETT*	0.02 mg/kg = 0.03 ml/kg
4.2% NaHCO₃	0.5 mmol/ml	i.v.	1 mmol/kg = 2 ml/kg
8.5% NaHCO₃	1 mmol/ml	i.v.	1 mmol/kg = 1 ml/kg (0.04 mmol Ca²⁺/kg)
10% Calcium gluconate	100 mg/ml (0.225 mmol Ca²⁺/ml)	i.v.	20 mg/kg = 0.2 ml/kg (minimum total dose 0.5 ml)
Diazepam	5 mg/ml	i.v./i.m./p.r.	0.25 mg/kg = 0.05 ml/kg slowly May be repeated after 5 min
Flecainide	10 mg/ml	i.v.	2 mg/kg over 15 min
Frusemide	10 mg/ml	i.v.	1 mg/kg = 0.1 ml/kg
Glucagon	1 mg/ml	i.m.	0.02 mg/kg = 0.02 ml/kg
25% Glucose	0.25 g/ml	i.v.	0.5 g/kg = 2 ml/kg
Hydrocortisone	100 mg/ml	i.v./i.m.	4 mg/kg = 0.04 ml/kg
2% Lignocaine	20 mg/ml	i.v./ETT*	1 mg/kg = 0.05 ml/kg
20% Mannitol	0.2 g/ml	i.v.	1 g/kg = 5 ml/kg over 30 min
Naloxone (adult prep)	0.4 mg/ml	i.v./i.m.	0.01 mg/kg = 0.025 ml/kg
Naloxone (infant prep)	0.01 mg/ml	i.v./i.m.	0.01 mg/kg = 1 ml/kg
Paraldehyde		p.r.	0.3 ml/kg diluted 1 : 1 with arachis oil
Phenytoin	50 mg/ml	i.v.	10 mg/kg = 0.2 ml/kg over 20 min

— Defibrillate with DC cardioversion (2 J/kg).
— Paediatric paddles (4.5 cm) pressed firmly onto conducting gel pads below the right clavicle and over the apex are preferred.
— If gel pads are not available, smear electrode jelly over the paddles rather than on the child's chest (to prevent current arc across the chest surface).

If defibrillation is not effective, follow the sequence in Table 2.8. If asystole follows defibrillation, continue basic life support for 1 min before resorting to drugs to induce fibrillation again (see (d) above). Then repeat the sequence in Table 2.8.

f. *Ventricular tachycardia.* Defibrillate as above (this is also effective in supraventricular tachycardia with aberrant conduction, which may be difficult to distinguish, so no harm is done).

Give lignocaine (1 mg/kg = 0.05 ml/kg of 2% solution) i.v.

g. *Supraventricular tachycardia.* SVT rarely presents as a cardiorespiratory arrest but it is the commonest tachyarrhythmia in childhood and may result in acute and severe cardiac failure with pallor, a rapid feeble pulse and hypotension, and breathlessness. Vagal stimulation is rarely effective in these circumstances and the treatment of choice is:

Table 2.8 Defibrillation

---

1. Basic life support — airway
                       — breathing: hyperventilate to correct acidosis and hypoxia
                       — external cardiac massage
2. Defibrillate (2 J/kg)
3. If still no pulse, restart ECM and ventilation and recharge defibrillator. After 15 chest compressions, stop ECM and read ECG.
   If still in ventricular fibrillation:
4. Defibrillate (2 J/kg)
   As for 3.
5. Defibrillate (4 J/kg)
   As for 3.
6. Give lignocaine (1 mg/kg = 0.05 ml/kg of 2% solution) i.v. and flush, or via ETT.
7. Defibrillate (4 J/kg)
   As for 3.
8. Give adrenaline (0.01 mg/kg = 0.1 ml/kg of 1 : 10 000 solution) i.v. and flush or via ETT.
   As for 3.
9. Defibrillate (4 J/kg)
   As for 3.
10. Give NaHCO₃ (1 mmol/kg = 1 ml/kg 8.4% solution) i.v.
    As for 3.
11. Defibrillate (4 J/kg)
    See 'when to stop', p. 15

(i) Adenosine: 0.05 mg/kg by rapid i.v. bolus. Repeat at 2-min intervals and increase dose by 0.05 mg/kg each time until effective or maximum dose of 0.3 mg/kg is reached.

(ii) Flecainide i.v: 2 mg/kg over 15 min.

(iii) DC cardioversion as for ventricular fibrillation (Table 2.8) but with the defibrillator set to 'synchronous' trigger. Give O_2 by mask and diazepam (0.25 mg/kg = 0.05 ml/kg of the 5 mg/ml diazemuls solution) i.v. slowly. DC cardioversion is more dangerous if the child has had digoxin.

Subsequent management

Once initial resuscitation has been undertaken and the child stabilised, obtain a full history. Do not overlook the possibility of drug ingestion. Pass NGT and aspirate the stomach, checking for any blood or tablets.

BASELINE ASSESSMENT

Document the following as soon as basic life support has been initiated:

1. Vital signs:
   a. pulse
   b. respiratory rate
   c. arterial blood pressure
   d. deep rectal temperature
   e. presence of cyanosis

2. Consciousness level. The GCS should be used (Table 2.9).

3. Muscle tone — increased
   — decreased
   — asymmetrical

4. Reflexes
   a. pupillary light reflex
   b. Doll's eyes reflexes
   c. gag reflex, if not already intubated
   d. deep tendon reflexes — brisk
      — absent
      — asymmetrical
   e. plantar reflexes

   Abnormalities of deep tendon and plantar reflexes are difficult to interpret after epileptic fits.

5. Auscultate the heart and chest and palpate the abdomen for generalised distension or organomegaly. Pneumothorax and ruptured viscus may occur after major trauma.

6. Look for obvious limb fractures. Blood at the urethral meatus or a palpable bladder suggests pelvic fractures. If the child is a victim of major trauma, avoid moving the neck and stabilise with a collar.

Table 2.9 Glasgow Coma Scale

Eye opening	1 = None
	2 = To pain
	3 = To speech
	4 = Spontaneous
Best motor response	1 = None
	2 = Extensor response to pain
	3 = Abnormal flexion to pain
	4 = Withdraws from pain
	5 = Localises pain
	6 = Obeys command
Best verbal response	1 = None
	2 = Incomprehensible sounds
	3 = Inappropriate words
	4 = Appropriate words but confused
	5 = Fully orientated

Notes:
1. Maximum score = 15.
    Score ≤ 8 is serious — admit to ICU.
2. Spontaneous extensor posturing (decerebrate) scores 2 and spontaneous flexor posturing (decorticate) scores 3 on the motor scale.

Modification of verbal response score for younger children:

2 – 5 years	< 2 years
1 = None	1 = None
2 = Grunts	2 = Grunts
3 = Cries or screams	3 = Inappropriate crying or unstimulated screaming
4 = Monosyllables	4 = Cries only
5 = Words of any sort	5 = Appropriate non-verbal responses (smiles, coos, cries)

INITIAL INVESTIGATIONS

Most of these can wait until the child has been transferred to ICU.

1. Whole blood glucose should be measured as soon as practical during resuscitation, by heel prick if venous access is impossible. Reflomat < 2.0 mmol/1: give 25% dextrose 2 ml/kg i.v. bolus and start dextrose (5%) infusion.
2. Plasma Na^+, K^+ and urea.
3. Plasma Ca^{2+} if there are seizures or arryhthmias.
4. WBC and platelet count.
5. Clotting studies (see Ch. 14) if there is purpura, haematemesis or malaena, known liver disease or known coagulopathy.
6. Blood cultures.
7. Save an extra aliquot of blood for further investigations which may not be available immediately.
    — Plasma (heparinised sample) for NH_3, LFTs, creatinine and toxicology.
    — Serum (clotted sample) for crossmatch or acute viral titres.

8. Attach a urine bag:
   a. to assess whether urine is being passed;
   b. to obtain a specimen for microscopy and culture;
   c. to save urine; a toxicology or metabolic screen may be relevant subsequently.
9. CXR; all children who require resuscitation should have a CXR which includes the neck and upper abdomen to look for:
   a. pneumothorax, pneumomediastinum and pneumopericardium;
   b. rib fractures or haemothorax;
   c. consolidation or collapse suggesting infection or foreign body;
   d. abnormal cardiac shadow or pulmonary oedema;
   e. free gas under the diaphragm suggesting perforated viscus;
   f. position of ETT, central lines and NGT. Ideally, the tip of the ETT should be halfway between the tips of the clavicles and the carina.
10. Cervical spine X-rays should be taken before the child is moved. X-rays for other fractures, including skull fractures, rarely influence immediate management.
11. Arterial blood gas; if the child is pink (whether breathing spontaneously or being ventilated) and already receiving $NaHCO_3$, blood gases will not alter immediate management. Placement of an arterial catheter is easier when a normal pulse volume has been restored.
12. LP; this depends on the age of the child, the previous history, the clinical picture, and the possibility of raised ICP. Papilloedema is a late sign of raised ICP. A normal peripheral WBC and the absence of fever do *not* exclude the need for LP.

POST-RESUSCITATION CARE

The management of specific causes of arrest are discussed elsewhere.

TRANSFER OF THE CHILD

All children who have required resuscitation should be admitted to an ICU or the high dependency area of a ward. *Before transfer* ensure that the child is accompanied by:
a. enough trained personnel to carry out resuscitation again in transit;
b. a working suction system and appropriate suction catheter;
c. a generous O_2 supply which has already been turned on;
d. an ECG monitor and defibrillator;
e. an intact supply of drugs for resuscitation;
f. a working laryngoscope and ETT of the appropriate size, a bag-and-mask ventilation system, and the means of connecting

either of these to the O_2 supply.

Keep the child warm during transit.

MONITORING

In the ICU, monitoring may include:

a. Apnoea alarm.
b. ECG monitor.
c. Saturation monitor (pulse oximetry) if added inspired O_2 is required.
d. Intra-arterial cannula if ventilation is required. If this is unsuccessful, capillary blood gases can be used in conjunction with pulse oximetry. Transcutaneous O_2 electrodes are unreliable beyond the neonatal period.
e. Urine output. Urinary catheterisation should not be necessary routinely.
f. Regular recording of:
   (i) pulse
   (ii) respiratory rate
   (iii) BP
   (iv) core temperature
   (v) consciousness level
   (vi) pupillary size and reflexes

Placement of a central venous catheter should be considered early as reliable venous access is crucial and repeated blood sampling may be necessary. Regular NG aspiration, mouth and eye care, and frequent turning are essential for the unconscious or paralysed child.

Supportive management

HYPOTENSION

If sinus rhythm has been restored and the circulating volume is normal or elevated (ideally the CVP should be measured to be >4 cm above the sternal angle), but the BP remains below the 5th centile for age (see Figs A.1–A.3, pp 364–366), start an i.v. infusion of dopamine or dobutamine at 5 µg/kg/min. This may gradually be increased to 15 µg/kg/min but may adversely affect renal function at higher doses.

CEREBRAL OEDEMA

This is common after a period of anoxia. Raised ICP should be treated if symptomatic (seizures, hypertension and bradycardia, apnoea). If there is any suspicion that the cause is bleeding, abscess, tumour or hydrocephalus, a CT scan must be arranged urgently.

1. Hyperventilation ($PaCO_2$ 3.2–3.5 kPa) will decrease raised ICP by decreasing cerebral blood flow.
2. Low arterial BP and high CVP (especially with CPAP or PEEP) decrease cerebral perfusion pressure.
3. Mannitol 5 ml/kg of 20% mannitol (1 g/kg) i.v. over 30 min will transiently decrease ICP provided the kidneys are making urine. If renal failure is suspected, 2.5 ml/kg of 20% mannitol can be given.
4. Dexamethasone 0.5 mg/kg i.v. may help transiently if the raised ICP is due to a tumour.

SEIZURES

Treat as for status epilepticus (see Ch. 12) but if the child is already ventilated, max. doses of anticonvulsants should be given sooner than later. A cerebral function monitor (continuous EEG analyser) is necessary to detect seizures in a paralysed child. Seizures may be manifest in a sedated child by periods of
a. tachycardia
b. apnoea or cyanosis
c. eye flickering
d. grimacing or mouthing

Drowning

Basic life support must be given as above but there are particular problems. Try to ascertain:
1. Duration of immersion; the heart may be restarted even after 2 hours under water.
2. Fresh/salt water; hyponatraemia (see p. 23) and red cell haemolysis are more likely with fresh water. Hypokalaemia (see p. 25) can occur after both.
3. Water temperature; hypothermia has a protective effect although it may itself induce resistant ventricular fibrillation.
4. Initial neurological and cardiorespiratory status and any change since resuscitation commenced.
5. The length of time resuscitation has already been given. Particular pitfalls in resuscitation after drowning are:
   a. Difficulty of clearing the airway of water, criteria for intubation are as for basic resuscitation but suction should be repeated frequently.
   b. Concealed trauma to head or neck.
   c. Resuscitation should be continued for up to 1 hour and until the core temperature is above 35°C.
   d. If resuscitation is successful, progressive hypoxia may occur due to pulmonary oedema. A common response is to give diuretics but the treatment of choice is to ventilate

with PEEP (up to 20 cmH$_2$O) and expand the plasma
volume with colloid to maintain an adequate cardiac output despite this high level PEEP.

e. Pneumonia is common, particularly if the water was
polluted or the child vomited, and the pathogens may
be unusual. Tracheal swabs and blood cultures should be
taken before antibiotics are given.

f. Rapid rewarming is undesirable and may cause hypotension. Icepacks may be required to limit the rate to
1°C/h.

The prognosis is worst with:
1. low or deteriorating GC score
2. raised ICP
3. flat EEG
4. other organ failure

When to stop resuscitation

1. Young infants are often brought to casualty with SIDS but
with resuscitation still being attempted. If there is already
fixed staining of the skin and rigor mortis, resuscitation should
be discontinued (see Ch. 21).

2. Fixed dilated pupils do not warrant cessation of resuscitation
per se. Pupillary size can be influenced by raised ICP, drugs
and electrolyte imbalance, all of which are reversible.

3. If there is no cardiac output after 30 min, resuscitation should
be stopped, unless:
   a. the core temperature is < 35°C
   b. electrolytes remain very abnormal
   c. there is a definite history of drug ingestion

The shorter the delay before the start of basic life support, the more
likely resuscitation is to be successful. Duration of initial resuscitation and eventual outcome are not related. If resuscitation is
unsuccessful, see Ch. 21 for further investigations, counselling the
parents, and the role of the coroner.

3

Fluids, electrolytes and acid–base balance

Fluids

Dehydration

CAUSES

— The commonest cause is diarrhoea and/or vomiting.
— Rare but important causes include diabetic ketoacidosis, diabetes insipidus, adrenal insufficiency and heatstroke.

ASSESSMENT

Three patterns are recognised:
— hypotonic: serum Na^+ < 130 mmol/l
— isotonic: serum Na^+ 130–150 mmol/l
— hypertonic: serum Na^+ > 150 mmol/l

CLINICAL FEATURES (see Table 3.1)

Beware of hypertonic dehydration, where there is mainly intracellular dehydration while ECF volume is relatively well maintained. Therefore, clinical features are different. Skin may

Table 3.1 Estimation of dehydration

Degree of dehydration	Symptoms
Mild (i.e. the child has lost 5% of his/her bodyweight)	Thirsty, alert, restless
Moderate (wt loss = 6–9%)	Irritable, increased thirst, dry mucous membranes, fontanelle and eyes may be sunken, reduce tissue elasticity, peripheral vasoconstriction, tachycardia, absent tears, decreased urine output
Severe (wt loss = ≥10%)	Severe shock, moribund, absent tears, hyperirritable to lethargic, low BP

have a doughy feel, eyes may be normal and fontanelle not sunken (may feel full). Irritability, muscle hypertonicity and convulsions may occur.

MANAGEMENT

Initial investigations

Take blood for Na^+, K^+, urea, osmolality and blood sugar.

Monitoring therapy

Fluid and electrolyte replacement is based on estimations of deficits and ongoing maintenance requirements. Assess the child and monitor biochemistry frequently.

Monitor:
1. pulse and BP.
2. serum — Na^+, K^+, urea, creatinine and osmolality (Ca^{2+} and glucose if required)
3. urine — Na^+, K^+, urea and osmolality
4. total input and output of fluids (and electrolytes if necessary) preferably by flow sheet
5. accurate monitoring of weight change with therapy can be very helpful

Indicators of decreased vascular volume (and ECF) may include:
1. tachycardia, decreased BP, decreased CVP, increased respiratory rate
2. decreased peripheral perfusion
3. metabolic acidosis
4. increased haematocrit, increased serum osmolality
5. increased blood urea and creatinine
6. decreased urine output, increased urine osmolality

These variables are seen to revert towards normal with appropriate rehydration and management.

Does the child need hospital admission?

>5% dehydration and/or the need for i.v. fluids suggest admission. Other factors, such as social, failure of outpatient management, and the differential diagnoses should be considered.

Oral or intravenous fluids?

All children with ≥10% dehydration need parenteral fluids. Children with <10% dehydration may be offered a trial of oral fluids while observed in hospital. Give small, regular volumes of an isotonic glucose/electrolyte solution (e.g. Dioralyte). If not adequate/possible give fluids i.v.

Intravenous therapy

Shock. Common to all 3 types of dehydration. If present, the child requires urgent rehydration. Give 10–20 ml/kg PPF or 0.9% saline over the first 30–60 min. This is discussed in Ch. 2, p. 5.

Table 3.2   Maintenance fluid and electrolyte requirements (mmol/kg per 24 hours)

Body weight	ml fluid/24 h	Na+	K+
<10 kg	100–120/kg	2.5–3.5	2.5–3.5
10–30 kg	60–90/kg	2.0–2.5	2.0–2.5
>30 kg	40–90/kg	2.0	2.0

Most conveniently given as 0.18% NaCl and 4% dextrose solution with added KCl.
This does not give sufficient calories but will prevent ketosis.

Maintenance requirements. These are required in addition to fluids needed for correction of dehydration. Body fluid requirements correlate best with body surface area for children > 10 kg (see Table A.3 (p. 367) for surface area calculation). Normal water requirement is about 1500 ml/m^2 per 24 hours. However, for rapid calculation a general rule for maintenance fluid is:

  100 ml/kg for the first 10 kg bodyweight
  50 ml/kg for the next 10 kg bodyweight
  20 ml/kg for the weight above 20 kg

  Example. A 30-kg child requires:
  100 ml/kg × 10 kg = 1000 ml for the first 10 kg
  50 ml/kg × 10 kg = 500 ml for the next 10 kg
  20 ml/kg × 10 kg = 200 ml for the last 10 kg
  This gives a total of 1700 ml per 24 hours

NB. Fever — increase fluids (i.e. H$_2$O) by 12% for each °C rise in temperature.
Hypothermia — decrease fluids (i.e. H$_2$O) by 12% for each °C reduction in temperature.
Appropriate maintenance fluid and electrolyte requirements based on weight are shown in Table 3.2 and types of intravenous fluids are shown in Table 3.3.

HYPOTONIC DEHYDRATION (Na+ <130mmol/l)

— Circulatory compromise appears early.
— Usually occurs when enteric losses are replaced with low solute fluids (e.g. water).

Table 3.3   Types of intravenous fluids

	Na+ (mmol/l)	Cl− (mmol/l)	K+ (mmol/l)	Glucose (g/100 ml)
0.9% saline	156	156	—	—
0.45% saline + 5% dextrose	78	78	—	5
0.18% saline + 4% dextrose	30	30	—	4
5% dextrose	—	—	—	5

— Seizures are uncommon, even with marked hyponatraemia.
  Lethargy is common.

Management

1. Fluid for resuscitation if required (e.g. 10–20 ml/kg plasma).
2. Fluids after resuscitation
   a. Calculate or estimate the total fluid deficit and electrolyte
      deficit. Subtract the amount given during resuscitation.
   b. If asymptomatic, give half of the remaining deficit and
      maintenance fluids and electrolytes in the first 8 hours and
      the other half over 16 hours.
   c. Estimate continuing losses e.g. vomitus or diarrhoea, and
      replace (for electrolyte contents see Table 3.4).
      Example. A 10-kg child with 10% dehydration has a serum
      Na$^+$ of 120 mmol/l and no ongoing fluid loss.
      1. Fluid requirements:
               Total volume needed to replace deficit = 10% of 10
               kg = 1 litre
               Maintenance fluid = 100 ml/kg × 10 = 1 litre
               Ongoing loss = nil
               Total volume needed over 24 hours = 2 litres
      2. Sodium requirements (deficit):
      The total exchangeable pool of Na$^+$ is approximately 0.6 l/kg
      (60%) of bodyweight. Thus the amount of Na$^+$ needed to
      restore the plasma concentration to normal (135 mmol/l) in a
      depleted patient can be calculated from the formula:
      a. Total body (Na$^+$ deficit) = 0.6 × bodyweight (in kg) ×
         (135–current serum Na$^+$) + fluid loss (in litres) × current
         serum Na$^+$ concentration (per litre).
               Na$^+$ deficit = 0.6 × 10 × 15 + 1 litre × 120
                             = 90 + 120
                             = 210 mmol of Na$^+$
      b. Maintenance = 2 mmol/kg per 24 hours = 20 mmol
         Total Na$^+$ in 24 hours = 230 mmol
      Therefore 2 litres of fluid are required containing total of
      approximately 230 mmol Na$^+$ in 24 hours (115 mmol Na$^+$/l).

In practice, the 2 litres and Na$^+$ may be given:
1. As 0.9% saline (156 mmol/l) or plasma to correct shock (e.g.
   10–20 ml/kg) and then change to,
2. 0.45 saline + 4% dextrose (Na$^+$ = 80 mmol/l); if shock is not
   present omit step 1.

NB. Add KCl to fluids as soon as the child has passed urine
(maintenance dose = 2.5 mmol/kg per 24 hours (provided
hyperkalaemia is not present).
   Metabolic acidosis is a common accompaniment due to
peripheral circulatory shutdown and intestinal loss of HCO$_3^-$.

Rehydration usually corrects acid–base balance and correction with HCO_3^- is rarely indicated.

With severe metabolic acidosis (HCO_3^- < 10 mmol/l) half-correction may be beneficial where:

$$\text{deficit (mmol } HCO_3^-) = \text{bodyweight (kg)} \times 0.3 \times \text{base deficit}$$

NB. Correction of acidosis may exacerbate hypokalaemia. Therefore, monitor K^+ levels.

ISOTONIC DEHYDRATION

For a given weight loss symptoms will be less than those for hypotonic dehydration.

Treatment
Similar to that for hypotonic dehydration.

> **Example.** A 10-kg baby presents with gastroenteritis and physical signs suggesting 10% dehydration. Serum Na^+ = 140 mmol/l. Estimated daily loss as diarrhoea = 400 ml. The volume and type of fluid required to correct the dehydration are:
>
> 1. Current volume deficit (10% of 10 kg) = 1 litre of fluid with a Na^+ content of 140 mmol.
> 2. To provide maintenance (100 ml/kg per 24 hours) = 1 litre of fluid and maintenance Na^+ at 2 mmol/kg per 24 hours (20 mmol).
> 3. To replace continuing daily losses (in this case estimated at 400 ml) = 0.4 litres of fluid. Diarrhoea contains approximately 45 mmol Na^+/litre (see Table 3.4). Thus continuing losses = 20 mmol Na^+ per 24 hours.
>   Therefore, the total *volume of fluid required* from the above is 2.4 litres.
>   The *Na* + *required* per 24 hours is 180 mmol.
> Therefore 2.4 litres of fluid containing 180 mmol of NaCl should be infused over a 24-hour period.

In practice, initial Na^+ as normal saline (0.9%) is given for re-

Table 3.4 Composition of body fluids (mmol/l)

	Na^+	K^+	Cl^-	HCO_3^-
Diarrhoea	50	40	40	40
Small bowel	130	15	110	20–40
Biliary	130	5–15	100	40
Gastric	50	10–15	150	0
Blood	140	4–5	100	25
Pancreas	140	5–10	50–100	100
Urine	Wide variations with intake			

suscitation (10–20 ml/kg). Fluids are then given as 0.45% saline (>78 mmol/l) plus 5% dextrose.

NB. KCl requirements of 2.5 mmol/kg per 24 hours are added once the child has passed urine.

HYPERTONIC DEHYDRATION ($Na^+ > 150$ mmol/l)

It is difficult to estimate the degree of dehydration. Assume a 5% deficit unless the child is clinically shocked, in which case he is at least 10% dehydrated.
— Check U & E, osmolality, glucose and Ca^{2+}.
— Hypocalcaemia occasionally needs correction with calcium gluconate.
— Hyperglycaemia is not uncommon with hypertonic dehydration. It is rectified with correction of fluid balance. Insulin has no place.
— Add KCl supplements as indicated once urine is passed.

NB. Regular U & E and osmolality measurements are needed to monitor rehydration.

Treatment

The plan is to replace total fluid deficit slowly over at least 48 hours. Aim to lower the serum Na^+ by approximately 10 mmol/l per 24 hours. Rapid correction may cause cerebral oedema.

1. **Immediate.** If shock is present infuse 20 ml/kg plasma or 0.9% saline over 20–30 min.

2. **1–4 hours.** There is controversy over the most suitable fluid. We use 0.45% NaCl/5% dextrose at 10 ml/kg/h. This should induce a good urine output allowing addition of maintenance KCl to the infusion.

3. **4–48 hours.** Maintenance fluids and water deficit.
   Calculate the water deficit. This may be estimated by knowledge of the serum osmolality and present body water.
   Normal body water
   $$= \text{present body water} \ \times \ \frac{\text{present osmolality}}{\text{normal osmolality (290)}}$$
   Present body water = present weight (kg) × 0.6
   Water deficit = normal body water − present body water
   Example. A dehydrated 10-kg child has an osmolality of 350 (Na^+ = 165).

   $$\text{Water deficit} = 10 \text{ kg} \times 0.6 \times \frac{350}{290} - (10 \text{ kg} \times 0.6)$$
   $$= 7.2 - 6$$
   $$= 1.2 \text{ litres}$$

The fluid used may be 0.45% NaCl/5% dextrose or 0.18% NaCl/4% dextrose.

Estimate maintenance as described previously.

Add maintenance KCl once urine has been passed.

Run infusion at a steady rate, do not try to correct the water deficit rapidly, i.e. correct over at least 2 days.

4. **Acute severe salt poisoning.** This requires peritoneal dialysis (especially if serum Na^+ is > 175 mmol/l) or frusemide diuresis (1 mg/kg) replacing urine output with 10% dextrose. Check Na^+ regularly (2–4-hourly). Administration of frusemide may be repeated. Always discuss with the consultant.

Inappropriate ADH secretion

Causes. Meningitis, head injury, neurosurgery, chest disease, e.g. severe infection, asthma.

Such patients are usually receiving parenteral fluids and as their ability to excrete decreases with increasing ADH, dangerous dilution and hyponatraemia may occur.

Clinical indicators. Weight gain, fluid retention, decreased urine output, irritability, decreased consciousness.

Laboratory findings. Hyponatraemia, low plasma osmolality (< 270 mmol/kg), high urine osmolality, high urinary Na^+ (≥ 40 mmol/).

The most common error in recognising inappropriate ADH secretion is the failure to realise that urine osmolality need only be inappropriately raised compared with plasma osmolality.

Treatment
1. Anticipate and prevent, i.e. restrict fluid intake to 50% of maintenance in early meningitis or head injury. Careful monitoring of plasma and urine osmolality and electrolytes in situations where inappropriate ADH may occur.
2. If present, fluid restriction is the best treatment. Loss of bodyweight with a slow rise in serum Na^+ and osmolality indicates improvement.
3. For acute hyponatraemia with severe CNS symptoms, treatment with hypertonic saline is needed as described below.

Electrolytes

Sodium

HYPONATRAEMIA (Na⁺ < 130 mmol/l)

Aetiology
Common causes include: diarrhoea, excessive salt-free infusions, inappropriate ADH secretion, water intoxication. Uncommon causes include: ARF, CRF, congestive heart failure, high environmental temperature. Rare causes include: adrenal insufficiency, cirrhosis, CF and excessive sweating.

Management
Symptomatic hyponatraemia (Na⁺ usually < 125 mmol/l): may be seen even with a serum Na⁺ of 130 mmol/l if the drop in serum Na⁺ has been sudden.

Regardless of cause (water excess or Na⁺ loss) the aim is to raise Na⁺ concentration quickly to stop symptoms.

Use hypertonic saline 2.7% (= 465 mmol/l) to deliver approximately 5 mmol/kg Na⁺ over at least 1 hour.

> **Example.** An irritable lethargic child with a serum Na⁺ of 120 mmol/l and no volume deficit. Bodyweight = 10 kg.
> Na⁺ deficit = 10 kg × 15 mmol/l deficit × 0.6 (volume of distribution of Na⁺ in water) = 90 mmol
> To raise Na⁺ by 5 mmol/l quickly needs 5 mmol/l × 0.6 × 10 kg = 30 mmol Na⁺
> Dose of 2.7% saline = *30 mmol Na⁺*
> 2.7% NaCl = 0.465 mmol Na⁺/ml
> = 60 ml over 1–3 hours

Following acute correction the child may become more acidotic. NaHCO₃ may be given mixed with the hypertonic saline to supply HCO₃⁻ and some of the Na⁺. Monitor acid–base status. Following acute treatment try to raise Na⁺ *slowly* to normal levels over at least 24 hours.

Asymptomatic hyponatraemia: see p. 19.

HYPERNATRAEMIA

See hypertonic dehydration, above.

Diabetes insipidus
Caused by deficiency of ADH, it may also be due to renal unresponsiveness (nephrogenic).

Aetiology. Includes head injury, neurosurgery, histiocytosis, meningitis, encephalitis, sickle cell disease and idiopathic causes.

Diagnosis. Suggested by persistent polyuria and polydipsia. The other major causes of polyuria to consider are diabetes mellitus, renal disease and excessive water intake.

Laboratory features.
1. Massive urine volume, over 3 l/m^2 per 24 hours
2. Dilute urine (osmolality 50–150 mmol/kg)
3. Low urine Na$^+$ (< 20 mmol/l)
4. High plasma Na$^+$ (> 145 mmol/l)
5. High plasma osmolality (> 295 mmol/kg)

Acute treatment. Diabetes insipidus may develop acutely, e.g. after surgery for a craniopharyngioma. If acute and severe, manage in ICU. Always discuss with consultants involved.
1. Calculate the fluid deficit from clinical assessment, electrolytes and fluid balance. In severe diabetes insipidus, fluid volume replacement is best estimated by adding insensible loss to the previous urine output over 1 hour (insensible water loss = 500 ml/m^2/per 24 hours). Dehydration, if present, should be corrected rapidly over 6–12 hours.
2. Type of fluid: use 0.18% (or 0.45%) saline/4% dextrose with 1 g (13 mmol) KCl to each 500-ml bag.
3. Regular measurements of plasma U & E and osmolality are essential.
4. In certain situations, steroid secretion will be inadequate in coping with the stress of the fluid and electrolyte disturbances. Consider steroid cover.
5. There is a tendency to give excessive DDAVP which is a dangerous practice and may cause gross hyponatraemia and, possibly, fits. However, DDAVP may have to be used to control fluid balance. This may be given nasally in a dosage of 2.5–10 μg (0.025–0.1 ml) depending on age and administered by a Rhinyl device. Beware of excessive doses. The most important marker of appropriate therapy is plasma osmolality which can be used to adjust the DDAVP dosage.
   Example. Plasma osmolality < 280: reduce DDAVP dose by 50%.
   Plasma osmolality 281–294: maintain dosage.
   Osmolality > 295: increase DDAVP by 50%.
   Also see Table 3.5.

Occasionally a child is passing several litres of urine daily whose losses have been replaced on an hourly basis. If a reasonable dose of DDAVP is being given and the child is well hydrated, cut back the fluid input for 30–60 min to establish if fluid diuresis is due to excessive fluid input. Do not give massive doses of DDAVP without consultation and without such a trial.

Table 3.5 Fluid and electrolyte balance in deficient and excessive DDAVP doses

	Deficient DDAVP	Excessive DDAVP
ECF volume	↓	↑
Plasma Na^+	↑	↓
Plasma osmolality	↑	↓
Urine volume	↑	↓
Urine Na^+	↓	↑
Urine osmolality	↓	↑

Management of this problem can be difficult, discuss with the consultant on call.

Diabetes insipidus screening test (as below). Rule out renal disease; if diabetes insipidus is confirmed assess full pituitary function and for CNS disease, i.e. CT scan, etc.

Water deprivation test.
1. Weigh the child at the start of the test.
2. Blood for Na^+, osmolality (ADH if available).
3. Urine for osmolality and specific gravity.
4. Stop fluid intake for no more than 6–7 hours in infants, 12–16 hours in older children.
5. Repeat blood and urine sample at 8 hours, check bodyweight.
6. Continue if tolerated and repeat sample at 12 and 16 hours and check weight.
7. If there is no urinary concentration, give 5 µg of DDAVP intranasally.
8. Collect mixed urine sample and a further blood sample at this time. Failure to concentrate urine and plasma osmolality to >300 mmol/kg suggests diabetes insipidus. A response to the DDAVP suggests pituitary ADH deficiency. No response to DDAVP and failure to concentrate, suggests nephrogenic diabetes insipidus.

NB. Compulsive water drinking may mimic symptoms but there is usually urinary concentration with water deprivation.

Potassium (1 g KCl = 13.3 mmol KCl)

Daily requirement = 2–3 mmol/kg.
Dangers of an abnormal K^+ level are exacerbated by abnormalities of Ca^{2+} in the opposite direction.

HYPOKALAEMIA (K^+ < 3.4 mmol/l)

Causes include diarrhoea or vomiting, diabetic ketoacidosis, starvation, renal tubular defects, diuretic therapy and inadequate i.v. therapy.

Symptoms
Muscle weakness, paralytic ileus, cramps, lethargy and confusion:
— may be associated with a metabolic alkalosis
— ECG: low voltage T wave, U wave and prolonged QT may be seen (best seen in ECG lead II)

Treatment
Treat the underlying cause:
— oral potassium supplements
— KCl added to i.v. fluids as necessary
The maximum 1-hour i.v. dose is 0.5 mmol/kg administered slowly by a doctor with ECG monitoring into a major vein.

KCl concentrations of > 40 mmol/l may cause phlebitis.

HYPERKALAEMIA (K^+ > 5.5 mmol/l)

Causes include renal failure, sudden oliguria, massive haemolysis, congenital adrenocortical hyperplasia, tissue necrosis and destruction.

Toxic effects

Cardiac. ECG shows an increased PR interval, widened QRS complexes, a depressed ST segment and peaked T waves. Heart block and ventricular fibrillation may occur.

NB. Hypocalcaemia, acidosis or hyponatraemia exacerbate toxic effects.

Treatment (see Ch. 10, p. 160)
Treat the underlying cause. If serum K^+ is > 7 mmol/l or ECG changes/arrhythmias are present:
1. Correct acidosis with 2 mmol/kg $NaHCO_3$ i.v. over 20 min.
2. Give calcium gluconate (10%) 0.5 ml/kg
3. Resonium A 0.5 g/kg p.o. or p.r.
4. If hyperkalaemia persists give glucose and soluble insulin: 2 ml/kg 25% dextrose (0.25 g/ml) plus 1 unit insulin (actrapid)/4 g glucose. These methods should allow time for institution of dialysis to be assessed.

Chloride

Plasma concentration = 99–105 mmol/l.
Abnormal losses with vomiting (i.e. pyloric stenosis), CF and

diuretic therapy may lead to metabolic alkalosis. Replacement is as NaCl.

Calcium

Normal plasma level = 2.15–2.70 mmol/l in neonates $Ca^{2+} < 1.7$ mmol/l = hypocalcaemia. Active calcium is in its ionised form. Acidosis increases Ca^{2+}. Alkalosis decreases Ca^{2+} and may cause tetany (e.g. with hyperventilation).

HYPOCALCAEMIA

Causes
Rickets, renal compromise, hypoalbuminaemia associated with liver disease or nephrotic syndrome, hypoparathyroidism and pseudohypoparathyroidism, drugs (e.g. frusemide, HCO_3^- and corticosteroids), exchange transfusions, Di George syndrome and hypomagnesaemia.

Symptoms
Shvosteck and Trousseau's signs positive, carpopedal spasm and seizures. ECG may show a prolonged QT interval relative to rate.

Investigations
Symptomatic hypocalcaemia needs treatment followed by investigations (see below). If asymptomatic, determine plasma Ca^{2+} on more than one occasion with the patient fasted before undertaking complex investigations. Avoid venous stasis when taking blood.

Take a fasting blood sample for:
1. Plasma Ca^{2+}, PO_4^{3-}, alkaline phosphotase, total protein and albumin
2. Creatinine, U & E (to exclude a renal cause)
3. Serum Mg^{2+}
4. Ionised Ca^{2+} (if available)
5. Serum PTH
6. Plasma vitamin D metabolites: 25-HCC 1,25-DHCC
7. 24-hour urine for Ca^{2+}, PO_4^{3-}, creatinine and hydroxyproline.
   NB. Always interpret plasma Ca^{2+} in relation to protein concentration.
8. ECG
9. CXR and wrist X-ray

Interpretation
1. With regards to parathyroid disease or disorders of vitamin D metabolism (N = Normal):

$Ca^{2+}\downarrow$	$PO_4^{3-}\uparrow$	PTH low/indetectable	Hypoparathyroidism
$Ca^{2+}\downarrow$	$PO_4^{3-}\uparrow$	PTH $\uparrow$	Pseudohypoparathyroidism
Ca^{2+} N/$\downarrow$	$PO_4^{3-}\uparrow$	Alkaline phosphatase	Rickets

2. With regards to rickets:

— Nutritional (vitamin D deficiency) rickets	Plasma 25-HCC	↓
	PTH	N/↑
— Vitamin D dependent rickets (type II)	Plasma 25-HCC	N
	Plasma 1,25–DHCC	↓
	Plasma PTH	↑/N
— Vitamin D dependent rickets (receptor defect)	Plasma 25-HDC	N
	Plasma 1,25-DHCC	N
	Plasma PTH	N
— Vitamin D resistant (hypophosphataemic) rickets	Plasma 25-HCC	N
	Plasma 1,25-DHCC	N
	Plasma PO_4^{3-}	↓↓
	Plasma PTH	N

Treatment

Treatment of the neonatal patient and the older child with hypocalcaemia are discussed here.

A. Neonatal.

1. Hypocalcaemia in asymptomatic babies on i.v. infusions only. Add Ca^{2+} 1 mmol/kg per 24 hours to the infusion as 10% calcium gluconate (4.4 ml/kg per 24 hours). (Avoid scalp veins; leak into tissues causes necrosis.)

2. Symptomatic hypocalcaemia (Ca^{2+} is < 1.5 mmol/l). Treat orally (safer). Indication for i.v. see below.
   a. Feed breast milk or low PO_4^{2-} formula.
   b. Give oral Ca^{2+}: 1 mmol/kg per 24 hours as 10% calcium gluconate (4.4 ml/kg per 24 hours).
   c. Calciferol 1000 u per 24 hours p.o. for rickets.

For severe convulsions, heart block or failure, give 0.2 ml/kg of 10% calcium gluconate diluted in 0.9% saline (5 ml) i.v. over 10–15 min under ECG monitoring. Extreme caution is needed to avoid tissue necrosis.

B. Older child with tetany or convulsions.

1. If tetany is due to hyperventilation, causing alkalosis, rebreathing into a paper bag may help.

2. Give 2 ml/kg i.v. of a 10% calcium gluconate solution slowly with ECG monitoring. If heart rate decreases, slow down or stop infusion.

3. When tetany has cleared the child can be maintained on calcium gluconate at 200 mg/kg per 24 hours p.o. in 4–6 divided doses.

An i.v. bolus will only transiently increase serum Ca^{2+} levels. Continuous i.v. administration may be associated with phlebitis, subcutaneous calcification and cardiac arrhythmias. It should be reserved for critical situations.

Treat the underlying cause.

HYPERCALCAEMIA (Ca^{2+} > 2.75 mmol/l)

This is uncommon in childhood. The hypercalcaemia should be confirmed on 3 occasions when the child is fasting prior to investigations.

Aetiology

Idiopathic hypercalcaemia of infancy (William's syndrome), primary hyperparathyroidism, secondary hyperparathyroidism, vitamin D and vitamin A toxicity and immobilisation. Leukaemia and sarcoid.

Symptoms

Nausea, constipation, weight loss, polyuria, polydypsia, head-aches, renal stones and bone pain.

Investigations

1. Plasma: PO_4^{3-}, alkaline phosphatase, Ca^{2+}, protein, albumin, creatinine, Na^+, K^+, Cl^-, pH and serum PTH.
2. Urine: 24-hour collection for Ca^{2+}, PO_4^{3-}, creatinine, hydroxyproline and cAMP.
3. X-rays, including skull and pelvis.

A normal or detectable PTH in the presence of hypercalcaemia indicates hyperparathyroidism.

Treatment of acute hypercalcaemia

1. 0.9% saline infusion + 1 mg/kg frusemide
2. Restrict dietary Ca^{2+}
3. Glucocorticosteroids are also useful in decreasing Ca^{2+}.

Acid–base balance

Blood gas analysis (See Tables 3.6 and 3.7)

METABOLIC ACIDOSIS (pH < 7.35, HCO_3^- < 18 mmol/l, base excess negative)

Causes include hypoxia, shock, septicaemia, metabolic disease (inborn errors of metabolism), HCO_3^- loss in diarrhoeal stools, renal failure, diabetes melitus, acute liver failure, salicylate poisoning, renal tubular acidosis.

The anion gap is the difference between serum cations (Na^+) and anions (i.e. $Cl^- + HCO_3^-$) and is normally 12 mmol/l. If metabolic acidosis is due to HCO_3^- loss alone, the anion gap changes

Table 3.6 Acid–base problems

	pH	HCO$_3^-$	↓PCO$_2$	Body compensation
Metabolic acidosis	↓	↓	N	↓PCO$_2$; acidic urine
Respiratory acidosis	↓	N/↑	↑	Acidic urine
Metabolic alkalosis	↑	↑	N/↑	↑PCO$_2$; alkaline urine
Respiratory alkalosis	↑	N/↓	↓	Alkaline urine

Table 3.7 Normal blood values

	pH	PCO$_2$	HCO$_3^-$
Arterial blood	7.38–7.45	4.5–6.3	23–27
Venous blood	7.35–7.40	6.0–6.6	24–29

little since Cl⁻ rises proportionately. In lactic acidosis (e.g. secondary to anaerobic metabolism in shock) the large anion gap reflects accumulation of the anion.

Treatment

A mild degree of metabolic acidosis needs no therapy as it improves once the fluid and electrolyte balance is corrected.

In severe acidosis, HCO$_3^-$ replacement will usually be necessary. The amount required can be calculated:

mmol of HCO$_3^-$ required = 0.3 × bodyweight × base deficit

To avoid lowering K⁺ it is suggested that no more than half the calculated amount be given immediately as 8.4% NaHCO$_3$ (infused over 30–60 min) and the remainder, if necessary, be given over several hours with careful monitoring of serum K⁺. Beware of HCO$_3^-$ leak into the tissues causing necrosis when given i.v.

METABOLIC ALKALOSIS (pH > 7.43, HCO$_3^-$ > 25 mmol/l, base excess positive)

Involves either gain of a strong base or HCO$_3^-$ or loss of a fixed acid, e.g. loss of HCl as in pyloric stenosis or from K⁺ deficiency as in diuretic therapy. In K⁺ deficiency H⁺ ions move intracellularly to replace K⁺ and are also lost in the urine because of distal tubular H⁺ secretion in exchange for reabsorbed Na⁺.

Treatment

Involves correction of dehydration with fluids containing adequate amounts of NaCl and provision of KCl, so that distal tubules can secrete K⁺ and conserve H⁺ in exchange for reabsorbed Na⁺. Often, 3–6 mmol K⁺/kg bodyweight will be required over 24 hours.

Fluid management in pyloric stenosis

Example. A 3-kg baby with pyloric stenosis with clinical signs indicating 10% dehydration.

Na^+ = 131 mmol/l, K^+ = 2.5 mmol/l, Cl^- = 70 mmol/l, HCO_3^- = 38 mmol/l

Fluid requirement: volume deficit of 10% of 3 kg (300 ml) is replaced with 0.9% saline (with 40 mmol/l KCl once urine is passed) over the first 12 hours. Check blood sugar by BMstix during saline infusion. The first 60 ml of 0.9% saline is given rapidly to treat shock. The whole day's maintenance fluid requirement (300 ml) is then given as 0.18% saline/4% dextrose with 40 mmol/l KCl over the following 12 hours. With less severely affected babies 0.45% saline/ 4% dextrose with added KCl will suffice.

RESPIRATORY ACIDOSIS (pH < 7.35, PCO_2 raised)

Caused by retention of CO_2 and consequent increase in H_2CO_3. This is due to inadequate pulmonary ventilation. The high CO_2 can only be corrected by improving alveolar ventilation (e.g. mechanically).

In acute respiratory acidosis, available buffering mechanisms and renal compensation are minimal. Thus, pH falls as CO_2 increases.

In chronic metabolic acidosis, by acidifying the urine the kidney can raise extracellular HCO_3 to 40 mmol/l or more to compensate. Usually neonates are incapable of this adaptation and will remain severely acidotic with RDS.

RESPIRATORY ALKALOSIS: (pH > 7.43, PCO_2 < 4 kPa)

Results from hyperventilation and consequent blowing off of CO_2.

Causes include hyperventilation with hysteria, mechanical ventilation, Reye's syndrome, early salicylate intoxication and hypermetabolic states. Rapid correction of metabolic acidosis can also lead to respiratory alkalosis.

Acute respiratory alkalosis may cause tetany and makes the patient feel light-headed. This may be treated by rebreathing into a paper bag.

4

Nutrition

Daily requirements of water, calories, Na^+, K^+, Ca^{2+}, PO_4^{3-} and iron are shown in Table 4.1.

Individuals vary greatly in intake and frequency of feeds. Adequacy of nutrition is best judged by demonstrating normal growth and development.

Feeding newborn infants

1. WHICH MILK?

a. Breast feeding is to be encouraged in all infants, the exception being extremely low birthweight infants who require a low birthweight formula (e.g. Osterprem, LBW Cow & Gate, LBW SMA or Prematil). In these infants, EBM (10% of total) may be added to the formula milk if the mother wishes to breast feed subsequently. It may also protect against infection and later atopy.

b. Where breast feeding is not being used babies should be fed on one of the milks that conform to the Department of Health standards which are:

	Whey based formula	Casein based formula
Wyeth	SMA Gold	SMA White
Farley	Ostermilk	Ostermilk 2
Milupa	Aptamil	Milumil
Cow & Gate	Premium	Plus

The whey based formulas are the closest to breast milk and are the milks of choice. Casein based formulas are no more satisfying. The Department of Health recommends continuing infant formula until 1 year of age. The use of a follow-on formula, e.g. Progress, has no advantage over continuing a baby milk. Formula milk may be changed to full cream undiluted pasteurised cow's milk at about 12 months.

Table 4.1 Daily nutritional requirements

Age	Water (ml/kg)	kcal/kg	Protein (g/kg)	Na+ (mmol/kg)	K+ (mmol/kg)	Ca2+ (mmol/kg)	PO43- (mmol/kg)
1 day	60–90	115	2.2	2–3	2–3	1.5	1.5
2 days	90–120	115	2.2	2–3	2–3	1.5	1.5
10 days	120–150	105	2.0	2–3	2–3	1.5	1.5
3 months	140–160	105	2.0	2–3	2–3	1.5	1.5
6 months	130–160	105	2.0	2–3	2–3	1.5	1.5
9 months	125–145	105	2.0	2–3	2–3	1.5	1.5
1 year	120–135	100	1.8	1–3	1–3	1.5	1.2
2 years	115–125	100	1.7	1–3	1–3	1.5	1.2
4 years	100–110	85	1.5	1–3	1–3	1.0	1.2
6 years	90–100	85	1.5	1–3	1–3	1.0	1.2
10 years	70–85	85	1.25	1–3	1–3	0.7	0.9
14 years	50–60	55	1.0	1–3	1–3	0.7	0.9

2. HOW MUCH MILK?

a. Fullterm infants

The first feed should be given as soon as possible after birth using breast milk or milk formula of the mother's choice. Babies should be fed on demand. Newborn infants usually need feeding every 2–4 hours.

Fluid requirements are:

day 1 40 ml/kg
day 2 60 ml/kg
day 3 80 ml/kg
day 4 110 ml/kg
day 5 150 ml/kg

For the bottle fed baby divide the volume to allow 3–4 hourly feeds. Infants should have regained their birthweight by 10 days of age.

Infants weighing 1.5–2.5 kg at birth

Feed within 1 hour if small for gestational age. Fluid requirements are:

day 1 60 ml/kg
day 2 90 ml/kg
day 3 120 ml/kg
day 4 150 ml/kg

May be increased to 180 ml/kg of breast milk or formula feed if weight gain is poor. Route: breast, bottle or NG — depends on maturity of the infant.

Infants weighing < 1.5 kg at birth

Low birthweight formula is suggested. Consider oral or NG feeds if there are no respiratory problems. The volume may be increased to 180–200 ml/kg if weight gain is inadequate. Feeds may be given continuously via NGT. If poorly tolerated, consider hourly intermittent NG feeds with NGT on free drainage. Ensure bowels open 12-hourly with the use of the tip of glycerine suppositories if necessary. If oral or NG feeds are not tolerated, give i.v. 10% dextrose:

60 ml/kg on day 1. If enteral feeding cannot be introduced, increase i.v. fluids to 90 ml/kg on day 2, 120 ml/kg on day 3 and 150 ml/kg on day 4.

If enteral feeding is not established by day 5 consider nasojejunal feeding or TPN.

Weaning

Iron fortified cereals are recommended when the child is 4–6 months old, initially one teaspoonful before milk feeds. The frequency and amount is then gradually increased. Other foods are increased one at a time, e.g. fruits, rusks, vegetables, bread. The food should gradually change from smooth purées to mashed, minced and then diced. This will encourage chewing. At 12 months the child should be taking a diet similar to that of the family. Milk should be reduced to a daily maximum of 700–900 ml. A cup should then be used instead of bottle feeds. A cup may be introduced from 6 months.

Vitamin drops are recommended for all babies from 6 months to 2 years and preferably to 5 years.

Common feeding problems

CONTRAINDICATIONS TO BREAST MILK

These include:
1. HIV-positive mother
2. Galactosaemia
3. Maternal chicken pox starting within 4 days of birth. The mother may express and commence breast feeding when all the lesions are crusted.
4. Maternal medication: drugs that are contraindicated during breast feeding include amiodarone, antineoplastic drugs, bromocriptine, chloramphenicol, cimetadine, clemastine, cyclosporin A, dapasone, ergot and ergotamine, gold salts, indomethacin, iodides, lithium, high-dose oestrogens, phenindione, all radioisotopes, tetracyclines, thiouracil, high-dose vitamins A and D, and sulphonamides (in jaundiced infants).

NB. Analgesics, anticonvulsants and antihistamines are not contraindications to breast feeding but may cause drowsiness in the infant and delay establishment of feeding.

Oral steroids and antithyroid drugs do not contraindicate breast feeding but the infant should be followed carefully. Maternal thyroxine will not harm the baby, provided the mother is euthyroid, but may interfere with neonatal screening tests for hypothyroidism.

GASTRO-OESOPHAGEAL REFLUX IN THE BREAST FED BABY

Small episodes of reflux (possets) are very common and usually require no treatment. If reflux is a problem thickening the feeds can be helpful. Infant Carobel (0.1–0.3 g) mixed with a small amount of water or breast milk may be given as a paste by spoon during a breast feeding session. Gaviscon may be given in a similar way but has the disadvantage of having a high sodium content.

GASTROENTERITIS IN THE BREAST FED BABY

Increase frequency of breast feeds for mild gastroenteritis. With moderate gastroenteritis breast feeds can be alternated with Dioralyte, or breast milk expressed diluted and given by bottle, spoon or tube.

GASTRO-OESOPHAGEAL REFLUX IN BOTTLE FED INFANTS

Thickened foods may help. Try:
1. Carobel 0.1–0.3 g added to the prepared formula.
2. Infant Gaviscon 1–2 g/120 ml added to the prepared formula.
Carobel is preferable as infant Gaviscon has a high sodium content.

CONSTIPATION IN INFANCY

This is common. If the child is well increase fluid intake with boiled water or diluted fruit juice. If the child has weaned encourage fruit, vegetables and cereals. If the child is unwell or if constipation persists see p. 138.

FREQUENCY OF STOOLS

May vary from each feed to every few days. Colour varies from green to yellow. Toddler stools often contain undigested food.
NB. Very pale stools in a jaundiced baby suggest biliary atresia; check for unconjugated bilirubinaemia immediately.

PARENTAL CONCERN REGARDING THE AMOUNT OF FEEDS

Parents are often worried that the baby is not getting enough, especially if he is breast fed. Take history of both maternal health and feeding pattern. Watch the baby feeding if necessary. Examine the child and plot height and weight on a centile chart. If weight gain is adequate and no abnormalities are detected, reassure. Arrange further follow-up by health visitor or GP.

TRANSIENT LACTOSE INTOLERANCE

Usually seen following gastroenteritis. Diarrhoea persists following re-introduction of usual milk formula. Lactose is demonstrated in the stool (Clinitest is positive and Clinistik negative in lactose intolerance). It is not usually necessary to stop breast milk. If bottle fed, changing to a lactose-free formula for 2–3 weeks will allow recovery.

VITAMIN C DEFICIENCY

Causes scurvy and can occur in those not given vegetables/fruit and fed on cow's milk.

Presents with pallor, irritability, bruising, petechiae, bleeding from gums and subperiosteal haematoma.

Treatment

200 mg of ascorbic acid per 24 hours in one dose.

VITAMIN D DEFICIENCY

See p. 27.

COW'S MILK HYPERSENSITIVITY

See p. 128.

Special dietary products

ENERGY SUPPLEMENTS

These can be added to feeds, breast milk, infant formulas or preterm formulas in order to increase the energy value.
1. Glucose polymers: used in preference to glucose as it has much lower effect on osmolality and taste. Usually starts with 1% and increase in 1% increments to a maximum of 3%. Brand names: Polycal, Maxijul, Caloreen (all 4 kcal/g).
2. Fat emulsion: vegetable oil emulsified with water (50 : 50). May be used instead of or as well as a glucose polymer. Usually increased in 1% increments. Brand names: Calogen-LCT (4.5 kcal/g), Liquigen-MCT (4.2 kcal/g).
3. Combined fat and carbohydrate: glucose polymer and vegetable oil combined in the form of an emulsion or oil. More balanced than either fat or carbohydrate alone. Brand names: Duocal powder — added in 1-g increments (4.7 kcal/g), Duocal liquid (1.5 kcal/ml).

NB. With all energy supplements care must be taken not to keep increasing the quantities without taking into account the effects of not increasing protein.

SPECIAL FORMULAS

The most commonly available products we use are discussed here.

Soya milks

Soya based feeds using a glucose polymer as the main carbohydrate source. The following are all suitable: Formula S, Isomil, Ostersoy, Prosobee, Wysoy. Used for cow's milk protein intolerance. Can be used for lactose intolerance and galactosaemia.

Galactomin 17 is preferred in secondary lactose intolerance where an already traumatised gut may be sensitive to new proteins. For the same reason peptide based feeds are also used, e.g. nutramigen as Galactomin is still whole protein.

Neocate

An aminoacid based feed using a glucose polymer and a blend of vegetable fats to produce an aminoacid profile similar to that of breast milk. Used only when peptide based feeds are not tolerated.

Pregestimil

Hydrolysed casein feed from which lactose is removed and re-placed with a glucose polymer. It also has a proportion of its fat as medium chain triglyceride (MCT) which increases osmolality. Used in the treatment of multiple malabsorption following surgery or resection, whole protein sensitivity where use of MCT may be desirable.

Nutramigen

Hydrolysed casein feed from which lactose is removed and re-placed with a glucose polymer. Suitable for lactose intolerance where a degree of whole protein malabsorption is anticipated.

Pepdite/Prejomin

Hydrolysed meat and soya protein feeds which are lactose free and contain no MCT. Thus osmolality and palatability are better. Indications as for Pregestimil.

Galactomin 17

Casein based feed from which lactose is removed and replaced with glucose polymers. Suitable for transient or primary lactose in tolerance, galactosaemia and galactokinase deficiency.

Nutrition in the failure to thrive child (see p. 130)

1. For catch-up growth the calories required are:
$$\text{kcal/kg} = \frac{120 \text{ kcal/kg} \times \text{median weight for current height}}{\text{current weight (kg)}}$$
2. Increase protein intake by 1.5–2 times.
3. Check for deficiencies in iron, zinc, and vitamin D. Supplement with multivitamins including zinc.
4. With moderate FTT encourage intake to meet catch-up growth. With severe FTT it may be appropriate to encourage normal intake with frequent small meals initially (up to 10 days) and then increase towards catch-up goals.
5. High calorie and protein foods should be used.

Suggested laboratory monitoring of nutritional status in various conditions

In addition to a clinical nutritional assessment, certain laboratory tests may be helpful in monitoring:

1. **Inflammatory bowel disease.** FBC and film (MCV), albumin, ferritin, PO_4^{3-}, Ca^{2+}, Mg^{2+}, Cu^{2+}, Zn^{2+}, folate, vitamin B_{12}, vitamins A, D, E, K and somatomedin C.

2. **Chronic liver disease.** LFT, serum albumin, NH_4^+, vitamin A, D and E, Zn^{2+}, PT and PPT, and total lipids.

3. **Renal failure.** Serum total protein, albumin, and transferrin. Serum urea, Na^+, K^+, Cl^-, HCO_3^-, Ca^{2+}, PO_4^{3-}, and Mg^{2+}. Creatinine and urea clearance and daily urine volume, fasting blood glucose, serum triglycerides, cholesterol and HDL, FBC and total lymphocyte count. Left wrist X-ray.

4. **Short bowel syndrome.** FBC differential and film. U & E, serum Ca^{2+}, PO_4^{3-}, creatinine, LFT, iron and iron binding capacity, Serum Cu^{2+}, Mg^{2+}, Zn^{2+}, vitamin B_{12}, folate, 24-hour urine collection for electrolytes. If stoma is present measure total stool volume and electrolytes.

Eating disorders

ANOREXIA NERVOSA

Diagnostic criteria for statistical purposes are:
1. Refusal to maintain normal bodyweight.
2. Loss of > 25% of original bodyweight.
3. Disturbance of body image.
4. Intense fear of becoming fat.
5. No known medical illness leading to weight loss.
Medical complications may include:
1. Fluid and electrolyte disturbances: hypokalaemia, metabolic alkalosis, chronic hypovolaemia, postural hypotension, secondary hyperaldosteronism, increased urea.
2. Vitamin and mineral deficiencies: decreased Ca^{2+}, Mg^{2+}, PO_4^{3-}, Zn^{2+}. Iron deficiency is rare.
3. Endocrine abnormalities: delayed onset or interruption of pubertal development, amenorrhoea, disturbed hypothalamic–pituitary–adrenal axis function, decreased T_3, decreased conversion of T_4 to T_3, increased basal GH, decreased ADH secretion.

4. Haematology: anaemia, leukopenia, thrombocytopenia.
5. Miscellaneous: mitral valve prolapse, hypothermia, bradycardia, arrythmias, constipation, renal calculi.

BULIMIA

Diagnostic criteria are:
1. Recurrent episodes of binge eating.
2. At least three of the following: consumption of high caloric, easily ingested foods during a binge; termination of binge by abdominal pain, sleep or vomiting; inconspicuous eating during a binge; repeated weight fluctuations of more than 4.5 kg.
3. Awareness of abnormal eating pattern and not being able to stop voluntarily.
4. Depressed mood after binge.
5. Not due to anorexia nervosa or any physical disorder.

Medical complications include:
Menstrual irregularities, Ipecachuanha poisoning, hypokalaemia (diuretic or laxative induced), acute gastric dilatation or rupture, oesophagitis, Mallory–Weiss tears, oesophageal rupture, aspiration pneumonia.

CRITERIA FOR HOSPITALISATION IN PATIENTS WITH ANOREXIA NERVOSA OR BULIMIA

1. Severe metabolic disturbance, e.g. pulse < 40/min, temperature < 36°C, systolic BP < 70 mmHg, hypokalaemia (< 2.5 mmol/l despite oral K$^+$ supplements).
2. Weight loss > 30% of index bodyweight.
3. Severe depression, psychosis or suicide risk.
4. Severe binging and purging.
5. Failure to maintain outpatient weight contract.
6. Family crisis, need to confront patient and family denial.
7. Exclusion of differential diagnosis.

Total parenteral nutrition

A child who cannot maintain nutrition adequate for his metabolic needs is a candidate for TPN, e.g. in protracted diarrhoea, oesophageal injury and postoperatively.

TPN may be given via a central or peripheral line under strict aseptic conditions. Central lines are preferable.

Regimens for TPN should be determined with the aid of the pharmacy department in each hospital.

NB. TPN should be commenced cautiously.

NUTRITIONAL COMPONENTS REQUIRED FOR PARENTERAL NUTRITION

Protein

Vamin 9 glucose is a solution of all essential and non-essential aminoacids. Glucose is present as a 10% solution.

Vamin 9 glucose contains the following per litre: 9.4 g nitrogen (60 g/protein), 50 mmol Na^{2+}, 20 mmol K^+, 2.5 mmol Ca^{2+}, 1.5 mmol Mg^{2+}, 55 mmol Cl^-, 650 kcal total energy, 400 kcal non-nitrogen energy.

Carbohydrate (in the form of glucose)

5% glucose	200 kcal/l
10% glucose	400 kcal/l
20% glucose	800 kcal/l
50% glucose	2000 kcal/l

Monitor blood glucose. Reduce the infusion rate if blood glucose is > 9.7 mmol/l or glycosuria is > 0.5%. Glucose solutions of over 10% are unsuitable for peripheral veins.

Fat

Provided in the form of Intralipid. High in essential fatty acids and has a low osmolality. Available as 10% and 20% solutions providing 1.1 kcal/ml and 2 kcal/ml respectively. Restrict the fat intake to 2 g/kg per 24 hours. Do not give intralipid if plasma bilirubin is > 170 μmol/l or if the child has an uncontrolled infection. If the flow rate of infusions falls behind, the flow rate of intralipid must not be increased due to the risk of 'fat overload'.

Intralipid is given over 18 hours per day in order for the serum to clear before blood sampling.

Vitamins

Water soluble vitamins are given as Solvito N. This is added to the aminoacid/glucose solution mixture which must then be protected from light.

Solvito N provides the following per vial: vitamin B_1 3 mg, vitamin B_2 3.6 mg, nicotinomide 40 mg, vitamin B_6 4 mg, pantotheric acid 15 mg, biotin 60 μg, folic acid 400 μg, vitamin B_{12} 5 μg, vitamin C 100 mg.

Fat soluble vitamins are given as Vitalipid N infant in the dose recommended; 1 ml/kg per 24 hours (max. 10 ml per 24 hours) is recommended up to the age of 11.

Sodium

Added in the form of NaCl and requests should be for the total amount per kg for 24 hours. Pharmacy should deduct any already provided by other solutions.

Potassium

Usually added in the form of potassium acid phosphate and requests should be for the total amount required per kg for 24 hours. Pharmacy should deduct any already provided by other solutions.

Minerals

Given to supplement the insufficient amounts present in Vamin 9 glucose. Most other minerals are provided by Pedel, 5 ml/kg in 24 hours in infants up to 10 kg added to the aminoacid/glucose solution. Pedel (5 ml) provides Ca^{2+} 0.75 mmol, Mg^{2+} 125 µmol, Fe^{2+} 2.5 µmol, Zn^{2+} 0.75 µmol, Mn^{2+} 1.25 µmol, Cu^{2+} 0.375 µmol, F 3.75 µmol, I 0.04 µmol, P 375 µmol, Cl 1.75 µmol.

Addamel in a dose of 0.2 ml/kg per 24 hours is usually used in children > 10 kg as it is more concentrated and avoids large fluid volumes and a high sorbitol load. It is not suitable in the long term.

Ca^{2+} and PO_4^{3-} are often required in higher quantities; owing to problems with precipitation discuss with pharmacy.

Increased needs for some trace elements, e.g. in diarrhoeal states, should be anticipated, e.g. Zn^{2+} and Cu^{2+}. Trace element mixtures should only be given when renal function is established.

INCOMPATIBILITIES

It is not advisable to infuse drugs at the same site as TPN. Wherever possible the line should be reserved for TPN. Pharmacy should be contacted before any additions are made to the bag or line.

LABORATORY MONITORING OF TPN

1. Prior to start: blood for FBC, U & E, creatinine, HCO_3^-, LFT including Ca^{2+}, PO_4^{3-} and alkaline phosphatase and blood sugar.
2. First week of TPN: daily — U & E, creatinine, lipaemia, blood glucose 6-hourly.
   Days 2 and 5 — bilirubin (conjugated and total), albumin.
   Urine — daily urinalysis including glucose, electrolytes on days 2 and 5.
3. Second week onwards:
   Mon, Wed, Fri — U & E, creatinine.
   Mon, Fri — albumin, glucose.
   Mon — LFT, FBC, Ca^{2+}, PO_4^{3-}, alkaline phosphatase.
   Daily — urinalysis.
4. Microbiology: daily swabs from the lines. When febrile, peripheral and line (if possible) blood cultures and urine culture. LP only if clinically indicated.
5. Haematology: as above. FBC when febrile. When bleeding, oozing check clotting screen and FDPs.

6. Biochemistry, when clinically indicated:
   Plasma — acid–base, Mg^{2+}, Zn^{2+}, Cu^{2+}, aminoacids, NH_3, triglycerides, FFA and selenium.
   Urine — organic acids.

COMPLICATIONS

Infection. Meticulous aseptic care is needed. Bacteria and fungi are the infecting agents. Repeated peripheral and line cultures are required. If sepsis is confirmed the central venous line should be withdrawn. Give antibiotic or antifungal agents as indicated.

Hypoglycaemia. A dangerous complication occurring if TPN is stopped suddenly. Wean patients off TPN gradually.

Hyperglycaemia. Common in patients with sepsis, renal disease and in neonatal patients. Reduce infusion rate or concentration if necessary.

Acidosis. Results from a large protein load. More common with prematurity or renal disease. Acid–base disturbances generally result from the underlying medical condition and not from TPN.

Hypocalcaemia. If symptomatic (see p. 27) begin Ca^{2+} replacement using a separate i.v. solution. Do not add to the TPN solution as this may cause precipitation.

Hypomagnesemia. Increase the Mg^{2+} concentration in the TPN solution.

Hypophosphataemia. Increase the PO_4^{3-} intake. A separate i.v. solution may be needed to avoid Ca^{2+}/PO_4^{3-} precipitation in TPN solution.

Hyperlipaemia. Results from excess intralipid administration.

Hyperammonaemia. Decrease the protein content of TPN.

Hepatic problems. Abnormal LFTs are common during TPN. Hepatomegaly may be found (liver biopsy shows fatty changes). Cholestatic liver disease often develops in premature infants. Rule out infections and mechanical cause of liver dysfunction. Avoid excessive calories or protein intake.

Copper, zinc, selenium and iron deficiency. Supplements are required. Discuss with the pharmacist/dietitian.

Bone demineralisation. Provide adequate Ca^{2+}, PO_4^{3-} and vitamin D.

Essential fatty acid deficiency. Provide a minimum of 2–5% of total calories as linoleic acid.

TECHNICAL COMPLICATIONS

Arrythmias. May occur due to central catheter placement. Monitor heart beat immediately after insertion; repositioning of catheter may be required.

Venous thrombosis. Venous distension or oedema of the body part drained by that vein. Aspiration of blood will verify the catheter is patent; discuss with the consultant the instillation of a fibrinolytic agent (e.g. urokinase) or catheter removal.

Air embolus. Symptoms include sudden onset of respiratory distress and cyanosis. Clamp the catheter immediately. Place in the Trendelenberg position with the right side up.

Extravasation and tissue necrosis. Remove the line immediately. Consult the plastic surgeon on call.

Breakage of Silastic catheter. Clamp the catheter immediately. Using sterile technique attach an 18 or 20G Luer stub adaptor as a temporary repair measure. Unclamp and flush with normal saline. Repair with the appropriate kit.

Obstruction of the infusing system. The occlusion alarm on the pump sounds and TPN fluid does not flow to gravity. Check the system for kinks. If the catheter has clotted attempt to dislodge the clot by careful flushing with 1 ml of normal saline attached directly to the catheter hub using sterile technique. If unsuccessful discuss the use of a fibrinolytic agent with the consultant.

5

Growth

This chapter includes guide lines for initial investigation and treatment. If doubt exists or for details regarding treatment, consult the endocrinology team.

Growth centile charts for height, weight and OFC are given on pp 56–61.

Height

In children with tall or short stature always determine if the child's height is compatible with that of his parents:

1. Measure the heights of the mother and father.
2. For boys, add 12 cm to the mother's height; for girls, subtract 12 cm from the father's height.
3. The mean of the adjusted maternal and paternal heights is calculated (midparental height).
4. Follow the child's centile line to age 19 years on the chart. If it is within 8 cm of the midparental height, then it is compatible with that of parents.

ESTIMATION OF MATURE HEIGHT

The height at 3 years shows good correlation with mature height. J.M. Tanner developed the following formulas:

Height (cm) at maturity (male) = 1.27 × height at age 3 years + 54.9 cm

Height (cm) at maturity (female) = 1.29 × height at age 3 years + 42.3 cm

Tall stature

AETIOLOGY

Most commonly constitutional. Rare causes include GH producing tumours, Soto syndrome, Klinefelter syndrome, homocystinuria, Marfan syndrome and sexual precocity.

INVESTIGATIONS

1. Full history and examination.
2. Check bone age and previous growth record. Try to predict adult height.
3. Further detailed investigations are not always necessary but may include karyotype, urinary aminoacids, head CT scan, and GH suppression test.

Growth hormone suppression test

Required if autonomous GH hypersecretion is suspected.
— In a fasting child, collect baseline samples for blood glucose, insulin and GH.
— Give 1.75 g/kg of glucose p.o. (max. 100 g).
— Repeat blood test at 30 min, 1 hour, then hourly for 5 hours.

Interpretation. GH suppresses to an undetectable level in normal children. High basal GH levels which fail to suppress and sometimes a paradoxical rise in GH levels are characteristic of GH hypersecretion.

TREATMENT

1. As for the underlying cause.
2. Very occasionally, girls with constitutional tall stature may benefit from oestrogen therapy to arrest growth.

Short stature

Definition: height below the 3rd centile.

AETIOLOGY

1. Physiological
   a. familial short stature (healthy child with short parents)
   b. familial delayed puberty
2. Pathological disorders
   a. often associated with FTT (see p. 130)
   b. chromosomal (e.g. Turner syndrome)
   c. skeletal dysplasia
   d. endocrine problems (e.g. hypothyroidism, GH deficiency, Cushing syndrome).
   e. nutritional
   f. metabolic disorders
   g. chronic disease (e.g. renal failure).

Other causes include IUGR and iatrogenic causes (e.g. drugs, X-rays).

Endocrine causes are uncommon but most important as they are treatable.

INITIAL ASSESSMENT

1. Full history and examination including visual acuity and visual fields.
2. Accurate height, sitting height, OFC and weight.
3. Document puberty (see below) and measure testicular volume (Praeder orchidometer).

   The majority of children will not require detailed investigations if history, growth velocity and examination are normal.

Indications for further evaluation

These include:
1. Severe short stature (height < −2.5 SD)
2. Unexpectedly short (i.e. parents' heights suggest the child should be taller)
3. Progressive shortening
4. Signs and symptoms of chronic disease, e.g. renal or intracranial
5. Disproportionate growth with either trunk or limb shortening.

NB. The following increase the likelihood of GH or other hormone deficiency:

— normal birthweight and length with subsequent growth failure
— neonatal or later hypoglycaemia; prolonged neonatal jaundice
— micropenis and cryptorchidism
— relative obesity and increased skinfold thickness
— delayed dentition with bone age severely retarded below height age
— previous cranial irradiation treatment or pituitary area surgery
— a subnormal exercise provoked GH level (usually < 5 mu/l).

INVESTIGATIONS

Fast the child. Take a blood sample for:
1. GH, FBC, ESR, Ca^{2+}, PO_4^{3-} and alkaline phosphatase, creatinine, thyroid function tests and cortisol
2. Perform an exercise GH screening test

Exercise growth hormone test

— In a fasted child, collect baseline blood samples for GH
— Run the child up and down stairs for 20 min. The child should be tired but not exhausted; heart rate should not exceed 180/min
— Repeat the blood GH sample (t=20 min)

Interpretation.   A GH level > 15mu/l excludes GH deficiency. Lower values do not necessarily indicate GH deficiency.

3.   Consider chromosomal analysis (especially in girls)
4.   Request SXR with pituitary fossa views/CT to exclude craniopharingioma and left wrist X-ray to determine skeletal bone age.

If these tests do not reveal the cause of short stature, review at 3-monthly intervals. If height velocity falls below the 25th centile (corrected for skeletal maturation) over at least 6 months, further investigation is justified. This involves formal pituitary provocation studies (see p. 53). Refer to the endocrine unit.

Weight

Obesity

AETIOLOGY

Idiopathic: both genetic and environmental. Rare organic causes include hypothyroidism, Cushing's disease, Prader–Willi or Laurence Moon Biedl syndromes, pseudohypoparathyroidism and Turner syndrome.

MANAGEMENT

1.   Full examination and history, including 7 days' full dietary and calorie intake assessment. Accumulation of previous growth data.
     Further investigation is not usually necessary; however, the following tests may be used to screen for an organic cause.
2.   Bone age, serum Ca^{2+}, alkaline phosphatase and PO_4^{3-}, thyroid function tests, early morning serum cortisol after overnight dexamethasone suppression test.
3.   Avoid medications.
4.   Weight loss can only be achieved with calorie restriction and increasing exercise.

Puberty

Definition: a series of changes that leads to the acquisition of the ability to reproduce.

Stages of puberty

Five stages are described, stage 1 being the prepubertal stage. Different elements of puberty can develop at different times relative to each other.

BOYS: GENITAL DEVELOPMENT

Stage 1 = testes, penis and scrotum as in early childhood.
Stage 2 = scrotum and testes grow, skin of scrotum becomes coarser (mean age 12, range 10–14 years).
Stage 3 = lengthening of the penis with further growth of the testes and scrotum (mean age 13, range 12–16 years).
Stage 4 = penis broadens and glans develops, testes and scrotum darkens (mean age 14, range 12–16 years).
Stage 5 = adult stage.

GIRLS: BREAST DEVELOPMENT

Stage 1 = only nipples are raised.
Stage 2 = breast bud; breast and nipple raised as a small mound and areola enlarges (mean age 11.5, range 9–13.5 years).
Stage 3 = further enlargement of the breast and areola but without separation of their contours (mean age 12.5, range 10–14.5 years).
Stage 4 = areola and nipple project to form a mound above the level of the main breast (mean age 13.5, range 11–16 years).
Stage 5 = only the nipple projects.

PUBIC HAIR: BOTH SEXES

Stage 1 = no pubic hair.
Stage 2 = sparse growth of slightly pigmented, downy hair at the base of the penis or along the labia (boys mean age 12.5, range 11–15 years; girls mean age 11.5, range 9–14 years).
Stage 3 = hair darker and coarser, more curled, spreading sparsely (boys mean age 13.5, range 12–15; girls mean age 12, range 10–14.5 years).
Stage 4 = hair adult in type but does not include the medial aspect of the thighs (boys mean age 14.5, range 12–16 years; girls mean age 13, range 10.5–15 years).
Stage 5 = adult pattern involving medial aspect of the thighs.

Common problems

1. **Asymmetrical breast development.** Common during puberty and is benign. Reassure.

2. **Gynaecomastia in boys.** Common during puberty. Usually resolves spontaneously. Very rare causes include Klinefelter syndrome, drugs (e.g. steroids, cimetidine) and testicular/liver cancer. If examination is otherwise normal, reassure.

3. **Menarche.** Mean age 13, range 11–15 years. Periods are often irregular for the first 2 years. Reassure.

4. **Dysmenorrhoea.** Primary dysmenorrhoea (colicky menstrual cramps on day 1 of period) is common and may cause absence from school. There are 3 main approaches to treatment which may be tried in the following order:
   a. analgesics (paracetamol)
   b. prostaglandin inhibitors (i.e. mefenamic acid, 250–500 mg 6-hourly) after food
   c. the combined pill
   Reassurance and explanation are essential.

Delayed puberty

The differential diagnosis of delayed puberty should be considered when a girl over 14 or a boy over 15 years lacks any sexual characteristics, or when the adolescent has not completed maturation over a 5-year period.

AETIOLOGY

1. Familial (constitutional) delayed puberty
2. Chronic systemic disease
3. Endocrine causes, e.g. pituitary or thyroid disorders
4. Chromosomal disorders (e.g. Turner or Klinefelter syndrome)
5. Bilateral gonadal failure

DELAYED PUBERTY IN BOYS

1. Take full history and examination.
2. Measure testicular volume with an orchidometer.
3. Record bone age (left wrist X-ray).
4. Look for evidence of chronic systemic disease, e.g. renal failure, coeliac disease.
5. Consider the possibility of pituitary or thyroid disorder.

By far the most common cause is *familial (constitutional) delayed puberty* which is more frequent in boys than girls. The diagnosis is likely if:

1. There is a family history of late puberty and continuing growth into late teens.
2. The child is showing no adolescent growth spurt.
3. There is no abnormality on examination.
4. Bone age is behind actual age by 2–4 years (height plotted for bone age is appropriate).

Reassure that further growth will occur with time. Only refer for formal investigations if there is no sign of puberty or growth spurt by 14 years of age.

Further investigations

If diagnosis is uncertain, include:
1. Blood for FBC and ESR, U & E, thyroid function tests.
2. Measure plasma testosterone, LH and FSH. Elevated basal levels suggest primary gonadal failure.
3. Thyroid function tests and a combined test of anterior and posterior pituitary function (see p. 53) if there are other features suggesting pituitary dysfunction.
4. Check smell to exclude Kalman's syndrome.
5. Check karyotype (Klinefelter syndrome).

Treatment

Treat the underlying cause. If familial, reassure. For certain patients, temporary hormone replacement (oxandrolone or testosterone in boys and oestrogen in girls) may be warranted for psychological reasons; discuss with the endocrinologist. Replacement therapy is justified for genuine pituitary or gonadal endocrine deficiency.

DELAYED PUBERTY IN GIRLS

Usually managed by gynaecologists. The majority of girls have constitutional delayed maturation. For the remainder, chronic systemic, pituitary and thyroid problems must be borne in mind.

NB. Turner syndrome is not always accompanied by conspicuous signs. Consider if short stature is not corrected by bone age delay.

Precocious puberty

The age range for normal puberty is wide but girls commencing sexual development by the age of 6 or having menarche < 8 years, or boys commencing sexual development < 8 years, may be regarded as having precocious puberty.

AETIOLOGY

Causes include idiopathic, pituitary/hypothalamic disease, neuro-fibromatosis, tuberosclerosis, McCune–Albright syndrome, gon-adotrophin secreting tumours, ovarian tumours, testicular or adrenal tumours, exogenous oestrogens, androgens, anabolic steroids, and hypothyroidism.

PRECOCIOUS PUBERTY IN GIRLS

History should include drug exposure (e.g. steroid or androgen) and detailed family history (e.g. for neurofibromatosis, tubero-sclerosis). Cyclical vaginal bleeding is associated with true puberty.

Assessment

Perform full physical examination including BP to exclude hypertension. Virilisation indicates an adrenal cause. Examine the abdomen and perform a rectal examination to check for an ovarian tumour. A full neurological examination searching for an intra-cranial lesion is essential.

Investigations

1. Measure plasma LH, FH, FSH and oestradiol levels.
2. If there is inappropriate virilisation, perform plasma and urine adrenal androgen studies.
3. Thyroid function tests.
4. Bone age (advanced in precocious puberty, delayed in hypothyroidism).
5. SXR with pituitary fossa views/CT.
6. Abdominal USS or further examination if ovarian tumour is suspected.

Management

Encourage treatment of the child in an age-appropriate manner. Where appropriate, therapy is directed towards the underlying cause (e.g. intracranial, adrenal or ovarian pathology). Indications for drug therapy in the idiopathic group include unacceptable sexual development which is disordering the child's life, and accelerated skeletal development, bringing the problem of severely reduced adult height.

Cyproterone acetate (70–100 mg/m^2 per 24 hours) will slow pubertal changes and skeletal maturation. Discuss with an endocrinologist.

PRECOCIOUS PUBERTY IN BOYS

This is uncommon but very worrying.

Assessment

Take full history including drug exposure and detailed family history. Detailed examination must include:

1. Measurement of testicular size; symmetrical enlarged testes appropriate to the stage of puberty suggest true intracranial puberty; inappropriately small testes point to a false, and probably adrenal, cause for puberty; unilaterally enlarged testis usually indicates a testicular tumour.
2. BP measurement.
3. Full neurological and ophthalmological review.

Investigations

1. Measure plasma LH, FSH and testosterone.
2. LHRH test.
3. Measure plasma and urine adrenal antigen.
4. Thyroid function tests.
5. Wrist X-ray for bone age and SXR with pituitary fossa views.
6. Head CT scan is indicated in all boys with precocious puberty.

Management

Principles are similar to those for girls. Cyproterone acetate is useful in selective cases.

Pituitary function tests

Performed to detect diseases of hypothalamic/pituitary/gonadal/adrenal/thyroid axes.

INDICATIONS

Include investigations of unexplained short stature with retarded bone age, and of other endocrine deficiencies.

Screening tests for GH deficiency have been described above (p. 46). Definitive tests as described below should be discussed with the endocrinologist.

Children with short stature and delayed puberty should be primed with sex hormones prior to the GH stimulation test. In delayed puberty and a bone age of ≤ 10 years boys are given one dose of Sustanon (100 mg i.m. 3–5 days before the test) and girls are given ethinyl oestradiol (100 μg p.o.) each day for 3 days prior to the test.

Insulin tolerance test

This is a potentially dangerous procedure and must only be performed after adequate preparation in the presence of an experienced doctor. Adequate adrenal function is essential. A 9.00 a.m. or exercise-provoked cortisol value > 175 nmol/l should be demonstrated prior to the test. A subnormal cortisol value is a definite contraindication to insulin administration unless the child is also given hydrocortisone. Other contraindications to the test: a history of convulsions, previous hypoglycaemic episodes and diabetes mellitus.

1. The child must be fasted.
2. A direct reading system at the bedside (e.g. Reflomat) will enable continuous monitoring of blood glucose. Arrange with the lab. for immediate analysis of blood glucose levels also.
3. Insert a reliable i.v. line.
4. 25% dextrose must be available in a syringe to treat severe hypoglycaemia (1–2 ml/kg bodyweight 25% dextrose i.v.) (see p. 174).
5. Collect baseline samples at t = –30 and 0 min for blood glucose, GH, cortisol and prolactin.
6. Inject insulin bolus i.v. Usual dose of Actrapid is 0.1–0.15 u/kg bodyweight. Use 0.05 u/kg if pituitary insufficiency is strongly suspected.
7. Collect blood samples for glucose and GH at t = 15, 30, 45, 60 and 120 min and for cortisol and prolactin at t = 30, 60 and 120 min.

Hypoglycaemic symptoms usually occur 15–30 min after insulin injection. If severe, collect a blood sample immediately for cortisol, GH, prolactin and glucose, and give i.v. dextrose. Always give a meal after the test and keep under observation in hospital until completely recovered.

INTERPRETATION

Blood glucose should decrease by 50% of baseline values or there should be signs of hypoglycaemia (sweating, tachycardia, drowsiness, headache). Peak GH levels < 7 mu/l indicate GH deficiency. This is excluded with levels > 15 mu/l. Levels between these may indicate partial GH deficiency and require a second, different, test for GH, e.g. the oral Bovril test.

Thyroid stimulating hormone (TSH) stimulation test

The child does not need to be fasted.
1. Collect blood at t = –30 and 0 min for TSH, T_4, T_3 and prolactin.
2. Give TRH (200 µg or 7 µg/kg i.v. over 10 min).
3. Collect blood at t = 0, 30, 60 and 120 min for TSH and prolactin, and at t = 120 min for T_3 and T_4.

INTERPRETATION

Peak TSH levels (10–30 mu/l) occur at 30 min. An exaggerated delayed peak TSH response is suggestive of hypothalamic hypothyroidism. Elevated basal and peak levels are consistent with primary hypothyroidism. Hyperthyroidism is usually associated with suppressed TSH levels unresponsive to TRH stimulation.

Gonadotrophin-releasing hormone

The child need not be fasting.
1. Collect blood at t = −30 and 0 min for LH, FSH and oestradiol (girls) or testosterone (boys).
2. Give 100 μg LHRH (or 2.5 μg/kg i.v.).
3. Collect blood at t = 30, 90 and 120 min for LH, FSH and at t = 120 min for oestradiol or testosterone.

INTERPRETATION

Depends on the stage of puberty. An absent response suggests gonadotrophin deficiency, but this is unreliable in prepuberty and in the child with simple delayed puberty. An exaggerated response is obtained in precocious puberty (exaggerated for age) and in primary gonadal failure (e.g. Turner syndrome).

Combined test of anterior and posterior pituitary function

This involves the above three tests performed simultaneously, collecting samples as described. As the child is fasting for the test a baseline plasma and urine osmolality is usually sufficient to exclude diabetes insipidus.

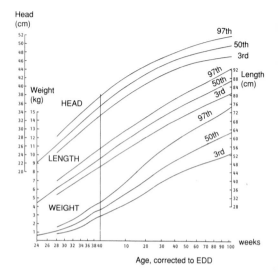

Fig. 5.1 Centiles for boys' weight, height and head circumference in the first 2 years of life.

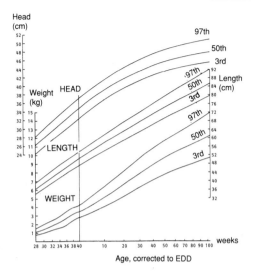

Fig. 5.2 Centiles for girls' weight, height and head circumference in the first 2 years of life.

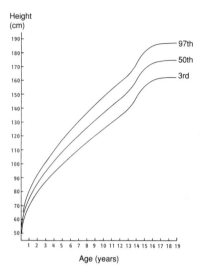

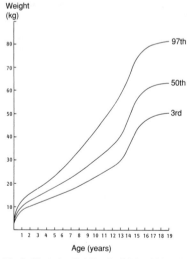

Fig. 5.3 Centiles for boys' height and weight from birth to 19 years.

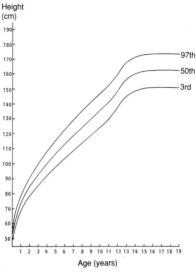

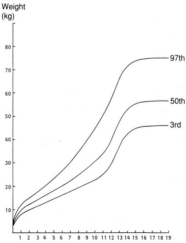

Fig. 5.4   Centiles for girls' height and weight from birth to 19 years.

a Head circumference (cm)

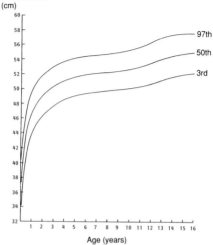

b Head
circumference
(cm)

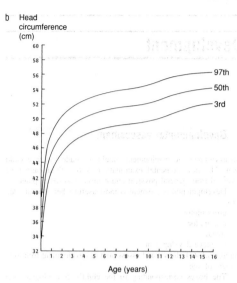

Fig. 5.5 Centiles for (a) boys' and (b) girls' head circumferences from birth to 16 years.

6

Development

An assessment of development should be made for each child seen. The developmental examination of the child cannot be divorced from general physical and neurological development.

Developmental assessment is most useful when it is divided into:

1. gross motor
2. fine motor
3. social
4. language development

Figures 6.1–6.4 allow rapid assessment of development from 0 to 5 years of age.

The boxes corresponding to the child's chronological age are filled in (horizontal axis) against the age related developmental items on the left. One box must be filled in for each item achieved.

90% of children will complete items above the black line. Those 10% scoring below the line should be reassessed within 1 month, and referral considered if they are still behind. Once suspicion regarding a child's development has been raised a paediatric consultation is required.

If developmental delay is confirmed a full multidisciplinary assessment is needed. The aims of this are to:

1. Promote optimal performance of the child
2. Involve parents in the assessment process
3. Arrange liaison between services offering help and support
4. Identify areas of delay and plan a management programme. Assessment of hearing (p. 280) and vision (p. 281) are detailed elsewhere.

PREMATURITY

A premature infant may not attain developmental milestones as quickly as a fullterm infant. Nevertheless a child born 4 weeks premature usually catches up by 1 year of age.

SYSTEMIC ILLNESS

Normal developmental milestones may not apply to infants and children with systemic illness, e.g. significant cardiac disease.

Language

The stages of speech and language development are shown in Figure 6.4.

ASSESSMENT

1. In a child with speech difficulty consider:
   a. general developmental delay
   b. hearing or visual defect (check hearing formally)
   c. neurological status (e.g. CP)
   d. environmental factors (e.g. poor stimulation)
   e. structural abnormalities (e.g. cleft palate, malocclusion of the jaw)
   f. psychiatric problems, e.g. autism
2. Speech therapists like to see children early.
3. If poor environment is thought to be the cause, consider the use of a toy library, home programme or day care.
4. Investigations are usually unnecessary. EEG is indicated if there is a history of epilepsy or if language has regressed.

With speech therapy the majority of children will manage in ordinary schools.

Common problems

Cerebral palsy

A permanent and non-progressive motor disorder due to brain damage before birth or during the first few years of life. The lesion is static but the clinical picture is not and the presentation reflects the part of the brain involved in motor control which is affected. Affects 2/1000 children.

The types of CP are:
1. Spastic (70%): monoplegia, hemiplegia (arm > leg), diplegia (both legs > arms), quadriplegia. There may be hypotonia initially.
2. Ataxic (usually truncal)

3. Dyskinetic
4. Mixed

AETIOLOGY

The causes listed below indicate an at-risk population which should be followed up, but at least 50% of the cases of CP will have no obvious predisposing cause.
1. Prenatal, e.g. intrauterine infections, drugs and placental dysfunction.
2. Perinatal, e.g. hypoxia, haemorrhage or infarction of the brain, hypoglycemia, meningitis.
3. Postnatal, e.g. meningitis or encephalitis, trauma, encephalopathies.
4. Very low birthweight babies.

FEATURES

1. Symptoms include parental concern about feeding, excessive quietness or irritability, poor vision or hearing, slow to sit, crawl or walk, or delayed developmental milestones.
2. Examine for signs of CP and aetiological clues:
   — microcephaly, hydrocephalus or abnormally shaped skull
   — spasticity, hypotonia, rigidity or ataxia
   — abnormal movements or posture, including fisting, athetosis, opisthotonus, scissoring of the legs
   — cataracts, retinitis pigmentosa, strabismus, blindness
   — deafness

DIFFERENTIAL DIAGNOSIS

This is enormous but revolves around whether:
1. there is purely a motor deficit, in which case the differential is of weakness (see Table 12.11) or ataxia (see Table 12.9);
2. there is associated mental impairment.

NB. Although CP is primarily a motor disorder, the following problems are commonly associated:
1. severe and moderate learning difficulties
2. 30% are epileptic
3. squint
4. sensorineural deafness and impaired language
Careful management of these disorders can enable the child to function at an optimal level.

ONGOING MANAGEMENT PROBLEMS

The consultant in charge of the child must be kept informed of any difficulties or changes in management.

Consider the following checklist at each 6-monthly appointment:

1. Do the parents know the diagnosis, prognosis and implication for future pregnancies?
2. What support do the parents have, family or otherwise?
3. Could any of the following professions help — health visitor, physiotherapist, occupational therapist and social worker? Vision and hearing should be formally assessed in every child and reviewed again as necessary.
4. The GP and, if at school, the teacher must be fully involved.
5. Dietitian and speech therapist involvement is needed for a difficult feeder or FTT. Obesity may occur due to immobility.
6. Are seizures adequately treated or overtreated (causing sedation)? Antispasmodic medication and night sedation may improve the quality of life.
7. Enuresis and constipation are common. Treat constipation as detailed on p. 138.
8. Orthopaedic advice for contractures and disabling foot equinus. Hip subluxation and eventual dislocation may occur. Early detection is important as soft tissue releases can be performed for hips that are at risk. Hip X-rays may be performed at 1-yearly intervals to monitor hip position.
9. Physiotherapy assessment is essential to prevent contractures. If these occur, tendon release may be advisable. Special shoes, splints, walking aids or wheelchair can be arranged through the physiotherapy department. Start physiotherapy by 6 months if possible.
10. Drooling can often be alleviated by techniques employed by speech therapists.
11. Dental health: especially important to obtain dental opinion if the child is irritable or in pain.
12. 'Chestiness'
    a. Exclude/treat GOR (this may also cause irritability and pain) as aspiration is common.
    b. Treat asthma if present. Inhaled beclomethasone dipropionate or budesonide may be given via a spacer device with a facemask attachment.
    c. Infection (see the section on pneumonia, p. 118).

Spina bifida cystica

DIAGNOSIS

The lesion is obvious.

INITIAL MANAGEMENT

1. Cover the defect with a sterile dressing soaked in saline.

2. Refer to the neurosurgeon who will discuss treatment (closure of the back) with parents.
3. Carefully monitor to detect the development of hydrocephalus as VP shunting may be required.
4. Urological assessment: urine for culture, renal USS to exclude hydronephrosis.
5. Orthopaedic assessment of hips and any musculoskeletal deformities present.

ONGOING MANAGEMENT PROBLEMS

Only those that may present to junior medical staff are considered here. Longterm management will be coordinated by the consultant in charge. Problems that the child may encounter should be discussed with this consultant whenever possible.

Subsequent admission will usually be for a specific operation or examination or for an acute or recurrent complication, e.g. shunt blockage or pressure sore.

1. Shunt problems
Blockage and infection are serious.
a. Shunt infection: this should be suspected in any child with a shunt who has recurrent shunt obstruction, fever, general malaise, headache, anaemia or splenomegaly. May mimic a UTI; therefore always send a urine sample.
b. Shunt blockage.

Symptoms. Drowsiness, headache, vomiting, fits. Occasionally shunt malfunction may be episodic or may occur over months with changes in school performance, personality or behaviour.

Signs. May include fontanelle tension, recent increase in head circumference in infants, deterioration in conscious state, focal neurological signs, change in BP, pulse and respiration.

If the upper end of the shunt is blocked, the pump depresses but does not refill. With a lower end block, the pump is difficult to depress. Disconnection may present as above or with local swelling. X-rays may demonstrate a disconnection.

Management. Refer to the neurosurgeon on call.

2. Renal problems
The aim is to preserve renal function and maintain continence:
a. UTI is common; if suspected (e.g. fever, vomiting, parental concern, irritability) obtain a bladder specimen by catheter or by suprapubic aspiration.

Older children may have an ileal conduit; urinary results from these are often difficult to interpret. The specimen is obtained by the double catheter method; a pure growth suggests infection but a mixed growth may not.

Investigations and treatment. Should be aggressive (see UTI, p. 155).

b. Bladder discharge in patients with ileal conduits; wash out daily with neomycin or Polybactrin via the urethral catheter. Systemic antibiotics are not usually necessary.

c. Continence, regular catheterisation. If problems arise discuss with the urologist.

3. Constipation

The goal in the management of the neurogenic bowel is for the child to be able to defecate at a time of his choosing and to be clean in between. Constipation and overflow incontinence should be prevented and treated with dietary advice, laxatives and bowel wash out if necessary (see p. 138).

4. Pressure sores

These occur in most cases with time. Avoidance is by occupational therapy assessment of pressure areas. Management of pressure sores: discuss with the consultant in charge and plastic surgeon.

5. Pathological fractures

May present as local swelling without pain. These are often of the femur secondary to osteoporosis. Consult the orthopaedic surgeon.

6. Epilepsy

Occurs in 15%. For management see p. 187.

7. Tethered cord

Suspicions should be aroused by loss of bladder and bowel control and loss of lower limb motor function. Consult the neurosurgeon.

8. Syringomyelia

Suggested by loss of upper limb function, especially sensory loss with preservation of motor function.

9. Basilar herniation

May cause central hypoventilation and require posterior fossa decompression.

10. Kyphoscoliosis

Check for presence. If unsure, assessment by the orthopaedic surgeons is indicated.

Mental handicap

The cause is currently impossible to define in a large number of children. Mild retardation (IQ 50–70) affects 30/1000 children and severe retardation (IQ < 50) affects 3/1000 children.

AETIOLOGY

1. Unknown in >20%.
2. Prenatal causes, e.g. chromosomal causes (e.g. Down's and fragile X syndromes), dysmorphic syndromes, intrauterine infections.
3. Perinatal infection (e.g. meningitis, encephalitis).
4. Postnatal infection, trauma, neurodegenerative disorders.

Many cases are associated with CP.

EVALUATION

It is reasonable to admit a child with mental impairment for investigation

a. to avoid missing a treatable cause and
b. to help with genetic counselling.

History

Pregnancy, drugs, labour, alcohol. Birth size, prematurity or perinatal problems. Family history for mental retardation and consanguinity.

Examination

Note specifically isolated microcephaly or megacephaly. Dysmorphic features should be recognised and evaluated. Full neurological examination, including Wood's light to exclude tuberous sclerosis. Hearing and vision should be formally assessed.

Investigations

It is important that none of the tests listed below be considered routine. It is beyond the scope of this book to discuss all possibilities. Where indicated, consultants in genetics, neurology, ophthalmology and dermatology may suggest further relevant tests.

Suggested investigations include:

1. **Mild mental handicap.** EEG; chromosomal analysis, including study for fragile X; creatinine kinase; plasma Ca^{2+}, plasma and urine aminoacids; thyroid function tests; lead levels; TORCH screen (for developmental delay in infancy); urine for metabolic screen; lead levels; fasting blood sugar. Further tests may be suggested clinically.

2. **Severe mental handicap.** As above plus CT brain scan; 24-hour urine for heparin sulphate and for free salycilic acid; skin biopsy for liposomal inclusions. Plasma aminoacids in the mother; LFTs.

3. **Profoundly retarded children.** As above plus ERG and plasma uric acid.

MANAGEMENT

1. Treatment of the medical cause if possible.
2. Parental counselling and early intervention should be coordinated by the consultant in charge or by the department of developmental paediatrics.

The late walking child

97% of children are taking 6 or more steps unaided by the age of 18 months. The remaining 3% fall into three groups:

1. Idiopathic late walkers account for > 90% of such children. They tend to have a family history of late walking and mobilise by bottom shuffling, rolling or creeping. They can also be hypotonic, have had late sitting or lax joints. They can be expected to develop normally.
2. Those with conditions that may present at this age with delayed walking, e.g.
   a. CP: spastic diplegia may present as late walking. Diagnosis is suggested by increased tone, difficulty in dorsiflexion of the feet and brisk reflexes.
   b. Mental handicap, late walking may be the first sign of global retardation.
   c. Congenital dislocation of the hip.
   d. Duchenne muscular dystrophy.
3. Those with previously diagnosed problems, e.g. CNS abnormalities, orthopaedic problems, Down's and other syndromes, neuromuscular conditions.
   Clues to neurological damage include — abnormal reflexes, head circumference below the 3rd centile, history of perinatal distress, delayed speech.

INVESTIGATIONS

If the cause is not obvious check plasma creatinine phosphokinase to exclude Duchenne muscular dystrophy.

The clumsy child

Definition: difficulty in learning and performing motor tasks (incidence 5–15%: boys: girls 4 : 1).

AETIOLOGY

Normal variant, delay in motor development, general developmental delay, perinatal asphyxia, hyperactivity.

Important but rare medical conditions include epilepsy, neuroblastoma, cerebellar tumours, acute cerebellar ataxia (e.g. post chicken pox), Wilson's disease, Friedreich's ataxia and hydrocephalus.

PRESENTATION

Children may have gross or fine motor difficulties, speech disorder, learning difficulties, problems with reading and writing. Laterality may be slow to develop. Older children may develop behaviour difficulties.

EXAMINATION

Full neurological examination to exclude minimal CP, progressive pathology or squint. Evaluate for emotional immaturity and hyperactivity.

Specific tests. Test fine motor skills (brick building, pencil grasp, pronation and supination of hand, threading beads), gross motor skills (standing on one leg, hopping, heel–toe walking, skipping, kicking a ball), movements of muscles involved in speech (i.e. blowing, whistling, tongue protrusion).

MANAGEMENT

Assuming a pathological cause has not been found:
1. Reassure the parents and child that he is not careless, lazy or dull and that things usually improve with time.
2. Encourage activities that the child can do well (e.g. swimming).
3. Training skills leads to improvement. Once a motor skill is learned it is retained. A graded series of tasks starting with what the child can do is helpful.
4. Involvement of teachers, occupational therapist, physiotherapist, speech therapist or educational psychologist in remedial programmes if required.

Common behaviour problems

Temper tantrums in toddlers

Full history is needed. Management depends on history. Reassurance can be given that the occasional tantrum in a young child (2–4 years) is commonplace and of no harm. Diverting the child's attention may abort a tantrum early in its course. However, it is almost impossible to reason with a toddler having a tantrum. In these circumstances advise the parent to pretend to ignore the behaviour, thus giving no reward. This is difficult and plans of how to do this may be needed, e.g. what to do if the tantrum occurs repeatedly in the supermarket.

Management must be consistent between parents and other care givers. Judicious use of 'time out' to give the child time to regain control may help. Locking the child in the bedroom may be frightening and is not recommended. Medication has no place in management.

Breath holding attacks

May occur in some children when they are frightened, annoyed or hurt.
1. Minor form: sudden cessation of breathing during the course of a spell of crying, usually brief and may be associated with cyanosis.
2. Severe form: may result in unconsciousness and convulsive movements and must be differentiated from true epilepsy by an accurate history. The characteristic sequence of events is provocation, crying, apnoea, rigidity, convulsive movements and stupor or loss of consciousness.
   Episodes commence between the age of 6 and 24 months and disappear spontaneously by about 4 years.
   Prognosis is excellent. No drug treatment is required. Parents need explanation and reassurance.

Sleep (night) terrors

A condition marked by repeated episodes of wakening from sleep in children aged 4–12 years. In a typical episode, the child sits up abruptly in bed, appears frightened and demonstrates signs of acute anxiety: dilated pupils, excessive perspiration, tachypnoea and tachycardia. This may last up to 10 minutes. The child is unresponsive to efforts to comfort him, until the agitation subsides as the child gradually wakens.

There is no memory of the event the following day. The course is variable, occurring in intervals of days or weeks and gradually resolves without treatment.

MANAGEMENT

Reassurance is essential. The condition is not associated with psychopathology in childhood. If symptoms are occurring very often and are very disruptive to the family a night sedative may be indicated for short periods.

Sleep walking

Onset is usually between 6 and 12 years, affects 1–6% of children and may last for several years.

The sleepwalker has a blank face, appears to stare and is unresponsive to the efforts of others to influence his sleep walking or to communicate with him. He can be awakened only with great difficulty.

Coordination tends to be poor and injury may occur from falls. The child may return to bed or fall asleep in another place.

Sleep talking may occur but articulation is usually poor. May be associated with night terrors.

On awakening from the sleep episode or the next morning the person has amnesia for the period. No specific psychopathology has been linked with this condition.

MANAGEMENT

Explanation and reassurance.

Sleeping difficulties

Parental worries include:
1. Amount of sleep: particularly when this does not match parental expectations. Newborns often have sleep/wake cycles of about 4 hours determined by hunger, though this may be very variable.

   By 12 weeks most have moved to a diurnal cycle and 50–70% are reported to sleep through the night.

   Older children may need only 8–10 hours sleep but may be

expected to sleep 12–14 hours.

2. Night waking: all children awaken briefly during the night and settle back to sleep.

    Night waking becomes less common with maturity — 20% of all 1–2-year-olds wake ≥ 5 nights a week, 14% of 3-year-olds wake ≥ 3 nights a week and 3% of 8-year-olds wake ≥ 3 nights a week.

3. Early morning waking: common in the 18–36-month age group. A combination of settling difficulties, night waking and early morning waking is common.

MANAGEMENT

1. Ensure regular meals, exercise, fresh air, etc.
2. Have a familiar routine at bed time, e.g. bath, warm drink, cuddly toy, bed time story, etc.
3. If the child comes into parents' bed, and this is not acceptable, quietly return the child to his own bed until the behaviour stops.
4. During the night, respond consistently. No change in lighting, no talking, resist giving drink.
5. If the child cries it is acceptable to go in every 5–10 min to check, but with minimal interaction between parent and child.
6. Move from unacceptable to desired pattern of behaviour in gradual small steps, e.g. move bed time forward in half-hour steps.
7. Positive reinforcement is useful in children > 3 years.
8. Drug treatment: not first line but useful in breaking the cycle of parental sleep deprivation. Short term only. Most useful in initiating sleep. Dose must be adequate as too little may have the reverse affect.

    Suggested dose: trimeprazine (Vallergan) 3 mg/kg.

Teething

Usually starts at 6 months. The diagnosis of severe illnesses has been delayed because symptoms have been incorrectly attributed to teething; teething does not cause fever, cough, convulsions or diarrhoea. It may cause some increase in restlessness, finger sucking and gum rubbing, dribbling and some change in feeding habits.

Examination of the gums reveals no change in the colour of the mucosa in one-third, slight erythema in one-third and marked erythema and small haemorrhages in the remaining third of infants.

TREATMENT

Reassure parents. Soften the diet if there is a reluctance to take hard food. Most infants need no help or treatment. However, an occasional dose of paracetamol, 'gum rub gel' or a teething ring may help in specific cases.

Tongue tie

Only very rarely causes genuine speech or feeding problems. As the tongue grows the tip becomes free. Frenectomy is only rarely required.

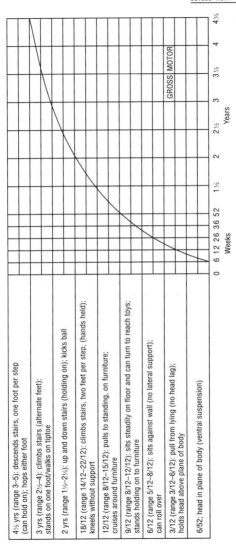

Fig. 6.1 Development of gross motor skills from 6 weeks to 4½ years.

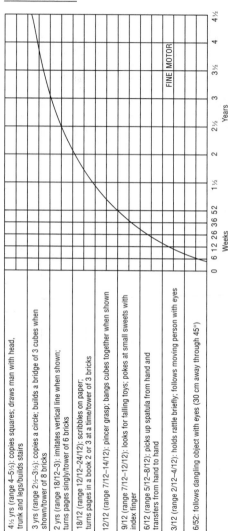

	4½ yrs (range 4–5½): copies squares; draws man with head, trunk and legs/builds stairs
	3 yrs (range 2½–3½): copies a circle; builds a bridge of 3 cubes when shown/tower of 8 bricks
	2 yrs (range 18/12–3): imitates vertical line when shown; turns pages singly/tower of 6 bricks
	18/12 (range 12/12–24/12): scribbles on paper; turns pages in a book 2 or 3 at a time/tower of 3 bricks
	12/12 (range 7/12–14/12): pincer grasp; bangs cubes together when shown
	9/12 (range 7/12–12/12): looks for falling toys; pokes at small sweets with index finger
	6/12 (range 5/12–8/12): picks up spatula from hand and transfers from hand to hand
	3/12 (range 2/12–4/12): holds rattle briefly; follows moving person with eyes
	6/52: follows dangling object with eyes (30 cm away through 45°)

Fig. 6.2 Development of fine motor skills from 6 weeks to 4½ years.

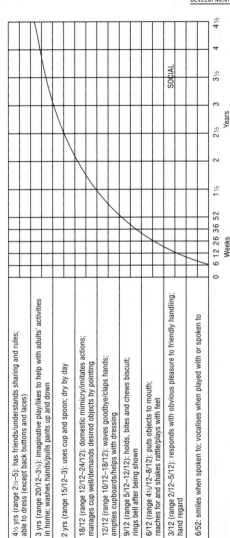

4½ yrs (range 2½–5): has friends/understands sharing and rules; able to dress (except back buttons and laces)

3 yrs (range 20/12–3½): imaginative play/likes to help with adults' activities in home; washes hands/pulls pants up and down

2 yrs (range 15/12–3): uses cup and spoon; dry by day

18/12 (range 12/12–24/12): domestic mimicry/imitates actions; manages cup well/demands desired objects by pointing

12/12 (range 10/12–18/12): waves goodbye/claps hands; empties cupboards/helps with dressing

9/12 (range 5/12–12/12): holds, bites and chews biscuit; rings bell after being shown

6/12 (range 4½/12–8/12): puts objects to mouth; reaches for and shakes rattle/plays with feet

3/12 (range 2/12–5/12): responds with obvious pleasure to friendly handling; hand regard

6/52: smiles when spoken to; vocalises when played with or spoken to

Fig. 6.3   Development of social skills from 6 weeks to 4½ years.

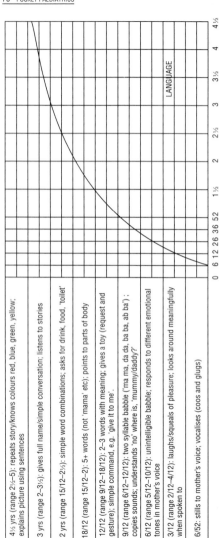

Fig. 6.4 Development of language skills from 6 weeks to 4½ years.

4½ yrs (range 2½–5): repeats story/knows colours red, blue, green, yellow; explains picture using sentences

3 yrs (range 2–3½): gives full name/simple conversation; listens to stories

2 yrs (range 15/12–2½): simple word combinations; asks for drink, food, 'toilet'

18/12 (range 15/12–2): 5+ words (not 'mama' etc); points to parts of body

12/12 (range 9/12–18/12): 2–3 words with meaning; gives a toy (request and gesture); simple command, e.g. 'give it to me'.

9/12 (range 6/12–12/12): two syllable babble ('ma ma, da da, ba ba, ab ba') ; copies sounds; understands 'no' 'where is', 'mummy/daddy?'

6/12 (range 5/12–10/12): unintelligible babble; responds to different emotional tones in mother's voice

3/12 (range 2/12–4/12): laughs/squeals of pleasure; looks around meaningfully when spoken to

6/52: stills to mother's voice; vocalises (coos and glugs)

7

Cardiology

Congenital heart disease (CHD)

Background

The commonest congenital abnormality (8 per 1000 livebirths and another 10 per 1000 with asymptomatic bicuspid valve). Over 15% have an extracardiac anomaly.

Postnatal presentation

CYANOSIS

$\frac{1}{3}$ of CHD — usually more complex. The major defects resulting in cyanotic CHD can be grouped by age of presentation — the two commonest causes are tetralogy of Fallot and transposition.

Detected within 48 hours

1. Transitional circulation (PFC) — associations are:
   a. No lung disorder — idiopathic
      — structural CHD
      — birth asphyxia
      — severe polycythaemia or haemolysis
      — hypoglycaemia and hypocalcaemia
   b. Lung disorder — MAS
      — pneumonia
      — RDS
      — congenital abnormality, especially diaphragmatic hernia
2. Transposition of the great arteries
3. Tricuspid atresia (with right-to-left shunt at the atrial level)
4. Total pulmonary atresia or severe stenosis (with or without intact ventricular septum)

Detected within the first week
5. Ebstein's anomaly (with right-to-left shunt at the atrial level)
6. AV canal defect

Detected after the first week
7. Tetralogy of Fallot
8. Total anomalous pulmonary venous drainage (unless obstructed when presentation is earlier)

ACYANOTIC

Represents the other $\frac{2}{3}$ and usually less complex. Present as:

A. Heart failure
Usually large left-to-right shunt or obstruction

Present within the first week
1. Hypoplastic left heart
2. Endocardial fibroelastosis
3. Aortic atresia or severe stenosis
4. Severe coarctation of the aorta

Present after the first week
1. VSD
2. PDA
3. More complex lesions, such as TAPVD, AV canal defect, truncus

B. Heart murmur
Seen in many infants in the first few days of life, innocent murmurs continue to be common throughout childhood. Significant CHD which may present as a murmur includes the six commonest acyanotic lesions:
1. PDA — murmur persists from neonatal period onwards
2. VSD — commonest CHD; heart failure at around 6 weeks, or murmur at any age . Murmur may be absent in the newborn period.
3. ASD — the murmur most commonly missed, usually detected in preschool or school child
4. PS
5. Coarctation of the aorta
6. LV outflow obstruction — AS or HOCM

Cyanosis, cardiac failure and cardiac murmur are the commonest presentations but the following may also suggest CHD:
1. Hypertension — coarctation; see also p. 95
2. Arrhythmias — see p. 90
3. Polycythaemia — if cyanosis not detected
4. Embolism or stroke — predisposed by right-to-left shunt, polycythaemia, SBE and hypertension

5. Atypical or recurrent chest infection — TAPVD, large ASD or VSD
6. SBE — see p. 92

Clinical diagnosis

SYMPTOMS

1. FTT or poor feeding
2. Symptoms of cardiac failure — sweaty forehead on feeding, slow to feed, rapid breathing
3. Cyanotic spells and squatting in Fallot's
   — cyanosis due to CHD is rarely accompanied by tachypnoea unless there is also cardiac failure
   — peripheral cyanosis in a neonate is common and normal

SIGNS

1. Cyanosis

Are there any signs of a non-cardiac cause?

a. respiratory disease
b. CNS depression
c. in the newborn, polycythaemia may be mistaken for cyanosis, as may trauma. Septicaemia and methaemoglobinaemia are other differentials

2. Pulses

Palpate both brachial pulses and *always* the femoral pulses (to exclude coarctation).

a. small pulse: cardiac failure, AS, shock
b. wide pulse: PDA, aortic regurgitation (very rare), septicaemia

Age (years)	Normal range for pulse (beats/min)
0–2	80–140
2–6	75–120
>6	70–110

3. Apex beat

a. CHD is more likely with isolated dextrocardia than with situs inversus of all viscera. The heart may be pushed to the right by left pneumothorax or left diaphragmatic hernia, or pulled to the right by collapse of the right lung.
b. Prominent LV most commonly due to a thin or febrile child. If genuine, think of LVH (VSD, AS, coarctation, PDA).
c. Prominent RV suggests RVH (PS, Fallot's, VSD).
d. Thrill at LSE (usually VSD but sometimes PDA if preterm) or suprasternal notch (AS).

4. Murmurs

a. *Innocent murmurs*: short, soft, systolic and do not radiate. The murmur may vary with position (e.g. venous hum). The child is asymptomatic, there are no other signs, and ECG and CXR (if done) are normal.

b. *Systolic murmurs:* ASD, VSD, AS, HOCM, coarctation.

c. *Diastolic murmurs:* always significant but rare.

d. *Continuous murmurs:* innocent venous hum is soft and low pitched. Harsh loud murmur continuing into diastole — think of PDA and coarctation.

Remember, absence of a murmur does not exclude CHD.

5. Heart sounds

a. A loud second sound is usually due to pulmonary hypertension. Don't worry about splitting of the second sound — very difficult for the inexperienced ear.

b. Definitely a single second sound — always CHD.

c. Definitely fixed split — ASD.

d. Pericardial rub — urgent USS for effusion.

Examine the child for dysmorphic features or associated congenital anomalies (15%). Hepatomegaly is an early sign of failure of either ventricle in infancy.

See Figs A.1–A.3 (pp 364–366) for BP. In the context of CHD, low BP suggests outflow obstruction or cardiac failure; high BP suggests coarctation (as does upper–lower limb difference of > 20 mmHg). Normal BP and no measured limb difference does not exclude coarctation.

Investigation

Many neonates have a murmur and the vast majority disappear with time. Only those who are symptomatic, cyanosed or have absent femoral pulses need urgent investigation. Investigations are more difficult to do and to interpret in the neonate so try to postpone them even if the murmur does not sound innocent (usually VSD or PDA). Therefore:

a. see the baby again at discharge. If the murmur is still present, follow-up at 6 weeks;

b. if still asymptomatic, thriving and isolated murmur at 6 weeks, see again at 3 months. If the murmur is still present, request ECG and CXR;

c. if ECG and CXR are normal, *make a decision* to either discharge or request USS if you can interpret it, or refer to the cardiologist for further assessment.

A. ECG (see Table 7.1 for abnormal values with age)

Voltage criteria for atrial and ventricular hypertrophy are better for monitoring progress than for arriving at a diagnosis. The common-est characteristic patterns are:

1. Right axis deviation

— secundum ASD (95% also have IRBBB, i.e. RSR[1] wave in V_1, and usually RVH)
— transposition
— RVH, including Fallot's
— hypoplastic left heart
— Ebstein's anomaly
— WPWS

2. Left axis deviation

— primum ASD (usually IRBBB, RAH and biventricular hyper-trophy)
— LVH
— AV canal defect
— cardiac pacing
— WPWS

Table 7.1a Electrocardiogram — axis and rhythm. Usually 1 mm duration = 0.04 sec, 10 mm amplitude = 1 mV

Axis	Compare the direction and size of R–S voltage in leads I and AVF
	If R–S is negative in I, axis is > +90° (abnormal outside the neonatal period)
	If R–S is negative in AVF, axis is superior (always abnormal)

Normal range	Age
+60 to +180°	1st week
+20 to + 120°	1 week–1 year
0 to +120°	1–3 years
0 to 90°	> 3 years

Rhythm	A P wave should precede every QRS
	Respiratory sinus arrhythmia is common in children

Max. P–R interval (sec)	Age
0.15	0–18 months
0.17	18 months to puberty
0.20	After puberty

QT interval may be prolonged in hypokalaemia, hypocalcaemia, hypothermia, myocarditis and as a familial cause of sudden arrhythmias (e.g. Lange-Neilsen syndrome). The interval varies with heart rate and must be corrected:

$$\text{QT corrected} = \frac{\text{QT interval (i.e. beginning of Q to end of T, in sec)}}{\sqrt{\text{R–R interval (i.e. cycle length in sec)}}}$$

Interpretation	The normal range of QT corrected is 0.35–0.45. If you are unable to calculate this, as a rough approximation the uncorrected QT should be <0.3 sec at 160/min and < 0.45 sec at 60/min

Table 7.1b Electrocardiogram — features of hypertrophy

Voltage criteria

Right ventricular hypertrophy	1.	R in $V_1 \geq 20$ mm at any age
	2.	S in $V_6 \geq 14$ mm first week
		≥ 10 mm 1 week–1 month
		≥ 7 mm–3 months
		≥ 5 mm > 3 months
	3.	R/S ratio in $V_1 \geq 7$ 0–3 months
		≥ 4 3–6 months
		≥ 3 6 months– 3 years
		≥ 2 3–5 years
		≥ 1 > 5 years
	4.	Persistence of upright T wave in V_1 after first week of life.
Left ventricular hypertrophy	1.	S in $V_1 \geq 20$ mm at any age
	2.	R in $V_6 > 20$ mm at any age
	3.	Inverted T waves in V_5 or V_6 at any age
	4.	Q wave > 4 mm in V_5 or V_6 at any age (also suggests septal hypertrophy as in the infant of a diabetic mother or HOCM)
Combined ventricular hypertrophy	1.	Total R + S ≥ 50 mm in V_3 or V_4 at any age
	2.	RVH as above + inverted T wave in V_6 (and usually upright T in V_1)
	3.	RVH and LVH by above criteria
Small ventricular voltages		Is the calibration correct?
	1.	Pericardial effusion, hyperinflation of lungs, or gross obesity
	2.	Hypothyroidism
	3.	Myocarditis or cardiomyopathy
Right atrial hypertrophy		P wave ≥ 3 mm any lead, any age
Left atrial hypertrophy	1.	Bifid P wave any lead, any age
	2.	P wave ≥ 0.1 sec in duration, any lead, any age

3. Superior axis

— cardiac failure and IRBBB = endocardial cushion defect
— cyanosis = tricuspid atresia (usually LVH also)

4. Right ventricular hypertrophy (RVH)

— VSD
— pulmonary atresia or severe PS and Fallot's
— primum ASD
— TAPVD
— transposition
— hypoplastic left heart
— truncus
— acquired cor pulmonale

Table 7.1c Electrocardiogram — morphology

Tall T waves (>30% of the R wave in a left-sided chest lead) — hyperkalaemia
Flat T waves — myocarditis, hypothyroidism
Inverted T waves — normal in III (horizontal heart); may also indicate myocardial ischaemia or pericarditis or endocardial fibroelastosis. See RVH and LVH above
Depressed ST segment — hypokalaemia
Elevated ST segment — myocardial ischaemia
Wide QRS complex (> 0.12 sec) — conduction defect or artificial pacing
Delta wave (slow upstroke of R wave) and wide QRS — WPWS

Table 7.1d Neonatal electrocardiogram

Neonatal pattern	1.	Axis is +60° to +180° at birth but +75° (average) by 1 month
	2.	The ECG is 'right dominant' at birth, i.e. voltages are larger in the right-sided chest leads and T waves are upright in V$_1$ initially. T waves invert in the right-sided chest leads after the first week and become upright again after puberty
	3.	Normal R wave progression (smaller on the right chest to larger on the left chest leads) occurs by 3 months

5. Left ventricular hypertrophy (LVH)

— VSD
— tricuspid atresia
— primum ASD
— coarctation
— PDA
— severe AS
— RV hypoplasia in the newborn

6. Right atrial hypertrophy (RAH)

— Fallot's (with RVH)
— Ebstein's anomaly (with IRBBB and RAD)
— tricuspid atresia
— obstructed TAPVD
— hypoplastic left heart
— primum ASD

7. Left atrial hypertrophy (LAH)

— primum ASD
— large PDA

8. Digoxin toxicity

— SVT, AV block, ventricular extopics or bigeminy

Remember that a normal or near-normal ECG does not exclude

significant CDH (e.g. transposition in the immediate newborn period).

B. CHEST X-RAY

1. Size
A cardiothoracic ratio of > 60% suggests hypertrophy or dilation of one or both chambers, or pericardial collection (fluid, pus, blood). The thymus is sail-shaped or has a scalloped edge and may persist up to 1 year on CXR.

2. Atrial enlargement
RAH is seen in pulmonary atresia without VSD and in Ebstein's anomaly.

LAH is hard to detect but may suggest congenital mitral stenosis or atrial myxoma (both rare).

3. Shape
— 'boot shape' = Fallot's or pulmonary atresia
— 'egg on side' and narrow pedicle = transposition
— 'cottage loaf' = supracardiac TAPVD

4. Situs
Dextrocardia is associated with an increased risk of CHD and Kartagener's syndrome.

5. Pulmonary vasculature
Difficult to assess.
a. Oligaemia — RV outflow obstruction
           — often accompanied by cyanosis as associated right to left shunt
b. Plethora — transposition (cyanosed as neonate)
           — obstructed TAPVD (usually cyanosed but present later)
           — large left-to-right shunt (e.g. VSD, ASD, PDA — not cyanosed)

A normal CXR does not exclude significant CHD (e.g. transposition) but consider non-cardiac causes of cyanosis and look for evidence of lung disease on CXR, or loops of bowel if a neonate.

C. ARTERIAL BLOOD GASES

The right radial artery is preferred (preductal).

1. In air
    a. Confirms cyanosis (as can pulse oximetry).
    b. $PaCO_2$ is usually normal in CHD but may be elevated if cyanosis is due to neurological or respiratory disease.
    c. If PaO_2 is normal but low saturation on pulse oximetry

(beware — the saturation from a blood gas machine is calculated, not measured) suggest methaemoglobinaemia.
d. Low pH is found in severe cardiac failure.

2. In 100% inspired oxygen (nitrogen washout or hyperoxic test)

Use an oxygen analyser to demonstrate that the FiO_2 is continuously > 90% for > 10 min. Ideally, use an indwelling right radial artery catheter. Transcutaneous PO_2 electrode on the right upper chest or a pulse oximeter on the right hand can also be used.

a. Normal child: PaO_2 rises above 50 kPa.
b. Methaemoglobinaemia: PaO_2 rises above 50 kPa but the child remains cyanosed. Treatment is by i.v. methylene blue.
c. 'Lung disease' or birth asphyxia: PaO_2 rises above 15 kPa unless there is severe lung disease, in which case $PaCO_2$ is also elevated and respiratory distress obvious, or PFC.
d. Common mixing: PaO_2 may increase by up to 1.5 kPa but never rises above 15 kPa (e.g. single ventricle or atrium or AV canal defect).
e. Large right-to-left shunt or transposition: PaO_2 is virtually unchanged. A hyperoxic test is only valid if ventilation is adequate. If there is any doubt (e.g. stridulous or floppy baby), results can only be interpreted following intubation and IPPV.

3. Pre- and postductal gases

Compare the right radial and low umbilical arterial, or transcutaneous PO_2 from the right chest and lower abdomen, simultaneously. Preductal PO_2 higher by ≥ 2 kPa is strongly suggestive of PDA with right-to-left shunt (e.g. in PFC).

D. ECHOCARDIOGRAM

Should only be considered after history, examination, ECG and CXR. USS can reliably diagnose almost all cardiac conditions causing cyanosis in the newborn.

Sedation of the infant is rarely necessary. Doppler aids detection of small shunts. USS in PFC demonstrates an anatomically normal heart with right-to-left shunt at atrial and ductal level.

E. CARDIAC CATHETERISATION

For diagnosis: defines complex lesions, pressures, gradients and shunt size. As intervention: atrial septostomy (transposition), balloon angioplasty of stenosis.

Management

1. Most children with a small VSD, ASD or mild PS or AS require no treatment (except antibiotic prophylaxis see p. 92).

2. Fallot's cyanotic spells — place the child in 'knee–elbow' position, give O_2 and i.v. morphine 0.1 mg/kg. If ineffective, give i.v. $NaHCO_3$ 1 mmol/kg and if there is still no improvement, give i.v. propranolol 0.1 mg/kg over 1 min.
3. Medical treatment of cardiac failure and endocarditis should be tried first; only consider surgery if medical treatment is ineffective.
4. In structural cardiac anomalies, surgery may be undertaken to totally correct the defect (e.g. coarctation, switch for transposition) or to palliate the symptoms (a shunt, PA banding, septostomy, valvotomy). Transplantation is also possible.

MEDICAL TREATMENT

A. General principles for the neonate with severe CHD

Do not defer supportive treatment while awaiting diagnosis. Stabilise the infant before transfer.

1. It is pointless to give O_2 unless a documented rise in PaO_2 is shown.
2. Correct hypoglycaemia, acidosis and hypothermia, all of which cause pulmonary vasoconstriction, impair myocardial contractility and exacerbate PFC.
3. Maintain plasma K^+ and Ca^{2+} concentrations in normal range.
4. Consider PGE infusion. Clinical improvement in 80% of all neonates with CHD, usually seen as increased PaO_2 within 15 min.

   a. *Cyanosed* — infant will benefit if pulmonary blood flow is duct-dependent.

      Infants with best response are:
      — <4 days old, very low PaO_2, normal pH
      — tricuspid atresia
      — pulmonary atresia or severe Fallot's
      Therefore always give PGE to neonates with PaO_2 < 5 kPa, poor hyperoxic response, and oligaemic CXR. Infants with little response are:
      — transposition
      — PFC
      — TAPVD (may get worse)
      If in doubt about the diagnosis, give PGE.

   b. *Acyanotic* — infant will benefit if systemic blood flow is duct-dependent. These infants are usually in heart failure because of obstruction of the left side of the heart. It may take 12 hours to see benefit (improved BP, urine output, acidosis).

      Infants likely to respond are:
      — aortic atresia
      — coarctation of the aorta
      NOT hypoplastic left heart as prognosis is very poor.
      Do not defer PGE, if indicated, to obtain USS.

Start i.v. infusion at 0.005 µg/kg/min and increase the rate in 0.005 µg/kg/min increments until effective or serious side-effects occur, or max. dose of 0.1 µg/kg/min is reached.

Side-effects of PGE.
— peripheral vasodilation and low BP
— fever, irritability and fits
— apnoea (15%) — more common in LBW, cyanotic CHD, dose > 0.01 µg/kg/min

Therefore, only use if IPPV is available, observe for at least 1 hour prior to transport, reduce dose in 0.005 µg/kg/min decrements once the desired effect is achieved.

5. Consider dopamine if there is clinically significant hypotension (acidosis, urine output < 0.5 ml/kg/h). Infuse i.v. at 5–10 µg/kg/min.

6. IPPV, with 6 cmH$_2$O PEEP, may be used as a treatment for severe heart failure.

B. Cardiac failure

Medical treatment may be longterm or to improve the child prior to surgery.

1. Nurse sitting up and do *not* restrict fluid (= calorie restriction). These infants may need ≥ 180 ml/kg per 24 hours of high-calorie feeds to thrive, if necessary by NGT continuous infusion.

2. Frusemide 1 mg/kg 12-hourly and spironolactone 1 mg/kg 12-hourly initially; avoids the need for unpalatable K$^+$ supplements. Both can be increased to 2 mg/kg 12-hourly.

3. If diuretics are insufficient, digoxin 5 µg/kg 12-hourly p.o. (check K$^+$ concentration) may help if there is low output but not if failure is associated with large shunt and dynamic heart. Rapid oral digitalisation is rarely essential but if the child is acutely ill, i.m. digoxin can be given 5 µg/kg 6-hourly for 24 hours and then 5 µg/kg 12-hourly i.v. or i.m.

   Therapeutic level = 1.5–3.0 nmol/l.

4. Oxygen and saturation monitoring for the child in severe failure.

The best guides to effective therapy are liver size and tenderness, respiratory and heart rates, and daily weight gain (too much is as undesirable as too little).

C. Cardiac failure due to PDA

Background. The infant is usually premature with large PDA. May manifest as inability to wean off IPPV rather than true failure.

Diagnosis. Bounding pulses, often cardiac thrill, loud continuous murmur under left clavicle (but may be LSE in neonate); hepatomegaly and tachypnoea are late signs of PDA.

Investigations.

1. Blood gases: normal (unless on IPPV) as shunt is left-to-right.
2. ECG: normal or LVH, LAH.
3. CXR: plethora and cardiomegaly.
4. USS: LA diameter : aortic root diameter > 1.2 : 1.

   PDA may be confirmed by 2-D echo, and Doppler.

   Treat if: asymptomatic and < 1 kg; on IPPV; or symptomatic.

Management.

1. *The newborn:* fluid restrict to 120 ml/kg per 24 hours and give 3 doses of indomethacin (0.2 mg/kg i.v.) and 3 doses of frusemide (1 mg/kg i.v.) 12 hourly.

   Contraindications to indomethacin are: platelets <75 000/ mm^3; abnormal U & E (may cause hyponatraemia and mild uraemia); PVH or other bleeding disorder; bilirubin near exchange level. This 3-dose regimen can be repeated after 48 hours if closure is incomplete or PDA recurs. May be effective up to 2 months postnatally but the success rate declines after 2 weeks.

2. *Older child:* PDA is always closed surgically irrespective of size because of very low surgical risk, less than that of endocarditis.

D. Arrhythmias

These must be distinguished from cerebral events (fits, emboli, transient ischaemic attacks, breath holding etc; see Ch. 12) and from the cyanotic spells of Fallot's. 12-lead ECG and 30-sec rhythm strip are essential.

1. **Supraventricular tachycardia** (SVT) is the commonest arrhythmia. Heart rate is very regular and > 180/min. QRS complex is usually normal (i.e. narrow) but P waves may be difficult to see.

   Associated with:

   a. previous cardiac surgery, especially involving the atria;
   b. underlying CHD (30%) especially Ebstein's anomaly;
   c. WPWS (easier to diagnose once reverted to SR);
   d. myocarditis.

   In over half, no cause is found.

   Presence of heart failure implies serious and prolonged SVT needing urgent treatment, especially in a baby, but if time allows, correct acidosis and potassium:

   a. give O$_2$ and check electrolytes;
   b. in a well baby, initial treatment should be vagal stimulation by iced water to the face. Attach the child to an ECG monitor, wrap in a towel, and immerse the whole face in iced water for 5 sec. The baby will be temporarily apnoeic so there is no need to obstruct mouth or nostrils. Effective in 90%.

If ineffective or the child is ill:

c. adenosine by rapid bolus via i.v. cannula 0.05 mg/kg followed by prompt saline flush. Increase the dose by 0.05 mg/kg increments at 2-min intervals until SR is restored (usually within 15 sec of bolus) or max. dose of 0.3 mg/kg is reached. Side-effects are few (bradycardia, flushing, pain) and last < 30 sec.

If adenosine is not available or is ineffective, next choices are:

d. flecainide 2 mg/kg i.v. over minimum of 15 min;

e. digoxin i.m. or i.v. (see p. 89) but this takes mean of 12 hours for effect. Should be avoided in WPWS as it may cause faster rate.

NEVER use verapamil — cardiac arrest may occur.

If the above are ineffective, or the child is moribund on presentation:

f. DC cardioversion is almost always successful. Ensure i.v. access, anaesthetist present, sedate with i.v. diazemuls 250 μg/kg over 2 min, O_2 by mask, disconnect ECG monitor (can monitor using paddles), place paddles and conducting gel or pad over apex and right sternal border, give *1 J/kg*. May require up to five repeat shocks at this energy. Correct acidosis.

Recurrence of SVT is common after all of the above treatments (up to 70%). Perform ECG and USS 24 hours after reversion to SR to exclude an underlying cause. Teach the parents how to feel and count the apex beat. Maintenance treatment may be required (digoxin 5 μg/kg 12-hourly, or amniodarone or propranolol 0.25–0.5 mg/kg 8-hourly).

2. Other arrhythmias.

a. *Complete heart block*
   — ventricular rate usually <60/min
   — often systolic flow murmur because of increased stroke volume
   — QRS may be narrow or wide
   — P waves are dissociated from QRS and usually faster (therefore sometimes confused with 2 : 1 block which is rare in children)

   Associated with: — previous cardiac surgery
                    — CHD
                    — maternal SLE (high anti-Ro antibody titre)
                    — familial type of congenital heart block

   May be asymptomatic. If Stokes–Adams attack occurs (abrupt loss of consciousness, without warning, and associated pallor), should be referred for permanent cardiac pacemaker.

b. *Ventricular tachyarrhythmias* — all rare. See Ch. 2 for ventricular fibrillation (Table 2.8).

Ventricular tachycardia following cardiac arrest or near-drowning or in inherited prolonged QT syndrome should be treated initially with 1 mg/kg lignocaine i.v. over 2 min, repeated up to 4 times, then 0.04 mg/kg/min (i.e. 40 μg/kg/min infusion gradually reduced by 0.01 mg/kg/min steps each 30 min.

E. Infective endocarditis

Background.

1. A child with a confident diagnosis of innocent murmur does not require antibiotic prophylaxis. If in doubt, give it as there may be bicuspid aortic valve or prolapsing mitral valve.

2. In most cases, there is underlying CHD

Greater risk of SBE	Very small risk of SBE
Small VSD	Secundum ASD
Fallot's	PS
AS	
PDA	
Palliative shunts	
Prosthetic valves	
Synthetic patch	

The risk persists after surgery (except following ligation of PDA).

3. In 30% of cases, there has been a recent surgical procedure presumed to cause bacteraemia (70% *Streptococcus viridans*; 20% *Str. faecalis*; consider staphylococci and fungi in the immunosuppressed or those with indwelling central venous catheters). Therefore, prophylaxis is required for:
   a. ear-piercing
   b. all dental treatment
   c. all ENT, respiratory, genitourinary and gastrointestinal surgery
   d. labour or termination of pregnancy
   If in doubt, give it.

Prophylaxis.

1. Rinse the mouth with phenolated mouthwash before dentistry.
2. Encourage regular cleaning of teeth and dental follow-up from an early age.
3. Antibiotics.

Procedure:

a. *Dentistry, ENT, respiratory tract*
   — amoxycillin p.o. 1 hour before: — 1.5 g if < 10 years
        — 3.0 g if > 10 years
   — if GA is required, give amoxycillin 4 hours pre-op and as soon as possible post-op
   — if the child is allergic to penicillin, erythromycin p.o. 1 hour before: — 0.5 g if < 10 years
        — 1.0 g if > 10 years

b. *GU or GI surgery*

— gentamicin 2.5 mg/kg i.v. and ampicillin 50 mg/kg i.v. at induction
— if allergic to penicillin, gentamicin 2.5 mg/kg i.v. and vancomycin 20 mg/kg i.v.

c. *Prosthetic valve or patch, irrespective of procedure*
— flucloxacillin i.m. 1 hour before: — 0.5 g if < 10 years
                                          — 1.0 g if > 10 years

and

— ampicillin i.m. 1 hour before: — 0.5 g if < 10 years
                                       — 1.0 g if > 10 years

Repeat both of the above 8-hourly for two doses post-op
— if allergic to penicillin, gentamycin 2.5 mg/kg i.v. and vancomycin 20 mg/kg i.v. for the same regimen of three doses

Diagnosis of infective endocarditis (acute and subacute).

Symptoms are often non-specific malaise and weight loss. Diagnosis may not be suspected if CHD is not known.

Signs are fever, anaemia, splenomegaly, vasculitis (Janeway's spots are painless haemorrhagic lesions on palms and soles), haematuria, cerebral abscess, fluctuating murmurs, pericardial effusion, cardiac failure due to valve incompetence, emboli.

The diagnosis is difficult and easily overlooked. Nevertheless, fever from other causes is much commoner.

Investigation of suspected infective endocarditis.

1. Every effort must be made to isolate an organism (six blood cultures with pristine technique) but treatment cannot be deferred for long (mortality 30%). Start treatment after three cultures if necessary. Stop any current antibiotics before taking cultures.
2. USS may suggest vegetations if cultures are negative *but a normal USS does not exclude SBE.*
3. Suggestive evidence is provided by blood counts and raised CRP or ESR. These provide a baseline against which efficacy of treatment may be judged.

Treatment

a. Initial 'blind' therapy: benzyl penicillin 50 mg/kg i.v. 4-hourly
gentamicin 2.5 mg/kg i.v. 8-hourly

Add flucloxacillin 25 mg.kg i.v. 6-hourly if there are clues to a *Staphylococcus* infection or if there is a prosthetic valve, graft, immuno-suppression or central line

If allergic to penicillin, vancomycin 20 mg/kg i.v. 8-hourly
gentamicin 2.5 mg/kg i.v. 8-hourly

b. Treat staphylococcal bacteraemia as endocarditis even if there is no murmur since healthy valves can be destroyed.

c. Once the organism is known, treat depending on sensitivities and as guided by in vitro cidal and inhibitory concentrations.

F. Other infections in the child with CHD

1. CHD is not a contraindication to any immunisation. Pertussis and measles are particularly dangerous in young children with CHD.

2. RSV bronchiolitis can cause serious respiratory disease in children with CHD. Admit and treat earlier than children without CHD (regular suction, NG feeding, O_2) to avoid IPPV. Nebulised Ribavirin may help.

3. Treat dental infection and superficial sepsis (e.g. abscess, impetigo, paronychia, etc.) very promptly and follow-up in case of SBE which may take 6 weeks to manifest.

4. In young children, it may be difficult to distinguish clinically and radiologically between 'chest infection' and cardiac failure. Fever is not a feature of failure per se (although sweating, tachypnoea and tachycardia are) and the liver may be pushed down by hyperinflation, e.g. RSV. If in any doubt, take blood cultures and NPA, FBC, viral titres and start broad-spectrum antibiotics *and* diuretics. The true diagnosis usually becomes obvious clinically or microbiologically within 48 hours.

Cor pulmonale and pulmonary hypertension

BACKGROUND

Commonest causes are *secondary pulmonary hypertension* (e.g. BPD, CHD, CF, neuromuscular disease, upper airway obstruction).

Primary pulmonary hypertension, which may be familial, is rare.

DIAGNOSIS

1. Symptoms and signs of the underlying condition. Many of these children are cyanosed at rest in air. Children with obstructed upper airway fail to thrive, snore, and are often difficult to wake for feeds in the morning (i.e. nocturnal hypoventilation and CO_2 retention). They may also present with acute apnoea ('near miss' SIDS) or chronic stridor.

2. Symptoms and signs of low cardiac output and inability to increase this during exercise, especially breathlessness and tachypnoea.

3. Cough and haemoptysis.

4. Signs of pulmonary hypertension (parasternal heave and loud or palpable second heart sound, P_2) and failure (particularly hepatomegaly).

INVESTIGATION

— To look for a cause of pulmonary hypertension
— To monitor efficacy of treatment
1. FBC (for polycythaemia)
2. Arterial blood gas in air (may be normal initially but very high HCO_3^- is clue to chronic respiratory acidosis)
3. CXR (dilated proximal PA, peripheral 'pruning', large heart, lung disease)
4. ECG (RVH, RBBB, RAH)
5. Echocardiography and Doppler studies
6. Lung function tests (exclude restrictive disease and determine whether any reversibility of obstructive disease); overnight saturation monitoring to detect upper airway obstruction.
7. Ventilation/perfusion scan — perfusion defect means angiography is needed

Right heart catheterisation and pulmonary angiography may be necessary to measure pressure.

ECG criteria for RVH are the most sensitive guide to monitoring the progression of pulmonary hypertension.

ACUTE MANAGEMENT

1. Treat the cause; ensure upper airway is adequate; nurse upright
2. Treat infection, especially respiratory
3. Diuretics
4. NG feeding
5. O_2 to maintain saturation > 90% if possible. Do not expect a normal $PaCO_2$. No not start IPPV on the basis of blood gases alone and consider first what will be the subsequent management if, as commonly occurs, the child cannot be weaned off IPPV. If IPPV is chosen, do *not* try to normalise blood gases.

Before embarking on treatment, consider the longterm prognosis. However, often acute treatment must be given while making a diagnosis. The outlook is poor in many of these conditions (for some a combined heart–lung transplant offers hope) and a senior colleague may elect not to treat cor pulmonale, infection or not to use IPPV.

Systemic hypertension

BACKGROUND

1. Underdiagnosed in children, and BP is infrequently and inadequately recorded. Childhood hypertension leads to end-organ damage.
2. See Figs A.1–A.3 (pp 364–366) for BP centiles with age.
3. Many children > 95th centile on initial reading will be normal but

all must be followed-up, even if asymptomatic, and at least simple investigations done if persistently > 95th centile for systolic *or* diastolic BP. There is familial aggregation of hypertension.

4. At most, only 1% will have BP consistently > 95th centile. Therefore, generalised screening for hypertension is not justified but the following 'at risk' groups should be screened yearly:

    a. previous BP > 95th centile
    b. any renal or urinary disease
    c. other known cause of hypertension (see below)
    d. first-degree relative with early onset essential hypertension (i.e. < 45 years)

    Screen more frequently if the BP is < 95th centile but symptoms suggest episodic hypertension.

5. The earlier the diagnosis, the better the outcome, especially as many are avoidable/correctable.

CAUSES (Table 7.2)

Table 7.2 Causes of acute and chronic hypertension in neonate and older child

Usually *secondary* to:		
Renal causes	1.	Reflux nephropathy
	2.	Obstructive uropathy
	3.	Glomerulonephritis
	4.	Congenital dysplastic kidney
	5.	Polycystic disease
	6.	Acute (usually 'nephritic') or chronic renal failure
Vascular causes	1.	Renal artery stenosis
	2.	Renal vein thrombosis
	3.	Coarctation of the aorta
	4.	Thrombosis following umbilical catheterisation
	5.	Hyperlipidaemias
Associated with tumours (hypertension often episodic)	1.	Neuroblastoma
	2.	Wilms' tumour
	3.	Phaeochromocytoma
	4.	Neurofibromatosis
Endocrine causes	1.	Congenital adrenal hyperplasia
	2.	Excess steroids — iatrogenic — endogenous (Cushing's and Conn's syndromes)
Neurological causes	1.	Raised ICP (see p. 195)
	2.	Stroke
	3.	Guillain–Barré syndrome
Miscellaneous	1.	Drug ingestion (accidental or iatrogenic)
	2.	Sickle cell disease and dehydration
PRIMARY essential hypertension		
Often strong family history		
Less likely to require urgent treatment		

DIAGNOSIS

Unless hypertension is acute or severe, symptoms and signs are rare (headache — see p. 190; fits; personal or family history of renal problem, UTI, hypertension; unexplained weight loss; increased pigmentation; cranial or adrenal bruits; absent femoral pulses; papilloedema). *Always*:
— measure the BP (see below)
— feel the femorals
— look at the fundi
    Measure the BP in every child who has a non-febrile seizure.

BP measurement

A. *Conventional mercury sphygmomanometer*
  1. Systolic is more accurate and reproducible than diastolic.
  2. Use the widest cuff that can be applied to the right upper arm (bladder should encircle $\frac{2}{3}$ of arm circumference arm).
  3. Measure after sitting or lying quietly for 3 min. Measure more than once at each visit and repeat at serial visits.
  4. Crying, eating, sucking, anxiety, venepuncture and exercise all increase BP.

B. *Other techniques*
In children under 5 years, automatic oscillometry ('Dinamap') or Doppler-assisted sphygmomanometry may be necessary. Direct intra-arterial measurement is the 'gold standard' but only used in ill children.

INVESTIGATIONS

See 'Background' (p. 95) for who to investigate. The younger the child and the more severe the hypertension, the more likely there is a secondary cause. Investigation and treatment must often be concurrent.

1. Urine tests

Always: urinalysis for blood, protein
          microscopy for cells and casts
          culture
Then consider: VMA : creatinine and HVA : creatinine ratios; send spot sample followed by 6–24-hour timed collection
          save frozen for steroid profile and toxicology

2. Blood tests

Always: FBC
          U & E, creatinine, HCO_3^-
          Ca^{2+}, PO_4^{3-}, albumin
Then consider: 17-OH progesterone; aldosterone, plasma renin

substrate and concentration; liaise with the lab. first as these may require to be taken 'on ice' or into inhibitors and ideally after 20 min lying quietly (with indwelling catheter)

3. CXR and ECG
— always.

Then consider: cardiac and abdominal/renal USS

MANAGEMENT

Principles
1. Have *you* measured the BP (correctly and serially)?
2. Is there a treatable cause?
3. Chronic hypertension can be treated with oral anti-hypertensives (Table 7.3).
4. Aim to reduce systolic and diastolic BP to < 95th centile for age and sex (see Figs A.1–A.3), side-effects of treatment permitting.
5. $\frac{1}{3}$ of desired BP reduction in *not less* than 6 hours; the remaining $\frac{2}{3}$ over the next 24 hours. *All* drugs in Tables 7.3 and 7.4 may cause relative or absolute *hypotension* which is as dangerous as hypertension.
6. a. start with vasodilator
   b. add beta blocker if ineffective or tachycardia
   c. add diuretic if still ineffective
   d. change to diuretic + captopril if still ineffective
7. In severe hypertension (child symptomatic, one measurement 50% greater than 95th centile, several measurements > 15 mmHg above 95th centile):
   a. insert an i.v. cannula for blood tests and drugs (see Table 7.4)
   b. consider a CVP line (child may be hypo- or hypervolaemic), intra-arterial line (continuous monitoring of BP)
   c. monitor urine output, vital signs, pupils, fundi and GC score
   d. try the drugs in the order they appear in Table 7.4, aiming for *gradual* BP reduction as in 5 above
   e. once BP is < 95th centile convert to oral treatment

Table 7.3 Oral antihypertensive drugs

Drug	Starting dose mg/kg per 24 h	Max. dose mg/kg per 24 h	Frequency	Possible disadvantages
Vasodilators				
Nifedipine	0.25	1.0	2 divided doses	Smallest tablet = 10 mg
Hydrallazine	1.0	8.0	3 divided doses	Tachycardia
Beta-blockers				
Propranolol	1.0	5.0	3 divided doses	Bronchospasm and decreased
Atenolol	1.0	4.0	24-hourly maintenance	exercise tolerance
Diuretics				
Frusemide	1.0	5.0	2 divided doses	Hypokalaemia
Spironolactone	1.0	3.0	2 divided doses	Hyperkalaemia if renal impairment
Angiotensin converting enzyme inhibitor				
Captopril	0.3	6.0	3 divided doses	Rarely neutropenia Caution with frusemide and in renal artery stenosis

Table 7.4 Emergency treatment of hypertensive crisis

Drug	Starting dose	Max. dose	Max. frequency	Onset	Duration	Possible disadvantages
Nifedipine, s.l.	0.2 mg	0.5 mg	2-hourly	10–30 min	3–12 h	Administering dose*
Hydrallazine, i.v./i.m.	0.2 mg/kg slowly	0.8 mg/kg slowly	hourly	10–30 min	2–6 h	Tachycardia
Diazoxide, i.v.	1 mg/kg slowly	3 mg/kg slowly	hourly	1–5 min	4–24 h	Tachycardia Nausea Hyperglycaemia
Labetalol infusion, i.v.	1.0 mg/kg/h	3.0 mg/kg/h	Onset rapid Increase by 1 mg/kg/h every 30 min until BP starts to fall			Contraindicated if heart failure, brady- or tachycardia, asthma
Sodium nitroprusside, i.v.	0.5 μg/kg/min	8.0 μg/kg/min	Onset immediate — needs intra-arterial monitor. Increase by 0.5 μg/kg/h every 5 min until BP starts to fall			Protect infusion from light

If tachycardia develops with any of the above drugs, start oral beta-blocker (propranolol; Table 7.3).
* (0.17 ml of liquid extracted with a syringe and 25G-needle from 5 mg or 10 mg capsule = 5 mg nifedipine).
Giving an antihypertensive 'slowly' means over 20 minutes minimum.

8

Respiratory medicine

Inspiratory stridor indicates obstruction in the larynx or upper trachea. With tracheal or subglottic lesions, expiratory stridor may also occur.

ASSESSMENT

Full history and examination is essential in every case. During the examination:

Do not use any instrument to depress the tongue in a patient with stridor as this may precipitate a respiratory arrest.

Do not lie the child flat as this exacerbates stridor.

The differential diagnosis of acute stridor is listed in Table 8.1. Croup and epiglottitis are the two common important causes. Dis-

Table 8.1 Causes of stridor

Acute	
Acute laryngotracheobronchitis ('croup')	Very common
Acute epiglottitis	Common
Bacterial tracheitis	Uncommon
Laryngeal foreign body (see Ch. 16)	Uncommon
Smoke inhalation	Uncommon
Diphtheria	Rare
Acute angioneurotic oedema	Rare
Retropharyngeal abscess (see Ch. 16)	Rare
Chronic	
Laryngeal (glottic and subglottic)	
Infantile larynx (laryngomalacia)	Common
Subglottic stenosis	
a. acquired	Common
b congenital	Rare
Subglottic haemangioma	Rare
Vocal cord palsy	Rare
Laryngeal webs	Rare
Cysts (e.g. posterior tongue)	Rare
Laryngeal cleft	Rare
Laryngeal papillomas	Rare
Tracheal; vascular ring, tracheal stenosis	Rare

tinction between them and their management are described below. Management of less common causes are also described either below or in Ch. 16.

ADMISSION TO HOSPITAL

The reason for admission with acute stridor is to identify the small number of children who will need intervention to maintain their airway. **All** children with a first episode of acute severe stridor or any child with stridor at rest should be admitted.

MANAGEMENT

This is discussed below under specific conditions. However, **when stridor is very severe**, when a clinical diagnosis of epiglottitis is made, or when stridor is due to a foreign body, direct laryngoscopy under GA is required. This should be performed by an anaesthetist skilled in intubating children with epiglottitis. Ideally an ENT surgeon should also be present to perform an emergency tracheostomy if intubation fails.

If a patient with stridor has collapsed and it is impossible to ventilate by bag and mask or to intubate, cricothyroid puncture can bring temporary relief (see Ch. 2. p. 3).

Specific conditions

Croup is the commonest cause of stridor, but must be differentiated from epiglottitis which is life threatening (Table 8.2). It may be clinically impossible to distinguish between epiglottitis and croup.

Table 8.2 Clinical features of help in distinguishing epiglottitis from croup

Epiglottitis	Croup
Rapid onset (within hours)	Slow onset
Weak or no cough	Croupy cough (barking)
Temperature > 38°C	Temperature < 38.5°C
Septicaemia	No systemic disturbance
Often severe stridor	Severe stridor less common
Drooling saliva	Able to swallow
Unable to eat or drink	Usually will swallow fluids
Weak voice	Normal voice
Any age	< 4 years
Expiratory snore	More frequent at night
Will often not move neck	

EPIGLOTTITIS

Rapid cellulitis of supraglottic tissues caused by *Haemophilus influenzae* type B. May occur at any age but is usually seen at 2–3 years.

Diagnosis

Presumptive diagnosis can be made clinically. Clinical features are listed in Table 8.2.

NB. Some children with epiglottitis have a temperature < 38.5°C and do not look sick.

The child must never be sent to the X-ray department for a lateral neck X-ray. This is not required for diagnosis and the child should be in an intensive care setting as there is a risk of respiratory arrest. Do not attempt to see the epiglottis or perform venepuncture, as these may precipitate complete obstruction. Do not lie the child flat.

Treatment

1. Intubation by a skilled anaesthetist; ideally an ENT surgeon is available when intubation is performed in case a tracheostomy is required.
2. Once intubated take blood cultures, FBC, and swabs of the epiglottis.
3. Give chloramphenicol (40 mg/kg i.v. stat, then 25 mg/kg 6-hourly i.v., then orally for 5 days).
4. Consider other foci of infection, e.g. pneumonia (p. 118), septic arthritis (see Ch. 13) or meningitis (see Ch. 12).
5. Consider bacterial tracheitis (see below) if the epiglottis is normal on direct inspection.

CROUP (see Table 8.2)

Stridor is caused by narrowing of the subglottic region. There are two types of croup; fortunately management is the same.

1. Viral laryngotracheobronchitis: infecting agents include parainfluenzae virus, RSV and adenovirus. Often preceded by an upper respiratory tract infection.
2. Spasmodic croup: tends to be recurrent and to come on suddenly at night with no preceding symptoms. These children are more likely to develop asthma.

Assessment

It may be helpful to classify the child on clinical grounds into one of three arbitrary groups.

1. Mild: barking cough, inspiratory stridor only when upset.
2. Moderate: as above but with suprasternal and sternal recession at rest. The child is not particularly distressed or anxious looking and is drinking reasonably well.

3. Severe: inspiratory and expiratory stridor at rest. Sternal and suprasternal recession.

NB. As the child becomes physically exhausted stridor and recession may decrease. Breath sounds over the chest may become reduced. The child looks anxious and distressed and may not want to drink. Early signs of hypoxia include restlessness, irritability, confusion and tachycardia.

Investigations
Rarely required. Lateral and AP neck X-ray are very occasionally indicated if there is something unusual in the pattern of stridor. Discuss with the consultant on call.

Management
Mist tents or steam inhalation for children have been very popular in the past; however, there is no proof that they are of any benefit in the management of croup. We do not recommend them.
1. Mild symptoms: most cases are very mild and can be managed at home. The child should return for admission if symptoms become worse or if the parents are worried.
2. Mild–moderate: admit and nurse the child in a quiet area under constant, calm supervision. Mother or father should stay until the child is settled. Ensure adequate oral fluid intake.
3. Severe:
   a. Notify the registrar immediately.
   b. Transfer to ICU.
   c. If the child's condition deteriorates with rising pulse rate (respiratory rate may rise or remain constant) and appearance of restlessness or cyanosis then give adrenaline 1 in 1000, 0.5 ml/kg/dose (maximum 5 ml) by nebulisation while transfer to ICU is arranged and the anaethetist summoned to assess the need for intubation.
   d. O_2 is not routinely given as it may hide cyanosis, masking impending arrest. Blood gases are not helpful in assessment.
   e. Indication for intubation is severe airway obstruction suggested by fatigue, hypoxia, restlessness, rising pulse and respiratory rates and cyanosis. **If the child is cyanosed he is likely to die suddenly.**

   NB. The ETT used should be a size smaller than the child would normally need to prevent subglottic damage (check with an experienced anaesthetist).
   f. Intubation may be required for several days. Dexamethasone 1 mg/kg may be given prior to intended extubation to improve the success rate of extubation.
   g. Consider systemic steroids.

Less common causes of acute stridor

These are included for reference. Also see Ch. 16 and the index for other causes.

BACTERIAL TRACHEITIS

Bacterial infection (*Haem. influenzae* or *Staph. aureus*) below the vocal cords. Initial clinical picture is often like croup but patients are more toxic. Epiglottitis is often suspected. Laryngoscopy may show pus below the vocal cords with mucosal oedema and mucopurulent membrane on the cords.

Treatment

1. Chloramphenicol 100 mg/kg per 24 hours i.v. in 4 divided doses (or cefotaxime) and flucloxacillin 50 mg/kg per 24 hours i.v. in 4 divided doses.
2. Patients may require intubation.

DIPHTHERIA

Very rare but consider if the child is unimmunised.

Inflamed tonsils and pharynx. Signs of infection. May be a thick grey membrane over the tonsils; removal may cause brisk bleeding. Airway occlusion may occur. Throat swab and blood cultures are needed.

Treatment

1. Endotracheal intubation may be needed for airway obstruction.
2. Penicillin 300 mg/kg per 24 hours i.v. in 6 divided doses.
3. Antitoxin i.m. as soon as possible.

SMOKE INHALATION

May cause severe respiratory distress and stridor. Symptoms may develop up to 12 hours after inhalation; thus any child with a history of smoke inhalation should be admitted for observation.

HYPOCALCAEMIA (see p. 27)

Consider Di George syndrome if stridor is due to hypocalcaemia and CHD is present.

URTICARIA, ANGIO-OEDEMA AND ANGIONEUROTIC OEDEMA

Urticaria is characterised by wheals of varying size, distribution and appearance (i.e. heat lumps, nettle rash). May be generalised, focal or confined to the mouth or face (angio-oedema). Occasionally the tongue and larynx may be affected and cause respiratory obstruction and arrest. Hereditary angioneurotic oedema causes intermittent non-pruritic oedema and may cause laryngeal obstruction and asphyxiation. Abdominal pain and diarrhoea may occur. To exclude hereditary angioneurotic oedema check C1 esterase levels (normal in 15%); if the latter result is normal, check C4 during an attack.

Management

Acute airway obstruction.

1. Children with angioneurotic oedema should go to casualty if any upper airway symptoms occur. Intubation or tracheostomy may be required for laryngeal obstruction.

2. Give hydrocortisone 10 mg/kg i.v. and adrenaline 0.1 ml/kg of 1 : 10 000 given slowly i.v. or less if the desired effect is achieved. If the child has hereditary angioneurotic oedema these drugs are not nearly as effective as when given for relief of urticaria and laryngeal obstruction seen in anaphylaxis and serum sickness; facility for immediate support of airway is required.

3. Purified C1 esterase inhibitor may be useful in an acute attack in hereditary angioneurotic oedema.

4. Androgens (e.g. danazol) markedly decrease the severity and frequency of attacks in the child with hereditary angioneurotic oedema.

Chronic stridor (see Table 8.1)

INVESTIGATION OF PERSISTENT OR RECURRENT STRIDOR

Patients with chronic stridor should be investigated to establish a precise diagnosis. The only exception is the normal child with typical features of infantile larynx in whom symptoms are mild. Initial investigation will depend on history.

Investigations to be discussed with the consultant should include:

1. CXR and lateral neck X-ray
2. Barium swallow
3. Direct examination of the airway (laryngoscopy and bronchoscopy) is indicated in most children with chronic stridor.

Foreign body in the bronchial tree

(For laryngeal and oesophageal foreign body causing stridor or a change in voice see pp 277–278). History may be obvious, i.e. coughing or choking episode while eating nuts or sucking small objects. However, the diagnosis is often delayed. Patterns of presentation with delayed diagnosis include wheezy bronchitis, failed resolution of acute respiratory infection, chronic cough, haemoptysis, lung collapse and respiratory failure.

CLINICAL FEATURES

Diminished breath sounds over whole or part of lung; wheeze.

DIAGNOSIS

1. May be on history alone as X-rays are often normal.
2. Obtain inspiratory and expiratory CXR. Air trapping on the side of the obstruction is usually more apparent on the expiratory film but may not be seen when the obstruction is partial. Check that the X-rays are actually inspiratory and expiratory by counting the ribs seen, especially in a young child. Fluoroscopy of the diaphragms may help in a child too young to comply with inspiratory and expiratory films.

TREATMENT

Admit all children with suspected foreign body inhalation.
1. Emergency mechanical efforts to dislodge a foreign body (i.e. the Heimlich manoeuvre) should be attempted only when air exchange is inadequate for life.
2. Nil by mouth from admission.
3. Laryngoscopy and bronchoscopy are needed to remove the foreign body. If the child has stridor then examination should be performed as a matter of urgency by the ENT surgeon as total obstruction may occur (see pp 277–278).
4. Physiotherapy, postural drainage or bronchodilators are not recommended. The foreign body may dislodge and become repositioned, causing complete obstruction.
5. If there are radiological changes preoperatively and the foreign body is removed, a repeat CXR is needed 24 hours later. Discharge if normal and clinical signs have resolved. Review in clinic.
6. If there are signs of associated infection or bronchoscopy shows associated infection treat with oral co-trimoxazole (or Augmentin) (i.v. antibiotics if unwell).

Whooping cough

Caused by *Bordetella pertussis*. The incubation period is 10–14 days and the child is infectious from 7 days after exposure to 3 weeks after the onset of typical paroxysms. Infants admitted should be isolated until they have had 10 days of erythromycin estolate.

DIAGNOSIS

A catarrhal phase with coryza and fever is followed, after 1 week by paroxysmal cough which may last up to 6 months. Vomiting may occur following paroxysms. In young babies an inspiratory whoop is often not heard and presentation may be with periods of apnoea.

INVESTIGATIONS

1. Postnasal mucus to virology for immunofluorescence (often only positive for the first week of the illness) and naso-pharyngeal swab to bacteriology for culture.
2. FBC for lymphocytosis.
3. CXR is usually normal (not always indicated).

COMPLICATIONS

Usually limited to infants < 6 months and include weight loss due to vomiting, petechiae, epistaxis, intraventricular haemorrhage, secondary bacterial infection and asphyxial brain damage.

IMMUNISATION

Provides some protection in 70% of patients and ameliorates illness in the other 30%. 70% of unvaccinated family contacts will develop the disease. See p. 224 for the immunisation schedule.

MANAGEMENT

1. The majority of children may be managed at home and re-viewed by the GP. Explain to parents that the cough may persist for several months.
2. Give erythromycin estolate 50 mg/kg/per 24 hours p.o. in 4 divided doses for 10 days. This is unlikely to modify the clinical course but will reduce the period of infectivity.
   Whether administration to susceptible contacts is of value is yet to be determined but consider in contacts < 1 year.
3. Admit to hospital all infants < 6 months for initial observation, infants with apnoea or frequent cyanotic attacks and all those with serious disease.
   a. Nurse in a quiet place with minimal handling.
   b. Infants are initially nursed in oxygen although this will not relieve hypoxia until the baby makes an inspiratory effort.
   c. Temporary ventilation may be necessary if the infant suffers from recurrent apnoeic or marked hypoxic spells.

Bronchopulmonary dysplasia

Chronic O_2 dependency following neonatal intensive care (> 30 days of O_2 therapy). Characterised by hypoxia, hypercapnia and O_2 dependence. CXR shows hyperexpansion and focal hyperlucency alternating with strands of opacification. Mortality is up to 30%. There is an increased incidence of SIDS.

Blood gases may show hypoxia and CO_2 level may be up to 10 kPa (75 mmHg); a high CO_2 may be considered acceptable if the child is well and not acidotic. If the child is hypoxic, inspired O_2 is needed to maintain O_2 saturation above 90%. Acute deterioration is not uncommon.

MANAGEMENT

Divided into maintenance treatment when stable and management of specific problems when the child's condition deteriorates.

Maintenance treatment

1. Ensure O_2 saturation is above 90% to prevent pulmonary hypertension. If an inspired O_2 concentration < 40% is needed, a nasal cannula may be used. For inspired O_2 > 40%, O_2 via a headbox is required. Beware nasal obstruction (e.g. due to a cold) if O_2 is given by a nasal cannula: prolonged hypoxia may occur due to decreased inspired O_2. Monitor O_2 saturation in patients receiving O_2 via a nasal cannula and change to a headbox if saturation is < 90%.
2. Nutrition is essential; aim for up to 150 kcal/kg per 24 hours.
3. Keep Hb > 11 g/dl.

Specific problems/treatment

NB. Deterioration may be due to more than one medical problem, e.g. infection combined with right-sided heart failure. If the child has deteriorated suddenly correction of hypoxia, antibiotics and diuretics may all be indicated.

Respiratory distress.
1. Prevent hypoxia (as in maintenance treatment above). Give extra O_2 if saturation falls during feeds or when upset.

   If the child's respiratory status has deteriorated nasal CPAP may stabilise the infant and avert the need for mechanical ventilation. Short-term ventilation is indicated if there is severe respiratory failure. Blood gases showing acidosis are particularly worrying.
2. Infection: for viral infection such as bronchiolitis some, but not all, units would consider ribavirin aerosol. In the systemically ill infant (i.e. fever, leukocytosis, additional changes on CXR) give broad spectrum antibiotics (e.g. ampicillin and flucloxacillin i.v.; add gentamicin if the child is sick or if his condition deteriorates) for a minimum of 5 days.
3. Wheeze: occasionally infants benefit from nebulised ipratropium bromide. Dexamethasone 0.25 mg/kg i.v. 12-hourly is

used in some centres and may improve respiratory function when there is increased CO_2 retention or inability to wean from IPPV.

4. CO_2 retention: a patient with a high $PaCO_2$ in the absence of oxygenation problems may have upper airway obstruction (usually subglottic stenosis). Bronchoscopy is needed to establish the diagnosis; discuss with the consultant.

Right-sided heart failure. This is secondary to pulmonary hypertension and may be severe. Keep O_2 saturation > 90%. Treatment with diuretics (frusemide 1 mg/kg 12-hourly and spironolactone 1 mg/kg 12 -hourly) is preferable to fluid restriction as the latter may result in calorie restriction.

Chlorthiazide 10–20 mg/kg 12-hourly may be preferable as frusemide can cause nephrocalcinosis.

Bronchiolitis

Most commonly (70%) due to RSV. Adenovirus may cause very severe bronchiolitis. Predominantly seen in the winter months.

CLINICAL FEATURES

Widespread fine inspiratory crepitations and wheeze are usually heard. Other features may include coryza, cough, pyrexia (usually < 38.5°C), apnoea, tachypnoea, recession, hyperinflation and cyanosis.

The threshold for admission should be low for infants < 4 months and those with heart or lung disease.

Remember that other conditions can present with a bronchiolitic-like illness, e.g. CF, cardiac failure, pneumonia, aspiration and congenital lung disease.

INVESTIGATIONS

1. Aspiration of postnasal mucus for immunofluorescence and culture.
2. CXR at presentation is performed on all infants with significant respiratory difficulty. Usually shows hyperinflation; patchy consolidation may be seen in 50%.
3. Blood gases are rarely needed for management of the child with bronchiolitis but are indicated in infants who are deteriorating and may require ventilation. In these infants arterial gases usually show hypoxia and a compensated respiratory acidosis.

MANAGEMENT

1. Predominantly nursing care. Isolate the child and insist on strict hand washing.
2. Monitor heart and respiratory rate.
3. Feeding: if respiratory distress is minimal and O_2 is not required, give frequent small regular oral feeds. If feeding becomes difficult or O_2 therapy is required, continual NG feeds may be given. All very sick infants should only be given i.v. fluids at two-thirds maintenance. Some units give i.v. fluids to all infants requiring O_2 therapy due to the risk of aspiration following NG feeds.
4. Humidified O_2 is given empirically via a headbox to cyanosed infants or infants with increasing respiratory distress until their condition improves. Aim to keep O_2 saturation > 90%.
5. Antibiotics: in sick infants who may possibly have septicaemia or bacterial pneumonia i.v. antibiotics (e.g. flucloxacillin and gentamicin) should be given until the clinical picture becomes clear.
6. Antiviral agents: ribavirin is only considered for infants with serious underlying heart or lung disease in our unit.
7. Ventilation: babies with fatigue, and severe respiratory distress often benefit from nasal CPAP which may obviate the need for full ventilation. Decisions about the need for CPAP and ventilation are usually made on clinical grounds; blood gases may be helpful to determine the level of acidosis.

Follow up

The majority of infants are not followed up even though up to 80% develop recurrent wheezing. Review those with extensive radiological changes, those who were very ill or who had unusual features (e.g. FTT).

Pneumothorax

AETIOLOGY

CF, trauma, IPPV, foreign body, post-thoracotomy and asthma (a rare cause in childhood unless due to ventilation). A lung cyst is the likely cause in unexplained cases.

DIAGNOSIS

Acute onset of respiratory distress. Infants and patients with CF may have minimal physical findings. Shoulder tip or chest wall pain may be felt. Order a CXR.

TREATMENT

1. If uncomplicated with no underlying lung disease, the pneumothorax may resolve spontaneously. Observation, initially in hospital, and follow-up CXR may be all that is required.
2. Needle aspiration may be life saving with a tension pneumothorax, followed by an intercostal drain. Aspiration is performed in the fourth intercostal space in the anterior axillary line (or second space in the anterior midclavicular line). The needle should be attached to a three-way tap and 20–50-ml syringe. Remove the needle following aspiration.
3. Chest drain: indicated for continuing air leak, underlying lung disease, in ventilated patients or when pneumothorax is likely to reaccumulate. Insert the drain under local anaesthesia; avoid the breast area. The end of the tube and water seal should be below the level of the patient's chest.

PNEUMOMEDIASTINUM

Common in asthma. Does not require treatment, only observation. The patient may develop signs of surgical emphysema.

PNEUMOPERICARDIUM

More common in neonatal patients with pulmonary interstitial emphysema. Only very rarely requires drainage (discuss with the consultant if time allows) with a needle attached to a three-way tap and 20-ml syringe and only if the patient is critically ill due to a compromised circulation. Insert the needle below the xiphisternum and aim for the left shoulder.

Cystic fibrosis

Autosomal recessive. Incidence: 1–2500 births. Characterised by diffuse chronic lung disease and insufficiency of pancreatic exocrine function.

COMMONEST PRESENTATIONS

1. Neonatal and sibling screening
2. Recurrent chest infections
3. FTT/steatorrhoea
4. Meconium ileus (15%)
5. Rectal prolapse

DIAGNOSIS

The sweat test (100 mg needed) is the definitive diagnosis and should be performed in an experienced laboratory. Upper limits of normal for Na^+ and Cl^- is 60 mmol/l.

COMMON PROBLEMS

Only those seen by resident staff are described.

Admission with exacerbation of chest infection

Antibiotics have often been changed to prevent deterioration as an outpatient (i.e. trial of oral chloramphenicol or ciprofloxacin for 2 weeks) and physiotherapy will have been increased. If admission is needed:

1. Notify the physiotherapist and dietitian.
2. Request pulmonary function tests (Table 8.3).
3. Order CXR if not done in the last 6 months.
4. Send sputum for culture and sensitivity.
5. Insert peripheral long line if possible. Give i.v. antibiotics; this will vary among units and patients. Our initial inpatient therapy is i.v. gentamicin and oral flucloxacillin. If response is poor or large amounts of sputum containing *Pseudomonas* are present, i.v. ticarcillin is added.
6. Inhalations: 2 ml nebulised propylene glycol diluent (or 0.9% saline) to aid physiotherapy or nebulised salbutamol if wheeze is present and improvement in lung function is seen following nebulisation of salbutamol.
7. Continue pancreatic enzymes and salt supplements.
8. Request weekly pulmonary function tests (see Table 8.3).
9. Do not repeat CXR unless there has been an unexpected deterioration.
10. Treat asthmatic symptoms if present with bronchodilators. Oral steroids are often required.

Keep in hospital until return to the previous state noted or until the condition plateaus, usually by 2 weeks. Usually discharged on Augmentin or Ceclor.

Table 8.3 Respiratory function tests

Height (cm)	FVC (2 SD range)	FEV$_1$ (2 SD range)	PEFR (2 SD range)
110	1.21 (0.9–1.5)	1.1 (0.9–1.3)	150 (110–190)
120	1.5 (1.1–1.9)	1.4 (1.1–1.6)	250 (150–250)
130	1.9 (1.4–2.4)	1.7 (1.4–2.0)	260 (190–320)
140	2.3 (1.7–2.9)	2.1 (1.7–2.5)	310 (230–390)
150	2.8 (2.0–3.5)	2.6 (2.1–3.0)	360 (265–455)
160	3.3 (2.5–4.2)	3.1 (2.6–3.7)	410 (300–520)
170	3.9 (2.9–4.9)	3.7 (3.0–4.4)	450 (340–580)

FVC = forced vital capacity; FEV$_1$ = forced expiratory flow volume; PEFR = peak expiratory flow rate.

Admission with meconium ileus equivalent

Distal intestinal obstruction due to faecal masses. May cause abdominal pain and vomiting. If the child requires admission:

1. Notify the dietitian, physiotherapist and consultant.
2. If the child has had frequent vomits, give i.v. fluids and nil by mouth.
3. If pain rather than vomiting is the problem give clear fluids.
4. Give oral laxatives (e.g. lactulose) and N-acetylcysteine (5–15 ml diluted in soft drink 8-hourly for 10 days). Consider oral Golytely (contraindicated if the child is obstructed).
5. Consider a disposable enema.
6. Consult the surgeon if symptoms are troublesome or if there is doubt about diagnosis. Intussusception or acute appendicitis must be considered.

Asthma

High index of suspicion. Treat with bronchodilators and inhaled steroid (e.g. budesonide or Becotide). Oral prednisolone is indicated for exacerbation.

Surgery

For elective surgery admit for assessment of chest. Increase physiotherapy and consider 'tune up' (see admission for respiratory exacerbation above). Intensive physiotherapy aided by adequate pain relief is needed to encourage cough postoperatively. Emergency surgery should not be delayed (e.g. acute appendicitis) but should be followed by intensive physiotherapy.

Immunisations

Insist on immunisation against pertussis and measles.

Nasal polyps

May require surgical removal but often recur. Try Beconase nasal spray.

Diabetes

Up to 10% of older children. Control is usually simple with insulin.

Hyponatremia

In hot weather give oral Na^+ supplements (2–3 mmol/kg).

Haemoptysis

Check blood clotting levels. Give vitamin K. Refer to a major centre as the child may need major vessel embolisation.

Cirrhosis

Occurs in up to 5%.

Malabsorption

Most children will need pancreatic supplements, e.g. Pancrease.

Asthma

INPATIENT MANAGEMENT OF ACUTE ASTHMA

Children with mild asthma can usually be managed at home. Children with moderate asthma should be admitted or observed until consistent improvement is seen prior to discharge (discuss with a senior colleague). All children with severe asthma should be admitted (see below).

Diagnosis and management

Mild attack. Audible wheeze but little distress; good air entry; peak flow > 50% predicted. Can usually be managed at home with inhaled bronchodilator (see outpatient management of asthma; ensure parents understand the treatment regimen and arrange follow-up by GP or hospital).

Moderate attack. Some respiratory distress; no cyanosis; good air entry with peak flow between 30 and 50% predicted.
1. Give nebulised salbutamol 0.03 ml/kg made up to 3–4 ml with saline; three inhalations may be given in the first hour (this is safe practice), then 2–4-hourly.
2. Give prednisolone 2 mg/kg per 24 hours p.o. in a single dose for 3 days.

Severe attack. Respiratory distress with use of accessory muscles. Wheeze may be minimal due to small tidal volume. The child may be cyanosed in air; palpable pulsus paradoxus (not always present); peak flow < 30% predicted. Observe in HDU or ICU.
1. Give O_2 by facemask.
2. Give salbutamol 0.03 ml/kg nebulised for 5 min via O_2 three times in the first hour then 1–2-hourly.
3. Insert an i.v. cannula.
4. Give i.v. steroids (e.g. hydrocortisone 4 mg/kg 6-hourly). Halve the i.v. steroid dose after 24 hours. Commence oral prednisolone 2 mg/kg once per 24 hours as soon as the child can manage; stop i.v. steroids and continue prednisolone for 3–5 days.
5. Give aminophylline 5 mg/kg as a bolus dose over 15 min; this dose may be repeated 6-hourly or the loading dose may be followed by an infusion of 0.7–1.0 mg/kg/h. Monitor serum levels.
   NB. If the child is taking oral theophylline omit the loading dose.

6. Give 50% maintenance fluids as 0.18% saline in 5% dextrose since increased ADH output may cause hyponatremia. Correct dehydration if present (see Ch. 3).
7. Although only very occasionally required, ventilation facilities must be available.

Improvement is expected in 6–12 hours. The i.v. line can usually be removed by 24 hours. Monitor progress with peak flow if possible (difficult if < 7 years). Gradually decrease nebulisations.

Review medications taken and inhaler technique prior to admission (often inadequate). Follow up in clinic.

Investigations

Usually none needed. CXR is commonly done at first presentation or if there is a discrepancy in physical signs over two hemithoraces. Pneumothorax is rare in childhood asthma.

Lobar/segmental collapse usually responds to treatment of attack and in some cases to physiotherapy.

Blood gases are usually only done on severely ill children who do not respond rapidly to initial therapy. A $PaCO_2$ > 7 kPa (50 mmHg) is of concern and patients should be in ICU.

OUTPATIENT MANAGEMENT OF ASTHMA

Asthma is very often undertreated. History suggesting this includes night time cough, wheeze or cough on exercise and recurrent exacerbation of wheeze. Examination is often normal between attacks. Peak flow charts can be useful in monitoring progress in children > 7 years.

Keep treatment simple. **It is essential that you know how to teach drug administration, check inhaler technique and encourage compliance on each visit.**

Treatment (For < 1-year-olds, see 'The wheezy infant')

1. Age 1–3.5 years.
   a. **Mild intermittent asthma.** Deliver Bricanyl or salbutamol using a spacer device with a facemask attachment (e.g. Nebuhaler with facemask or aerochamber) or use a paper cup (coffee cup method) as a spacer device (two actuations into cup, repeat × 3) or nebulised salbutamol 2.5 mg as required up to 4-hourly. Salbutamol syrup is much less effective.

   b. **Symptoms requiring prophylactic treatment.** Give bronchodilators (Bricanyl or salbutamol) as above plus nebulised 1% SCG 2 ml nebulised for 5 min 8-hourly. SCG may be given by MDI via a spacer with facemask, 1–2 mg 8-hourly.

   c. **Severe symptoms.** Consider differential diagnosis. Try two actuations of beclomethasone diproprionate 200 µg 12-hourly or one actuation of budesonide into a spacer device with a facemask attachment 12-hourly.

Nebulised budesonide is also available. Discuss such patients with the consultant.

2. Age 3.5–6 years.

   a. **Mild intermittent symptoms.** Beta-2 agonist as required, e.g. given by Turbohaler (Bricanyl; this is the easiest device to use or Diskhaler (salbutamol). Give prior to exercise if this induces asthma.

   b. **Symptoms requiring prophylactic treatment.** Beta-2 agonist as above plus Intal via Spinhaler (1 capsule 3–4 times per 24 hours) or MDI via a spacer (1–2 mg 8-hourly).

   c. **Continuing/severe asthma.** As above but substitute an inhaled steroid for SCG. Always give inhaled steroid via a spacer (larger dose to lungs). Two types of inhaled steroids may be given, either budesonide via Nebuhaler device (initial dose 200 µg 12-hourly or beclomethasone dipropionate via Volumatic (initial dose 200 µg 8-hourly device. Dose should be increased until symptoms are controlled. Very few children need oral steroids. Review management with specialist if oral steroids are considered. Give theophylline at night if nocturnal asthma cannot be controlled by improving maintenance medication.

3. Children over 6 years.

   Treat as for 3.5–6-year-olds; discourage the use of metered dose inhaler as good technique in clinic is often poor at home. Still administer inhaled steroids via a spacer device (administration should be supervised by parents). If inhaled steroids are required in low doses only, pulmicort (e.g. 200 µg 12-hourly) via a Turbohaler may be used.

Follow-up

Ideally by the same doctor. Both child and parents need continuing education and encouragement; the child should lead a normal active life. Check inhaler technique and compliance; discourage smoking. Difficult patients should have formal lung function performed (usually only reliable in children > 7 years) and be reviewed by a specialist.

The wheezy infant

These infants are considered separately as their response to conventional anti-asthma therapy is poor. Many of these children have asthma. It is essential to see the child when unwell and wheezing.

DIFFERENTIAL DIAGNOSIS

Includes asthma, viral bronchiolitis, postbronchiolitis wheeze (asthma), aspiration, bronchopulmonary dysplasia, airway or vascular malformations, mediastinal cysts and tumours, and underlying lung disease, including CF.

It is essential to distinguish stridor (see Table 8.1), which is an inspiratory noise, from wheeze, which is an expiratory noise.

INVESTIGATIONS

Baseline CXR. Further investigations as determined by history and examination.

TREATMENT

1. Observation; if well with mild intermittent wheeze only.
2. Treat GOR by thickening feeds, e.g. with Carobel (investigations see p. 35).
3. Nebulised ipratropium bromide (125 µg made up to 3 ml in normal saline, as required, up to 6-hourly) may give temporary benefit in some infants.
4. Beta-2 agonists are usually ineffective.
5. If symptoms are severe discuss differential diagnosis with the consultant. If asthma is diagnosed and severe try an inhaled steroid (e.g. beclomethasone dipropionate from metered dose inhaler; three 50 µg actuations of beclomethasone diproprionate into a spacer device with facemask attachment).

Pneumonia

It may be difficult to differentiate viral from bacterial pneumonia, especially as bacterial cultures are often negative.

The younger the child the less likely symptoms and physical signs are to be characteristic of pneumonia. A CXR in a sick young child may reveal extensive changes with minimal chest signs. Conversely CXR may be normal early in pneumonic illness when physical signs are present.

AETIOLOGY

Viral or bacterial, e.g. *Str. pneumoniae, Staphylococcus, Mycoplasma, Haem. influenzae.*

INVESTIGATIONS

1. Erect CXR. If pleural fluid is suspected, decubitus film can be helpful.

2. Take blood for cultures, viral serology and mycoplasma ELISA. Send a clotted sample to be stored for viral serology if indicated.
3. Send urine for bacterial antigen detection if available.
4. Collect postnasal mucus for virological study, immunofluorescence and culture.
5. If pleural fluid (parapneumonic effusions and empyema) is present:
   a. Nil by mouth.
   b. The fluid requires tapping by needle connected to a syringe by a three-way tap. This may be performed in a ward setting. If a small amount is present or loculation of fluid is possible, USS will guide aspiration and confirm loculation. Withdraw as much fluid as possible.
   c. If aspiration is difficult or recurrence occurs, a formal chest drain is required (ideally under GA); thoracotomy with breakdown of adhesions may be needed to free loculated fluid. Discuss with the surgical team. Send fluid for bacterial culture and microscopy, including analysis for acid-fast bacilli.
6. Consider Mantoux test.

TREATMENT

Antibiotics are indicated in all cases because of the difficulty making an aetiological diagnosis on clinical grounds. Many older children, if only mildly unwell, can be managed at home. Almost all children < 2 years should be admitted.

Outpatient management

If the child was previously well and is now only mildly unwell and can be managed at home, give oral antibiotics (amoxycillin if < 5 years and erythromycin if > 5 years to cover Mycoplasma). Arrange daily review and admit if improvement is not seen or is slow.

Inpatient management

1. If the child is unwell and requires admission treat with i.v. ampicillin and flucloxacillin. Lobar pneumonia in an older child may initially be treated with penicillin alone. If the child is very ill treat with i.v. flucloxacillin and chloramphenicol (or flucloxacillin and ceftazidime). For *Staph. aureus* pneumonia, give i.v. flucloxacillin and gentamicin. Vancomycin is indicated for methicillin resistant strains.
2. Give O_2 if the child is in respiratory distress or is cyanosed.
3. If i.v. fluids are given the rate should initially be 50% of maintenance once dehydration is corrected.
4. Review all children regularly. If the child has staphylococcal

pneumonia repeat CXR to exclude cyst formation and collection of fluid.

ANTIBIOTIC CHANGE

Indications:
1. If there is no improvement after 1–2 days or earlier for a deterioration in condition.
2. If bacterial culture shows that the antibiotic is inappropriate. Treatment is for a full 2 weeks except for staphylococcal infection where oral flucloxacillin should be continued for 6 weeks following discharge.

FOLLOW UP

Review in the outpatient clinic at 6 weeks with repeat CXR.

NB. It may take up to 6 months for the X-ray to return to normal.

Aspiration pneumonia

Often there is a history of GOR and vomiting or difficulty swallowing.

SYMPTOMS

Cough, rattely and wheezy breathing, tachypnoea with or without fever. If recurrent, it may cause FTT.

INVESTIGATIONS

1. CXR: young infants who lie supine tend to develop changes in the posterior parts of upper and lower lobes.
2. Barium swallow and oesophagogram may be indicated to identify swallowing difficulty, GOR or H-type fistula.
3. pH monitoring may detect reflux not seen on barium examination.

TREATMENT

Chemical and/or bacterial pneumonia can occur. Both anaerobic and aerobic organisms may cause infection. Continuous use of antibiotics prophylactically with recurrent aspiration has not proved beneficial and may lead to resistant organisms. If signs and symptoms develop after aspiration give penicillin initially (covers most anaerobes except *Bacteroides fragilis*). In severely ill patients, add chloramphenicol and metronidazole.

Apnoea in infancy

Definition: cessation of breathing for > 20 sec with or without colour change, bradycardia or hypotonia.

MANAGEMENT

1. Admit and observe for at least 24–48 hours.
2. Relate investigations to a detailed history and physical examination.
3. In the ill infant, consider a screen for sepsis first (FBC, suprapubic urine, blood cultures and LP).
4. Other investigations to be considered include:
   a. FBC
   b. routine U&E and Ca^{2+}, blood sugar
   c. nasopharyngeal aspirate for virology study and *B. pertussis*
   d. Cranial USS
   e. Barium swallow and/or oesophageal pH monitoring
   f. Urine for metabolic screen
   g. EEG
5. The need for an apnoea monitor at home should involve prior discussion with the consultant in charge.

MEDICAL INDICATIONS FOR MONITORING

1. Severe apnoeic episode requiring resuscitation.
2. Premature infants with apnoea beyond the expected birth date.
3. Families who have lost one or more infants with SIDS.
4. Infants with a tracheostomy.

9

Gastroenterology

Vomiting

CAUSES

Gastrointestinal

1. Reflux — 'normal' possetting
   — significant GOR
   — hiatus hernia
2. Infective — viral gastroenteritis
   — bacterial infection   } see Table 9.1
   — toxin food poisoning
3. Immunological — coeliac disease
   — cow's milk intolerance
   — other specific food allergies (e.g. fish, strawberries)
4. Inflammatory — appendicitis
   — mesenteric adenitis
5. Obstructive — pyloric stenosis
   — intussusception
   — volvulus
   — strangulated hernia
      — inguinal
      — umbilical
      — epigastric
   — Hirschsprung's disease
   — tumour
   — postoperative ileus

Systemic

1. Infective — any febrile illness
   — UTI in infants
   — following paroxysms of whooping cough
   — acute hepatitis
2. Neurological
   a. increased ICP — trauma
      — meningitis or abscess
      — tumour

    b.   migraine
3.   Metabolic — diabetic ketoacidosis
                — Reye's syndrome
                — many inborn errors of metabolism
4.   Ingestion — drugs (even at therapeutic doses)
               — poisons
               — post GA

ASSESSMENT

History

A dietary/feeding history is paramount:
1. Has vomiting been a problem since birth?
2. Does vomiting only occur soon after food?
3. Has vomiting only been a problem since weaning or the recent introduction of a new food into the diet?
4. Is there diarrhoea?
5. Do other family members have vomiting or diarrhoea?
6. Has the child or a family member been abroad (within the last year)?
7. Is the vomit green (Fig. 9.1)?

Constipation occurs in many febrile illnesses but is also a feature of obstruction. *Steatorrhoea* (smelly stools, difficult to flush) suggests malabsorption. *Abdominal pain* is not specific for a surgical cause of vomiting. Pain also occurs in:
— gastroenteritis
— peptic ulceration and oesophagitis
— renal tract infection (ask about dysuria, haematuria, enuresis)
— hepatitis (travel abroad or recent contacts)
— migraine (family history, or history of recurrent abdominal pain)
— diabetic ketoacidosis (polydipsia, polyuria, weight loss)
— iron ingestion (ask about drugs in the house or at the grandparents')

Examination

A full examination is necessary in all children. Look for fever (infection), anaemia (acute or chronic blood loss or chronic malabsorption), jaundice (pyloric stenosis, hepatitis).
1. Abdominal distension may occur in:
    — chronic constipation
    — gastroenteritis
    — coeliac disease
    — obstruction
    — ileus
    Only in the latter case are bowel sounds diminished.
2. Tenderness is more likely to be due to a surgical cause the

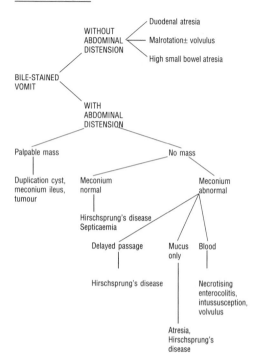

Fig. 9.1 Green vomit in an infant suggests mechanical obstruction until proved otherwise. In duodenal obstruction, stools may not be pale because of a Y-termination of the common bile duct (10%).

more localised it is, the more reproducible it is, and the further from the umbilicus it is.

3. Don't forget the hernial orifices and genitalia.
4. Rectal examination to look for:
    a. fissures exacerbating constipation.
    b. lax sphincter and loaded rectum of chronic constipation. Faecal 'rocks' may also be felt per abdomen, especially on the left side.
    c. tight sphincter and empty rectum of Hirschsprung's disease.
5. Whenever possible, examine the stools for blood, diarrhoea or steatorrhoea. Test the urine for blood or protein: if positive, urgent microscopy is required.

6. If an abdominal cause seems unlikely, look at the ears, throat and fundi.
7. Measure the height and weight of the child for evidence of a chronic problem.

Investigations

If the cause of vomiting is still not clear, consider:
1. urine microscopy and culture
2. FBC
3. U&E for evidence of dehydration, hyponatraemia or hypokalaemic alkalosis (pyloric stenosis)
4. blood sugar
5. blood cultures if febrile
6. stool specimens for both viral and bacterial culture
7. erect and supine AXR if there is localised tenderness or distention and constipation. Air–fluid levels may be seen in:
   — gastroenteritis
   — malabsorption
   — obstruction
   — ileus
8. in an infant between 2 and 10 weeks, consider a *Test feed* to look for pyloric stenosis, even if the vomiting is not projectile.

   Look for visible peristalis and *feel* (from the left side, palpate the right upper quadrant immediately lateral to the rectus sheath) for a pea-sized pyloric tumour

NB. One negative test feed or normal biochemistry does *not* exclude this diagnosis.

MANAGEMENT

Treat the cause if possible. However, two common and non-specific presentations which the junior doctor frequently has to manage are:
1. Chronic vomiting in a baby presenting to casualty or outpatients. Exclude cleft palate, Pierre Robin sequence and neurological abnormality.
   a. If the infant is well, growing along a centile, and the vomits are small, reassure the parents and explain that reflux will improve with time. If vomiting is still a problem at follow-up, try:
      (i) Carobel 1 scoop to 100 ml milk
      (ii) infant Gaviscon ½ sachet with feeds
      (iii) earlier introduction of solids and propping upright for 1 hour after feeds
   b. If the infant is falling away from the centiles, despite adequate intake, and no cause can be found, start Carobel and add infant Gaviscon to every feed but if the child has not regained the centile after 6 weeks of treatment, seek

the advice of a more senior colleague or arrange admission. A barium swallow or oesophageal pH monitoring may elucidate a cause:

(i) oesophagitis secondary to severe reflux
(ii) true sliding hiatus hernia
(iii) small tracheo-oesophageal fistula
(iv) oesophageal stricture
(v) achalasia
(vi) vascular ring or mediastinal mass causing compression

2. *Acute diarrhoea and vomiting.* Few children with gastroenteritis require hospital admission. If the child is < 10% dehydrated, stop all foods and drinks and give a water/dextrose/electrolyte mixture (e.g. Dextrolyte or Dioralyte) orally and frequently using volumes calculated as on p. 18. If there is no vomiting after 24 hours of rehydration with this therapy, restart normal diet. Reintroduction of milk (or a light diet in an older child) should be based on cessation of vomiting, not diarrhoea.

Advise the parents that:

a. loose stools may continue for 2 weeks
b. the child is infectious to others
c. scrupulous hand washing is essential while diarrhoea persists
d. a breast feeding mother must express to maintain her milk supply while the infant is restricted to the electrolyte/dextrose mixture.

If the child is ≥ 10% dehydrated, admit for rehydration and measure electrolytes. Intravenous rehydration is essential in the very ill and severely dehydrated child (see Ch. 3) but should otherwise be reserved for children who have failed a 6-hour trial of water/dextrose/electrolyte mixture.

Diarrhoea

It is difficult to define an absolute threshold of normality; breast fed infants have looser and more frequent stools, sometimes after every feed.

A. ACUTE DIARRHOEA

Whether or not there is vomiting, the commonest cause is gastroenteritis (Table 9.1). Fever may accompany gastroenteritis.

1. Gastrointestinal bleeding

Blood in the stools strongly suggests one of:

a. *Campylobacter jejuni*

Table 9.1 Infective causes of diarrhoea and vomiting

Viruses	*Bacteria*
Rotavirus	Enteroinvasive *E. coli*
Adenovirus	*Campylobacter jejuni*
Coronavirus	Salmonellosis (esp. *S. typhimurium*)
Astrovirus	*S. typhi* and *S. paratyphi*
Calicivirus	*Shigella* (usually. *Sh. sonnei*)
Parvovirus	*Vibrio cholera*
Echovirus	*Yersinia enterocolitica*
Following oral polio vaccine	
Protozoa	*Bacterial toxins* (usually 'food poisoning')
Giardia lamblia	Enterotoxic *E. coli*
Cryptosporidium	*Staph. aureus*
Entamoeba histolytica	*Bacillus cereus*
Malaria	*Clostridium*

b. shigella
c. amoebae
d. intussusception (3 months–3 years)
e. HUS
f. Meckel's diverticulum
g. ulcerative colitis

Small haematemeses, relatively common after vomiting, are presumably due to a small Mallory–Weiss tear or gastritis. Check Hb and clotting but no further investigation.

2. Fluid replacement

For the supportive treatment of gastroenteritis, see the sections on vomiting (p. 126) and on fluid balance in Ch. 3 (p. 18).

3. Specific chemotherapy

Kaolin or antispasmodics should be discouraged and antibiotics are only indicated as follows:

a. erythromycin for prolonged *C. jejuni* infection
b. ampicillin or co-trimoxazole for *Salmonella* bacteraemia or severe *Shigella*
c. metronidazole for *Giardia lamblia* or *Entamoeba histolytica*
d. vancomycin for *Clostridium difficile*

4. Prevention

Advise the parents of measures to reduce cross-infection in the home. If the child is admitted, barrier nurse in an isolation cubicle.

5. Complications

a. Recurrence of diarrhoea: warn the parents that loose stools may persist for 2 weeks.

b. Diarrhoea persisting beyond 2 weeks:
  (i) Transient lactose intolerance is common after gastroenteritis. Stool is positive with 'Clinitest' tablets (i.e. reducing substances). Try a lactose-free milk (Pregestimil or Wysoy). There may be a generalised disaccharidase deficiency, in which case Pregestimil is better.
  (ii) Transient protein intolerance. Normal stool pH and no reducing substances. Try a hydrolysed casein milk (Pregestimil) or soya-based milk (e.g. Wysoy or Formula S). Soya-protein intolerance may coexist with cow's milk intolerance.

B. CHRONIC DIARRHOEA (Table 9.2)

1. Distinguish between faecal overflow (see p. 138) and true diarrhoea by abdominal and rectal examination.

Table 9.2 Causes of chronic diarrhoea

Non-specific diarrhoea	Malabsorption	Inflammatory bowel disease
Normal growth Well child	Abnormal growth Anaemia Rickets Muscle wasting/hypotonia	Abdominal symptoms Bloody diarrhoea
1. *Irritable bowel syndrome* = 'toddler diarrhoea' Onset 6 months–2 years 'Peas and carrots' stools Rarely persists into school age Exaggerated gastrocolic reflex 2. *Postgastroenteritis* See above 3. *Giardiasis* Positive stool microscopy or duodenal aspirate	1. *Mucosal abnormality* Post gastroenteritis Cow's milk or soy milk protein intolerance Carbohydrate intolerance Coeliac disease Giardiasis Post cytotoxic drugs 2. *Pancreatic abnormality* CF 3. *Structural abnormality* Congenital lymphangectasia Blind loops Malrotation Tumours (especially lymphoma) 4. *Immunodeficiency* Hypogammaglobulinaemia Severe combined immunodeficiency syndrome 5. *Other inborn errors of absorption* Acrodermatitis enteropathica (zinc deficiency) Congenital chloridorrhoea	1 Crohn's disease 2. Ulcerative colitis 3. Chronic Campylobacter infection or dysentery

2. Inflammatory bowel disease is rare, even in older children and adolescents.
3. If growth is normal, toddler diarrhoea and post gastroenteritis/giardiasis should be distinguishable.
4. This leaves children with malabsorption, essentially coeliac disease, versus 'the rest'.

COELIAC DISEASE (GLUTEN-SENSITIVE ENTEROPATHY)

History

Usually < 2 years. Anorexia, vomiting and frequent, smelly, pale stools. Onset of symptoms after introduction of solids (usually 4–6 months; wheat, barley, rye and oats all contain gluten; corn and rice are non-toxic).

Examination

Anaemia
Short stature
Muscle wasting (buttocks most obvious)
Distended abdomen
Dermatitis herpetiformis (itchy vesicular rash, genitalia or buttocks, usually > 4 years).

Investigation

Jejunal biopsy. The definitive test.
1. Defer only if the child is very ill or clotting is abnormal.
2. Discuss histochemistry/electron microscopy with the histology lab. *beforehand.* Book 1 hour of fluoroscopy screening time in the X-ray department.
3. Starve for at least 6 hours. The child should have received at least 10 g of gluten per 24 hours for the last 2 weeks.
4. Give the following 1 hour before procedure:
   — Vallergan 4 mg/kg p.o. (max. 100 mg)
   — Chloral hydrate 40 mg/kg p.o. (max. 600 mg)
   — Metoclopramide 0.3 mg/kg p.o. (max. 10 mg)
   Give procyclidine (< 2 years 0.5–2 mg, > 2 years 2–5 mg, > 12 years 5 mg) if there is a dystonic reaction to metoclopramide.
5. Check that the Crosby capsule fires with suction, reload, and pass the capsule through a mouth guard and into the stomach.
6. Leave the child on his right side and the capsule should pass through the pylorus within 30 min. If not, pass a guidewire through the tubing or give metoclopramide 0.3 mg/kg i.v.
7. Once the capsule is in the jejunum, fire the biopsy six times, retrieve the biopsy specimen and aspirate any luminal fluid to look for *Giardia*.
8. The child may be admitted as a day case and can go home once he can sit or stand. No solid food until fully awake. The

Table 9.3 Causes of an abnormal jejunal biopsy

Villous atrophy
Coeliac disease
Temporary gluten intolerance
Cow's milk protein intolerance
Soy protein intolerance
Gastroenteritis
Giardiasis
Severe combined immunodeficiency
Cytotoxic chemotherapy

Other abnormalities
Agammaglobulinaemia (no plasma cells)
Lymphangiectasis (dilated mucosal lymphatics)
Abetalipoproteinaemia (distention of epithelial cells by fat)
Disaccharidase deficiency (absent on histochemical staining)

Giardia may be seen on microscopy (or organisms cultured) in gastroenteritis
or blind-loop syndrome.

---

parents should contact the ward if there is a haematemesis, abdominal pain, fever, or malaena.

Differential diagnosis of abnormal jejunal biopsy (Table 9.3). For absolute confirmation of gluten-sensitive enteropathy, three jejunal biopsies are recommended:
1. Initial biopsy — villous atrophy
2. Following clinical improvement on a gluten-free diet for 6 months — normal repeat biopsy
3. Following 6-week gluten challenge (or less if symptomatic) — villous atrophy recurs

Management
Abnormal biopsy: follow the scheme in Fig. 9.2.
Normal biopsy: other investigations are necessary.

Failure to thrive

1. Distinguish from acute weight *loss*, usually due to dehydration.
2. The cause of FTT is chronic and more often there is *inadequate weight gain* rather than actual loss. Hence, the child 'falls away' on a centile chart. Serial weights over 3 months are more reliable than single absolute measurements.
3. A common catch is that birthweight is an unreliable predictor of future weight and 'physiological down regulation' is common in the first 6 months of life.
4. In the older child, decreased height velocity is a more sensitive indicator of FTT than weight.

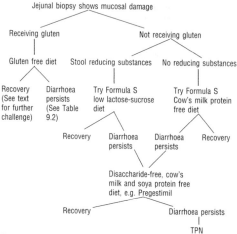

Notes:
1. The very ill child may need immediate resuscitation with plasma/blood transfusion and TPN until well enough for a trial of diet.
2. Introduce each new preparation by a graded increase in concentration. Diarrhoea may persist for several weeks. Try each stage for at least 1 week. Ideally, recovery should be proved by repeat biopsy.
3. Re-introduce potential provoking nutrients in the order lactose, protein, gluten.

Figure 9.2 Trial of diets for chronic diarrhoea. Specific vitamin and mineral supplements may also be required.

CAUSES

Almost any chronic paediatric condition can result in FTT but all causes act via one or more of the mechanisms in Table 9.4. In over half the cases, the cause is poor dietary intake.

HISTORY

1. Detailed history of the onset of FTT and growth prior to introduction of solids.
2. Past medical history.
3. Family history of short stature, CF, coeliac disease etc. Social circumstances. Who feeds the child?
4. Pregnancy history (?congenital infection), gestation and birthweight.
5. Detailed dietary history, both offered and taken. The mean

Table 9.4 Causes of failure to thrive*

Inadequate diet offered
Too little offered
Not offered often enough
Offered but deficient in calories, protein or vitamins

Inadequate intake
The 'fussy eater'
Anorexia due to an organic cause, e.g. coeliac disease
Cardiovascular, respiratory or neurological disease may render intake difficult despite good appetite

Vomiting
Diet is taken but not absorbed.
Severe reflux has the same consequence and may additionally cause oesophagitis
Chronic vomiting or reflux will lead to loss of appetite also

Malabsorption
Diet is taken in sufficient quantities but not absorbed: specific mucosal or exocrine problem

Increased requirements
Cardiac failure, respiratory failure and thyrotoxicosis result in increased basal energy expenditure

Decreased utilisation
Many dysmorphic children fail to thrive even with adequate intake. Endocrine FTT is due to inadequate utilisation of diet

* Several may occur simultaneously, e.g. CF

milk intake of thriving babies is > 150 ml/kg (2.5 oz/lb) per 24 hours during the first 6 months, with feeds at 3–6-hour intervals.

The diet of older children should be scrutinised by a dietician for calories, protein, vitamins, iron and Ca^{2+} intake.
6. Developmental milestones: motor delay is common.
7. Ask specifically about:
   a. vomiting
   b. diarrhoea
   c. abdominal pain
   d. shortness of breath, chronic cough (recurrent aspiration, CF)
   e. tiredness/cyanosis/sweating on feeding (cardiac failure)
   f. urinary frequency or excessive thirst (UTI, diabetes mellitus or diabetes insipidus)

EXAMINATION

1. Measure height, weight and OFC and plot on an appropriate centile chart using the child's decimal age.
2. Height of parents and siblings (see Ch. 5, p. 45).

3. Complete physical examination, including mouth, BP and fundoscopy.
4. Stool inspection and urinalysis.

The features in Table 9.5 suggest the child is constitutionally small. Serial weights should continue for 6 months but no other action is necessary.

If the child is failing to thrive, but is well, simple dietary advice may suffice. However, if at follow-up 6 weeks later there has been no 'catch-up', admit for a *trial of feeding* (Fig. 9.3).

A successful trial effectively excludes an organic cause for FTT and often requires hospital admission; 4 weeks may be needed to demonstrate the improvement effectively. If the trial is unsuccessful, the period of inpatient observation may direct the nature of further investigations (see Fig. 9.2 and Table 9.6).

Table 9.5 The constitutionally small child

1. Asymptomatic
2. Low birthweight for gestational age
3. Proportionally small (height, weight and OFC centiles similar)
   Asymmetrical growth patterns suggest particular causes:
   (a) OFC centile > height > weight suggests third trimester IUGR (usually followed by 'catch up' growth if diet is adequate) or nutritional FTT
   (b) OFC centile = weight > height suggests endocrine FTT
4. Normal height and weight velocities (i.e. growing parallel to but below the third centile)
5. Small parents

If not, look for evidence of:
— congenital infection
— fetal alcohol syndrome
— chromosomal abnormality
— dysmorphic features
— skeletal dysplasia

Gastrointestinal bleeding

In over 50% of cases in childhood, no specific cause is found.

A cause should be sought more vigorously in either the newborn (vitamin K deficiency) or an older child (portal hypertension and oesophageal varices), or if the bleeding is severe.

Haematemesis is more common than melaena, and if a small haematemesis occurs after previous bloodless vomiting, the cause is probably a small Mallory-Weiss tear. In the newborn, haematemesis may be swallowed maternal blood, and in an older child, the result of a nose bleed.

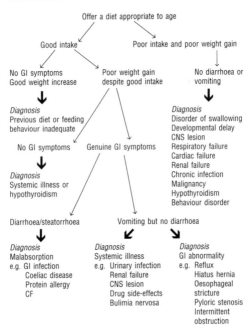

Fig. 9.3 Trial of feeding for failure to thrive.

Fresh blood p.r. is most commonly due to an anal fissure or bacterial enteritis. If not, consider:
1. clotting abnormality
2. intussusception (3 months–3 years)
3. volvulus
4. dietary protein allergy
5. inflammatory bowel disease
6. haemangioma or telangiectasia
7. sexual abuse or foreign body

Melaena suggests bleeding from stomach or small bowel:
1. clotting abnormality
2. peptic ulceration or gastritis
3. oesophageal or gastric varices
4. Meckel's diverticulum

In all cases:
1. Resuscitate first, if necessary. Give plasma or uncrossmatched blood 20 ml/kg if shocked.

Table 9.6 Investigation of failure to thrive

	Investigation	Probable diagnosis
Trial of normal diet in hospital for 2–4 weeks	Daily weights Inspect stools	Deprivation
Stools	Microscopy	Cysts of Giardia or Amoeba. Pathogenic E. coli, Shigella, Salmonella
	Reducing substances pH < 5.5	Disaccharidase deficiency
	Fat globules	Pancreatic disorder
Urine	Culture	UTI
	Glycosuria	Diabetes mellitus
	Proteinuria/haematuria	Renal failure
	Reducing substances other than glucose (Clinitest positive, Clinistix negative)	Galactosaemia
	Osmolality < 200 mosmol/l Specific gravity < 1.005	Diabetes insipidus
	Aminoacid and organic acid chromatography	amino- or organic aciduria
	Valinyl mandelic acid	Neuroblastoma
Sweat	Sweat Na^+ > 80 mmol/l on two occasions (provided > 100 mg of sweat)	CF
Blood	Hb, WBC, platelets and film	Anaemia
	Folate (serum and RBC)	Schwachman's syndrome Leukaemia
	Iron/ferritin/transferrin/TIBC	Iron deficiency
	Electrolytes	Chronic vomiting Diabetes insipidus Chloriddorrhoea
	HCO_3^-	Renal tubular disorder
	Creatinine	Renal failure
	Ca^{2+}, PO_4^{3-}, alkaline phosphatase	Rickets
	Conjugated bilirubin, liver function tests, albumin	Biliary or liver disease
	Clotting studies	Dietary deficiency, malabsorption or liver disease
	Thyroid function	Hypo/hyperthyroidism
	GH	Hypopituitarism
	Cholesterol	Abetalipoproteinaemia
	Immunoglobulins	Hypogammaglobulinaemia

Table 9.6 (continued)

	Investigation	Probable diagnosis
	Hypoproteinaemia	Dietary deficiency, liver disease, nephrotic or protein losing enteropathy
Jejunal biopsy	See p. 129	See Table 9.3
Radiology	CXR	Aspiration pneumonia, CF Cardiac failure
	Erect and supine AXR Consider barium meal and follow through	Malrotation Blind loop syndrome Crohn's disease Peptic ulcer Constipation Cystinosis
	Left hand and wrist	Bone age
Xylose absorption test	5 g oral xylose after 6-hour fast Take blood (fluoride tube) after 1 hour (xylose < 1.3 mmol/l = abnormal)	Small bowel mucosal abnormality
^{51}Cr albumin i.v.	Normally < 1% appears in next 4 days' stools	Protein losing enteropathy

2. Look for other bleeding sites, signs of portal hypertension, skin haemangioma.
3. Initial investigations:
   a. crossmatch blood
   b. Hb (initial Hb may not reflect serious blood loss)
   c. platelet count
   d. clotting screen
   e. evidence of chronic liver disease (see Table 9.10).
4. Involve a surgeon early. Proctoscopy for small rectal bleeds.
5. All children with head injuries or receiving intensive care should be given cimetidine 10 mg/kg 12-hourly by slow i.v. infusion.

Bleeding varices

In addition to the above:
1. Low threshold for insertion of central venous catheter. Keep CVP 1–2 cmH$_2$O relative to sternal angle. Avoid over-transfusion.
2. Pass an NGT and aspirate frequently.

Table 9.7   Causes of acute abdominal pain

Require early surgical referral	Abdominal cause but does not require immediate surgical referral	Systemic cause
Appendicitis	Gastroenteritis*	Any febrile illness but especially ENT infection
Peritonitis	Infantile colic*	
Intussusception	Ingestion	Lower lobe pneumonia
Volvulus	Constipation*	Abdominal migraine*
Strangulated hernia	Peptic ulcer (including	Diabetic ketoacidosis
Obstruction	*Helicobacter pylori*	Sexual abuse*
Trauma	associated gastritis/	Sickle causes
GI bleeding	ulceration)*	Porphyria
	Pancreatitis, including	Lead poisoning
	mumps	HSP
	Cholecystitis/cholangitis	
	UTI*, nephrotic syndrome	
	Urinary calculus*	
	Hepatitis	
	Dysmenorrhoea*	

* More common organic causes of recurrent abdominal pain

3. Treat hepatic encephalopathy (see management of acute liver failure, p. 140).
4. Triglycyl lysine vasopressin (Terlipressin) 0.3 u/kg i.m. 6-hourly, or vasopressin 0.3 u/kg i.v. over 15 min. Infusion may be continued at a lower dose but reduce if nausea, increased abdominal pain or hyponatraemia develops.
5. Passage of a Sengstaken Blakemore tube requires expert assistance.

Abdominal pain

A. ACUTE ABDOMINAL PAIN (Table 9.7)

The single most important question is — 'does this child require emergency surgery?' This is a clinical decision but pointers to a surgical cause are:

1. Signs of peritonism (fever, localised tenderness, including rectally, guarding, rigidity and absent bowel sounds). Appendicitis is the commonest cause but is rare < 2 years. Anorexia is usual and vomiting very common. The younger the child, the more vague the signs of appendicitis.
2. Signs of obstruction (vomiting, abdominal distension, high pitched bowel sounds and constipation — the rectum may or may not be empty).
3. GI bleeding.

Investigations

Consider:

1. Urine microscopy.
2. Urinalysis for glycosuria, proteinuria, haematuria.
3. FBC and WBC differential. Sickling test in African and Afro-Caribbean children.
4. Plain AXR (erect and supine).

B. RECURRENT ABDOMINAL PAIN

All of the causes of acute abdominal pain may recur but some are more likely than others (see Table 9.7, asterisks). However, at least 90% of children with recurrent abdominal pain do *not* have an organic cause. Functional abdominal pain ('periodic syndrome', 'abdominal migraine') is a positive clinical diagnosis and *not* a diagnosis of last resort after multiple investigations. Clues are:

1. child is otherwise healthy and thriving
2. good appetite and no diarrhoea or vomiting
3. episodes are relatively short and may coincide with environmental triggers
4. pain is periumbilical; there are no abnormal physical signs
5. family history of recurrent abdominal pain or migraine

If still in doubt, urine microscopy, FBC and ESR, and plain AXR should suffice to reassure you and the parents.

Constipation, soiling and encopresis

Whilst these are usually considered together, *encopresis* is a quite separate entity:

1. No organic abnormality.
2. No constipation. Therefore laxatives are not indicated.
3. Faeces are voluntarily passed in an unacceptable place, including the child's pants.

There is a significant emotional disorder in the child or in the family and this must be recognised early.

Soiling (involuntary passage of faeces) may be due to:

1. 'Developmental delay', i.e. the skill of toilet training has not yet been acquired.
2. A neurological abnormality, e.g. spina bifida.
3. Chronic constipation and overflow of liquid faeces.

The management of *constipation* is in two stages.

Firstly, exclude an organic cause (Table 9.8), and secondly, restore a normal bowel habit. Clues to an organic cause are:

1. Constipation since birth or delay in passage of meconium beyond 24 hours.
2. The more severe the constipation and the younger the child.
3. FTT or abnormal physical signs.

Table 9.8 Organic cause of chronic constipation

Gastrointestinal
Hirschsprung's disease (if necessary, exclude by rectal biopsy stained for
ganglion cells and cholinesterase)
Anal stricture
Anal fissure
Partial intestinal obstruction

Systemic
Hypothyroidism
Hypercalcaemia
Lead poisoning (associated with pica: anaemia and basophilic stippling on
blood film)
Renal tubular disorders (plasma HCO_3^- and urine pH)
Diabetes insipidus (urine osmolality; may need water deprivation test, see
p. 25)
Sexual abuse

* Organic causes are more likely in infants, especially if onset is from birth

4. Empty rectum or 'toothpaste sign' after p.r. exam (suggests
   Hirschsprung's disease).

MANAGEMENT OF CONSTIPATION WITHOUT AN ORGANIC CAUSE

Response to treatment is directly proportional to the confidence,
enthusiasm and persistence of the paediatrician.

ASSESSMENT

Detailed history of the onset of constipation (e.g. febrile illness or
visit to a relative), whether unremitting or alternating with periods
of normal bowel habit, the age and pattern of toilet training, and
the ambience of the domestic lavatory. A dietary history may
suggest the cause. A complete physical examination is essential,
including rectal examination and assessment of anal tone. Look
particularly for an anal fissure.

TREATMENT

1. Explain that the problem is common, treatable and not the
   child's fault.
2. Recommend increased fluids (especially fruit juice), brown
   bread instead of white, bran or high fibre breakfast cereals,
   cooking with vegetables and pulses.
3. Start *regular* faecal softeners, e.g. Lactulose 5 ml 12-hourly
   and increase by 5 ml 12-hourly every 4 days until the stools
   are soft.
4. Recommend that the child sits on the toilet for at least 5
   minutes after mealtimes.

5. Advise that a diary be kept.
   See the child with the diary again in 2 weeks. Be encouraging, even if there has been no result.
6. If there is no response, start regular laxatives, e.g. Senokot 2.5 ml 12-hourly which can be increased to 10 ml 12-hourly.
7. If there is still no response after a further 4 weeks, start behaviour modification (star chart) with 'rewards' which are appropriate to the child's age, sex and family circumstances. Follow-up at 2-week intervals and do not allow your enthusiasm to wane. If the child remains severely constipated despite 3 months of intensive outpatient treatment, arrange a brief admission for enema under GA (forcible use of suppositories or enema in a resisting child is harrowing for all concerned) and continue vigorous outpatient follow-up, including a home visit. If there is still no improvement, arrange an inpatient admission for nursing observation, dietary manipulation, behaviour assessment, and intensive behaviour therapy employing nursing staff and the hospital school. This is very rarely necessary.

Hepatosplenomegaly

The causes are legion but many are rare. The differential diagnosis can be narrowed by ascertaining whether there is enlargement of liver only, spleen only, or both (Table 9.9) and whether this is recent or chronic.

ACUTE LIVER FAILURE

Suggested by:
1. alteration of consciousness level
2. vomiting
3. hypoglycaemia
4. bleeding diathesis
5. jaundice and electrolyte abnormalities
6. enlarged and tender liver

Management
1. Identify and treat the underlying cause (Table 9.10).
2. Record baseline vital signs and Glasgow Coma score (see Ch. 2).
3. Avoid sedation. In the presence of liver failure, the dose of all drugs must be checked (see also Table 9.12).
4. Minimise encephalopathy:
   a. low protein diet; avoid TPN but
   b. maintain a normal blood glucose with i.v. dextrose if necessary

Table 9.9 Causes of hepatomegaly. Hyperinflation of the chest (asthma, bronchiolitis) may push the liver down but there is not true hepatomegaly

	Hepatomegaly	Hepatosplenomegaly	Splenomegaly
Infection	Viral hepatitis	Congenital infections Glandular fever	Subacute bacterial endocarditis Malaria
Congestion	Cardiac failure Biliary atresia	Portal hypertension due to a prehepatic cause — cardiac failure — pericarditis — Budd–Chiari syndrome	Portal hypertension — idiopathic extrahepatic portal vein obstruction — cirrhosis — previous portal sepsis
Haematological	Haemolytic disease of the newborn	Thalassaemia	Sickle cell disease in a young child (later splenic atrophy) Spherocytosis
Malignancy	Neuroblastoma	Leukaemia Lymphoma	
Metabolic	Reye's syndrome Galactosaemia Glycogen storage disorder Wilson's disease	Mucopolysaccharidoses	
Inflammatory	Early cirrhosis Juvenile chronic arthritis		

Table 9.10 Investigation of liver failure

	Abnormality	Diagnosis
Urine	Glycosuria	Haemochromatosis or CF associated with liver damage and diabetes
	Reducing substances	Galactosaemia
	Haematuria	Coagulopathy
		Hepatorenal syndrome
	Bilirubin but no urobilinogen	Biliary obstruction

Save urine for toxicology screen and chromatography for rare inborn errors of metabolism. Send for viral (CMV) and bacterial culture, and microscopy (infection may precipitate acute or chronic liver failure)

Blood	1. *FBC*	
	Hb and iron binding	Iron deficiency anaemia due to chronic GI bleeding. Iron overload in haemochromatosis Haemolytic anaemia due to hypersplenism
	WBC	Infection may precipitate acute on chronic liver failure
	Platelets	Low if DIC has supervened or there is hypersplenism
	2. *U&E*	
	Glucose	Hypoglycaemia commonly complicates liver failure and inborn errors of metabolism
	Electrolytes	Electrolyte abnormalities may precipitate liver failure or result from liver failure (usually hyponatraemia)
	Urea	May be low in severe liver failure (urea is synthesised in the liver) or high if ascites and vomiting cause hypovolaemia and prerenal failure
	3. *Tests of hepatocellular function*	
	NH_4^+	May be elevated in liver failure and is not specific for Reye's syndrome. Falsely elevated if sample is not fresh
	ALT or AST	Transaminases are elevated with liver cell damage
	4. *Tests of synthetic function*	
	Clotting studies	Both intrinsic and extrinsic paths are prolonged by deficiency of vitamin K dependent factors (II, VIII, IX, X) May occur rapidly
	Albumin	Synthesised in the liver but several days must elapse before levels fall significantly
	5. *Tests of excretory function*	
	Conjugated bilirubin	May be elevated in hepatocellular or obstructive jaundice (see urine)

Table 9.10 (continued)

	Abnormality	Diagnosis
	Unconjugated bilirubin	Only elevated in very severe liver failure or coexistent hypersplenism (haemolytic anaemia)
	Alkaline phosphatase	Note the wide and age-dependent normal range
		High levels suggest biliary obstruction
	Gamma-glutamyl transpeptidase	High levels suggest biliary obstruction
	6. *Evidence of infection*	
	Blood cultures	
	Hepatitis antigens and antibodies	See Table 9.13
	Also CMV and EBV	
	7. *Metabolic disorders*	
	Alpha-1-antitrypsin	Deficiency causes cirrhosis
	Plasma Cu^{2+} and caeruloplasmin	$\uparrow Cu^{2+}$ and $\downarrow$ caeruloplasmin in Wilson's disease
Sweat	Sweat test	CF leads to cirrhosis
Radiology	USS	Essential to exclude biliary obstruction and space-occupying lesion
Liver biopsy	See p. 145	

    c. purge the gut of blood and protein using oral lactulose (1 ml/kg 8-hourly)

    d. oral neomycin (15 mg/kg 6-hourly) to reduce gut bacteria.

5. Correct any coagulopathy. Give vitamin K_1 (phytomenadione) 0.3 mg/kg i.v. slowly routinely and FFP 10 ml/kg if there is active bleeding or to cover an invasive procedure. Crossmatched blood should always be available if there has been haematemesis, malaena or known varices.

6. Correct electrolyte imbalances, preferably by altering intake. Treat ascites by:

    a. restrict fluid intake to $\frac{2}{3}$ maintenance requirement

    b. restrict Na^+ intake to 1 mmol/kg per 24 hours

    c. give oral spironolactone (1–2 mg/kg 12-hourly) or i.v. potassium canrenoate (1–2 mg/kg 12-hourly — contraindicated in hyponatraemia) to combat hyperaldosteronism; avoid all other diuretics

    d. consider salt-poor albumin solution i.v. if serum albumin is < 25 gl and response to (a)–(c) is poor *but* do not expect to generate a negative fluid balance of more than 1% bodyweight in each 24-hour period. Avoid paracentesis unless infected ascites is suspected.

7. Mannitol 1 g/kg i.v. may temporarily reduce ICP.
    If more aggressive management is deemed appropriate (ventilation, ICP monitoring, renal dialysis, exchange transfusion, charcoal haemoperfusion), consider this early on and arrange transfer to a major centre.

CHRONIC LIVER FAILURE

Hepatomegaly or portal hypertension due to cirrhosis (Table 9.11) are suggested by:
1. spider naevi
2. palmar erythema
3. jaundice, anaemia or Kayser-Fleischer ring
4. purpura, haematemesis or malaena
5. enlarged and hard liver with non-tender splenomegaly
6. ascites and peripheral oedema

A mixture of these features may be seen in acute on chronic liver failure and obviously there may be other signs of the underlying cause.

Table 9.11 Causes of childhood cirrhosis

Hepatic (commonest)
1. Wilson's disease
2. Chronic hepatitis (following hepatitis B or as an autoimmune disorder)
3. alpha-1-antitrypsin deficiency
4. Drug induced (paracetamol overdose, chlorocarbon ingestion, isoniazid, methotrexate, halothane)

Post-hepatic
1. Biliary atresia and other anatomical anomalies of the biliary tree
2. Recurrent cholangitis
3. Inflammatory bowel disease
4. CF

Pre-hepatic (rarest)
Budd–Chiari syndrome

Management

Usually as an outpatient. The following may require attention:
1. Treatment of the underlying cause.
2. FTT:
    a. high-energy, high-carbohydrate, low-protein diet
    b. vitamin supplementation (particularly fat soluble vitamins A, D, E and K — use Ketovite liquid (B, C, E, folic acid) 5 ml per 24 hours and Ketovite tablets (A, D, B_{12}) orally, one tablet 8-hourly.
3. Coagulopathy: monitor PT as index of adequacy of vitamin K supplementation. Iron deficiency anaemia suggests chronic GI bleeding.

Table 9.12   Drugs to be used with caution in liver disease

Drug	Problems in liver disease
Magnesium trisilicate	Sodium load aggravates ascites
Gaviscon	Sodium load aggravates ascites
Diuretics	Hypokalaemia precipitates coma
Beta-blockers	Reduce dose as decreased first pass metabolism
Anticoagulants	Clotting already prolonged
Aminophylline	Reduce dose
Aspirin	GI bleeding and Reye's syndrome
Paracetamol	Reduce dose
Opiates	May precipitate coma
Anticonvulsants	Avoid valproate
	Dose of other anti-convulsant may need to be reduced
Chloramphenicol	Increased risk of bone marrow failure
Erythromycin	
Isoniazid	*Avoid:* increased risk of hepatosplenomegaly
Rifampicin	
Doxorubicin	
Methotrexate	Reduce dose

4. Biochemical rickets: monitor Ca^{2+}, PO_4^{3-} and alkaline phosphatase as index of adequacy of vitamin D supplementation.
5. Jaundice: monitor levels of unconjugated bilirubin. Cholestyramine (30 mg/kg 8-hourly orally) may be necessary for pruritus but may exacerbate fat-soluble vitamin and folic acid deficiency.
6. Monitor transaminase levels: look for causes of abrupt deterioration.
7. Ascites (see p. 143).
8. Haematemesis and melaena: advise the parents to seek urgent admission. Avoid aspirin and other non-steroidal anti-inflammatory analgesics (Table 9.12) Endoscopy and sclerotherapy (provided the coagulopathy can be corrected or covered with FFP) may avoid the need for surgery.

Liver biopsy

Should be performed only by an expert and only when the result may aid management:
1. Wilson's disease
2. chronic hepatitis (active or persistent)
3. conjugated jaundice without evidence of viral infection or anomaly of biliary tree
4. unconjugated jaundice without haemolysis (Crigler–Najjar syndrome)

Platelet count and PT should be checked, blood crossmatched and

Table 9.13 Causes of jaundice outside the neonatal period

Hepatocellular jaundice (mixed conjugated and unconjugated
hyperbilirubinaemia)
1. Infective — acute hepatitis
   (a) *Viruses*   *Blood test* (unless otherwise stated)
       Hepatitis A   HepA IgM
       Hepatitis B   HepB surface antigen ('Australia' antigen)
       Non-A, non-B hepatitis
       Epstein–Barr virus   Atypical mononuclear cells on blood film
       CMV   CMV IgM
                                          Urine culture
   (b) *Bacteria*
       Leptospira   Elevated antibody titre
       icterohaemorrhagiae   CSF lymphocytosis if meningism clinically
       (Weil's disease)
       Liver abscess   Positive blood cultures
   (c) *Protozoa*
       Toxoplasma gondii   Elevated antibody titre
2. Chronic hepatitis (all rare)
   Wilson's disease
   Alpha-1-antitrypsin deficiency
   Chronic active hepatitis (adolescent girls; positive autoantibodies)
   Chronic persistent hepatitis (80% HBsAg positive)
   Recurrent cholangitis
   Inflammatory bowel disease
   Drug induced (cytotoxic drugs, sodium valproate)
3. *Acute liver failure*
   Reye's syndrome (plasma NH_3 > 80 µg/100 ml)
   Acute viral hepatitis (rare)
   Paracetamol ingestion

Obstructive jaundice (conjugated hyperbilirubinaemia)
a. *Congenital anomalies* Biliary atresia
                          Bile duct stenosis
                          Choledochal cyst
b. *Gallstones* Chronic haemolytic diseases
                CF
                Chronic liver disease
c. *Cholecystitis*

Unconjugated hyperbilirubinaemia
1. *Haemolysis* (commonest). Think of infection and drugs as precipitants
   Congenital   Acquired

   a. spherocytosis   a. idiopathic
   b. sickle cell anaemia   b. HUS
   c. G6PD deficiency   c. *Mycoplasma* infection
2. *Inherited defect of bilirubin metabolism* (Gilbert's and Crigler–Najjar
   syndromes)

available, and consent obtained. The histopathologist *must be consulted before* the procedure regarding the need for samples for:
1. formalin fixation for light microscopy
2. unfixed core for frozen section
3. glutaraldehyde fixation for electron microscopy
4. snap freezing for enzyme studies

Jaundice

NEONATAL

See Ch. 19.

THE OLDER CHILD (Table 9.13)

Mixed hyperbilirubinaemia is more common and the cause is usually infective. Hepatitis A is the commonest in the UK and rarely requires hospital admission. Elevated transaminases precede jaundice. No longer infectious once jaundice appears. Urine is dark. Stools may be pale.

Conjugated hyperbilirubinaemia (pale stools and dark urine) is rare in childhood and always requires investigation: early USS to demonstrate biliary obstruction. Look for evidence of chronic liver disease (see Table 9.11).

10

Renal and genitourinary problems

Common presentations of renal disease

DYSURIA

Usually due to infection but also non-infectious urethritis, foreign body, calculi and passage of blood per urethra. In preverbal children, crying and drawing up legs during micturition suggests dysuria.

POLYURIA (Table 10.1)

Many of these disorders also result in enuresis, nocturnal or day and night. Frequency (frequent passage of small amounts of urine) may be confused with true polyuria but the cause is more likely to be infection, behavioural or neurogenic bladder.

Table 10.1 Causes of polyuria

Intrinsic renal disease	1. CRF
	2. Following relief of obstructive uropathy
	3. Nephrogenic diabetes insipidus (end organ insensitivity to ADH)
	4. Fanconi's syndrome
	5. Cystinosis
Metabolic or endocrine disorders	1. Diabetes mellitus
	2. Central diabetes insipidus (deficiency of ADH)
	3. Hypoadrenalism (initially salt-losing and polyuric; later hypovolaemic and oliguric)
	4. Vitamin D intoxication
Excessive water intake	Psychogenic polydipsia. Water deprivation results in passage of smaller amounts of concentrated urine (> 400 mosmol/l)

Table 10.2 Causes of haematuria

Non-glomerular	1.	Infection of any part of the urinary tract (urethritis, cystitis, pyelonephritis, including TB)
	2.	Hydronephrosis without infection
	3.	Stones
	4.	Foreign body or trauma
	5.	Coagulopathy
	6.	Sickle cell disease
	7.	Vascular anomalies
	8.	Cyanotic heart disease
	9.	Wilm's tumour
	10.	Menstrual blood
Glomerular		Red cell casts, white cell casts or epithelial casts on microscopy suggest a glomerular cause but absence of casts does not exclude glomerular problem. The greater the degree of proteinuria, the more likely the source of blood is renal.
	1.	Benign familial haematuria
	2.	Berger's disease (IgG/IgA nephropathy)
	3.	HSP
	4.	Glomerulonephritis
	5.	SLE
	6.	Alport's syndrome (hereditary deafness and nephritis)
	7.	SBE or shunt nephritis (infected CSF shunt)

HAEMATURIA (Table 10.2)

Test strips are extremely sensitive and detect red cells (5 RBC/mm^3 minimum) and free myoglobin or Hb (0.02 mg/dl minimum). Intact RBCs give a spotted reaction whereas free Hb gives a uniform green on the test strip.

Transient haematuria

Affects 4% of schoolchildren and it should be sufficient to take a full history and examination (especially for purpura, abdominal masses, BP, deafness and evidence of local trauma or abuse).

Persistent haematuria

May be macro-or microscopic but not a useful discriminator of seriousness and requires further investigation. As a minimum:
1. M, C & S of urine
2. check urine of other family members
3. blood tests — FBC, U & E and creatinine, ASOT, ANF
4. renal USS

If the history suggests calculi:
5. blood tests: Ca^{2+}, PO_4^{3-}, urate
6. plain AXR
7. 24-hourly urine collection for protein, calcium, creatinine, urate, oxalate and cystine

Table 10.3 Causes of glycosuria

Hyperglycaemia
1.	Persistent hyperglycaemia	Diabetes mellitus
2.	Transient hyperglycaemia	'Stress', febrile illness, following a seizure, steroids, i.v. glucose infusion

Decreased renal threshold (with normal blood glucose)
1.	Isolated renal glycosuria	May be hereditary
2.	Fanconi's syndrome	

False-positive Clinitest (presence in the urine of reducing substance other than glucose)
1. Galactose
2. Fructose
3. Alkaptonuria
4. Vitamin C, nalidixic acid, cephalosporins

Heavy proteinuria or heavy urate deposits may also give false-positive but *Clinistix* reagent strips are specific for glucose.

GLYCOSURIA

May present as polyuria, enuresis or on routine urinalysis (Table 10.3).

PROTEINURIA

Detected by reagent test strips which are very sensitive for albumin but may give false positive results if the urine specimen is old or if the dipstick is left in urine too long (Table 10.4). Haematuria is inevitably accompanied by proteinuria (trace — 0.5 g/l).

RENAL MASS

USS is helpful in distinguishing cystic and solid masses (Table

Table 10.4 Causes of proteinuria

Significant proteinuria = 0.1 g/m^2 per 24 hours but urinalysis sticks are very sensitive (1+ = 0.3 g/l, 4+ = 20 g/l)

Transient proteinuria	Affects 11% of school children 1. Fever 2. Exercise
Orthostatic proteinuria	Proteinuria is absent at night. Diagnosis is by sequential 12-hour collections. May be benign or reflect glomerular disease.
Persistent proteinuria	1. UTI 2. Nephrotic syndrome (> 1g/m^2 per 24 hours) 3. Glomerulonephritis

Table 10.5 Causes of a palpable renal mass

Intrarenal		
Solid	1.	Wilm's tumour
	2.	Renal vein thrombosis (usually haematuria)
	3.	Benign nephroma (rare neonatal problem)
	4.	Horseshoe kidney
	5.	Graft rejection
Cystic	1.	Hydronephrosis (due to reflux or anatomical or functional obstruction)
		May be accompanied by:
		a. no megaureter = PUJ obstruction
		b. megaureter = VUJ obstruction or VUR
		c. large bladder = bladder outlet obstruction
		d. prune belly syndrome
		A mass arising outside the urinary tract may also cause obstruction of the urinary tract
	2.	Single cyst (benign renal cyst)
	3.	Multicystic
		a. dysplastic kidney
		b. polycystic disease — infantile (autosomal recessive) onset — adult (autosomal dominant) onset
		(nephronophthisis, medullary sponge kidney and congenital nephrotic syndrome are other causes of multicystic kidney on USS but rarely present as abdominal mass)
Extrarenal		An adrenal mass (e.g. neuroblastoma) is difficult to distinguish clinically. A left 'renal' mass may be the spleen

10.5). Commonest causes of a child presenting because of a palpable mass are hydronephrosis and Wilms' tumour, and, in a neonate, hydronephrosis, multicystic dysplastic kidney or renal vein thrombosis.

ANTENATAL USS DIAGNOSIS

Urethral valves, PUJ obstruction, multicystic dysplastic kidney, infantile polycystic kidney. Obstructive uropathy or renal agenesis (Potter's syndrome) causes oligohydramnios and pulmonary hypoplasia.

Investigation of the genitourinary system

Urinalysis is quick, cheap and should be routine in all children, inpatient or outpatient, but tends to be neglected, whereas too many specimens are sent routinely for M, C & S (expensive test with high false-positive rate).

COLLECTION OF URINE SAMPLES

Always send the sample fresh to the lab.

1. 'Clean catch' midstream urine (MSU) specimen

Clean the perineum or prepuce and glans with sterile water. Provide the mother with a sterile container and explain that she should catch the middle portion of the stream, avoiding contamination of the top of the container with her fingers. Children > 2 years will often void on request, especially if encouraged to drink.

Superior to 'bag' urine; an alternative for general practice is to wet a dip-slide in the midstream.

2. 'Bag urine'

Clean the genitalia with sterile water and allow to dry. Attach a Hollister U-bag which allows urine to be withdrawn from the bag as soon as voided without having to remove the bag.

False-positive rate is high.

3. Suprapubic aspiration (SPA)

The 'gold standard' but very traumatic in children > 18 months. Attempt SPA if the bladder is defined by palpation, percussion or USS. If not, attach a U-bag, give a feed and wait 45 min before re-examining, unless the child is very ill and antibiotics cannot be delayed. Infants will often pass urine as the bladder is being palpated.

Scrub hands and use sterile technique as for LP. Assistant holds the infant firmly in the frog's legs position. Insert a 23G-needle and syringe vertically, immediately above the symphysis pubis, in midline, aspirating as you advance not more than 2.5 cm.

4. In-out catheterisation

Use only if a urine sample is essential and unobtainable by any other means. Use a fine NGT and sterile technique.

URINALYSIS

Colour

Normal urine is yellow — urobilinogen

Dark urine — normal but concentrated
— small amounts of blood cause smoky urine, larger amounts a frank red colour
— presence of clots suggests bleeding from lower tract (e.g. cystitis with platinum cytotoxics)
— free Hb or myoglobin cause dark red or black urine (e.g. malaria)
— conjugated hyperbilirubinaemia. Pale stools and dark urine of obstructive jaundice or hepatitis but *not* haemolytic jaundice

Coloured urine — drugs (e.g. rifampicin — orange; desferrioxamine — red or brown; methylene blue — green)

Cloudy urine — most commonly benign, due to PO_4^{3-} or urate crystals; bacteriuria or pyuria more significant

Concentration

Specific gravity — easily measured at the bedside

Osmolality — (laboratory determination) better index of renal concentrating ability

The relationship between these is *not* linear (Table 10.6) e.g. glycosuria increases SG by proportionately more than osmolality.

pH

Normal 4.6–8.0 depending on diet, but usually acidic (pH 5–6)

Alkaline urine (pH > 8.0) — urine infected with *Proteus* or *Pseudomonas*
— respiratory alkalosis
— metabolic alkalosis (including iatrogenic alkalinisation for salicylate overdose or tumour lysis syndrome) but not if hypokalaemic
— RTA (pH > 6 is abnormal in presence of metabolic acidosis)

Acidic urine (pH < 4.6) — starvation (ketonuria)
— urine infection
— respiratory acidosis
— metabolic acidosis (except RTA)
— hypokalaemic alkalosis

MICROSCOPY

Red cells

Normally < 3 RBC/mm^3 of uncentrifuged urine or < 2 RBC/high-power field of centrifuged urine (see Table 10.2).

White cells

Normally < 3 WBC mm^3 of unspun urine or < 5 WBC/high-power

Table 10.6 Measurement of urine concentration

Specific gravity	Osmolality (mosmol/kg)
1.002	100
1.005	150
1.010	300
1.020	600
1.030	1200

field of centrifuged urine. Infection can be present without WBCs and pyuria can occur without a positive bacterial culture (e.g. TB, appendicitis, calculi).

Epithelial cells
Normal

Organism
Bacteria or yeast — *always* abnormal but may be a contaminant.

Casts
Hyaline casts — normal but often increased in febrile illness, post-exercise, cardiac failure
Red cell casts — suggest glomerular disease
Granular casts — occur in acute and chronic renal failure
White cell casts — occur in glomerulonephritis and infection of upper tract
Epithelial casts — suggest tubular damage

Crystals
PO_4^{3-}, urate and oxalate crystals are common and usually of no pathological significance. However, crystalluria may also indicate *Proteus* infection, hyperuricaemia or cystinuria.

INVESTIGATION OF A SOLID RENAL MASS (see p. 151)

Most likely diagnoses are Wilms' tumour or neuroblastoma. In addition to abdominal USS:
1. Height and weight
2. FBC
3. U & E, creatinine, Ca^{2+}, PO_4^{3-}
4. LFT
5. Clotting studies
6. Screen for increased urinary catecholamines (found in 90% of neuroblastoma cases). 'Spot' sample for VMA : creatinine ratio: diagnostic if elevated but false negatives occur. 24-hour collection for VMA is more sensitive.
7. CXR

Further investigation may include bone scan, IVP, CT (if Wilms' tumour is suspected) and bone marrow biopsy (if neuroblastoma is diagnosed). Definitive histological diagnosis requires biopsy of mass.

DIAGNOSTIC IMAGING AND RENAL BIOPSY

The roles of these investigations are discussed as they relate to the conditions in the following sections.

Urinary tract infection (UTI)

BACKGROUND

The commonest nephrological problem in general paediatrics (3% of girls and 1% of boys during childhood).

Infection may cause symptoms (see below) or covert bacteriuria but we take a *proven culture-positive diagnosis of UTI* as:

a. any growth on culture of SPA

b. > 100 000 organisms/ml in pure growth from a *reliable* (see above) MSU or bag urine; ideally two consecutive growths of the same organism with identical sensitivities

Accurate diagnosis and treatment are important to:

a. alleviate symptoms

b. prevent renal scarring

c. detect underlying anomalies

d. avoid unnecessary investigation

DIAGNOSIS

Dysuria, abdominal pain, renal colic, frequency or retention, enuresis, offensive urine, vomiting, fever, loin tenderness or the non-specific acutely ill or chronically non-thriving child may all suggest UTI. The younger the child, the less specific the clinical features. Nevertheless, it is equally inappropriate to culture the urine of every child who vomits. Ask specifically about urine stream in boys.

Examination must include — BP
— abdominal masses
— genitalia and back for congenital anomalies
— growth centiles

ACUTE TREATMENT

Start antibiotics once urine is obtained. Treat empirically until sensitivities available and treat for minimum of 7 days.

If well — oral trimethoprim 4 mg/kg 12-hourly (avoid in neonate)
— or oral amoxycillin 15 mg/kg 8-hourly

If ill — i.v. ampicillin 25 mg/kg 6-hourly and i.v. gentamicin 2 mg/kg 8-hourly

Encourage oral or i.v. fluids and give analgesia. Check that urine culture is negative after 7 days' treatment.

INVESTIGATIONS

Every first proven UTI (see definition above) should be investigated, irrespective of the child's age or sex. Do not defer antibiotic treatment while awaiting investigations. Discharge on regular chemoprophylaxis (see below) until investigations are complete. Controversy persists over best combination (USS is especially operator-dependent) but one scheme is:

< 1 year — USS as inpatient
— MCUG after 6 weeks

If these suggest reflux, consider DMSA for degree of renal scarring.

If obstruction is suggested, consider DTPA to assess function of each kidney.

1–5 years — USS
— MCUG
— ±DMSA, DTPA as above
> 5 years — USS
— AXR

MCUG only if recurrent UTI and USS suggests reflux.

An IVU is not a routine part of this scheme (DTPA gives less radiation) but may be indicated in any age group to accurately define anatomy. The above investigations will show an anomaly in 30–50% (more commonly in boys), most commonly VUR.

PREVENTION

Conservative management:
Follow-up 3-monthly with urine culture and BP check.
1. Hygiene: clean perineum 'front to back'
2. No nylon underwear
3. Avoid constipation
4. Regular toileting and 'double micturition'
5. Chemoprophylaxis if (a) investigation shows abnormality
                       (b) no abnormality but frequent
                           recurrence (> 3/year)

   Oral trimethoprim 2 mg/kg at night
   or oral nitrofurantoin 2 mg/kg at night
   or oral nalidixic acid 20 mg/kg at night
Continue until infection-free for 2 years; some advocate continuing until repeat MCUG demonstrates that VUR has resolved.

PROGNOSIS

VUR accounts for 20% of adult dialysis. Worst scarring is already present by 1 year of age — hence need for prompt investigation protocol. 10% of children with renal scarring develop hypertension. VUR resolves spontaneously in 80% and chemoprophylaxis until resolution of VUR improves prognosis as much as surgical re-implantation.

Nephrotic syndrome

BACKGROUND

Rare (1/50 000) but 90% are due to minimal change nephropathy (rare < 1 year and > 8 years) which is steroid responsive and suggested by normal BP, normal creatinine, microscopic or no haematuria, highly selective proteinuria (IgG/transferrin clearances < 0.2), normal complement C3.

DIAGNOSIS

Triad of oedema (often ascites and pleural effusions), proteinuria (> 1 g/m² per 24 hours or > 0.05 g/kg per 24 hours) and hypoalbuminaemia (< 25 g/l). Also hyperlipidaemia.

INITIAL INVESTIGATION

1. Proteinuria > 1 g/m² per 24 hours
2. Serum albumin is often < 25 g/l
3. U&E, creatinine
4. Complement C3, ASOT, cholesterol

MANAGEMENT

Admit if it is the first episode or there are any complications.
A. Prepubertal, normal BP, no gross haematuria:
  1. Oral prednisolone 60 mg/m² per 24 hours (2 mg/kg per 24 hours), max. dose 80 mg per 24 hours in 3 divided doses
  2. Oral penicillin V 12.5 mg/kg 6-hourly prophylaxis against pneumococcal infection of ascites
  3. Do not restrict activity or fluids (see hypovolaemia below)
  4. High protein diet without added salt
  Urinalysis, weight, BP — daily; electrolytes — alternate days.
  If symptomatic effusions or weight increase is seen despite starting steroids, give:
  5. Oral spironolactone 1 mg/kg at night
  6. Salt-poor 20% human albumin 1 g/kg i.v. over 3 hours followed by frusemide 2 mg/kg i.v.
  Proteinuria is absent in most by 2 weeks (95% by 4 weeks). Stop diuretics and penicillin and discharge, reducing prednisolone by 10 mg/m² per 24 hours each week until the child is off steroids after 6 weeks. If proteinuria still persists by 4 weeks, refer for biopsy. In relapse (4+ proteinuria for 4 days), restart the steroid regimen at 60 mg/m² per 24 hours until the urine is protein-free for 4 days, then taper as above. More than two relapses in 6

months needs alternate day steroids at the lowest dose which maintains remission.
B. Pubertal or hypertension or raised creatinine or frank haematuria:
Renal biopsy before specific treatment of cause (e.g. idiopathic but not minimal change histology, SLE, hepatitis B, renal vein thrombosis, toxins).

COMPLICATIONS

1. Hypovolaemia — oliguria, abdominal pain, hypotension, tachycardia and uraemia suggest pre-renal failure exacerbating minimal change nephropathy. Give salt-poor 20% albumin 1 g/kg i.v. over 3 hours. If this results in normovolaemia but no diuresis, give frusemide 2 mg/kg i.v. Avoid using diuretics to induce a weight loss > 15 g/kg per 24 hours (negative fluid balance > 15 ml/kg per 24 hours) as hypovolaemia is likely.
2. Thrombosis — cerebral, renal vein. More likely if the child is hypovolaemic and haemoconcentrated. Measure PCV, treat as hypovolaemia and consider anticoagulation if symptoms persist.
3. Infection — abdominal paracentesis (right lower quadrant) and i.v. benzyl penicillin 50 mg/kg 6-hourly and gentamicin 2 mg/kg 8-hourly.

PROGNOSIS

For steroid-responsive disease — 30% have one attack, 30% have infrequent relapses, 20% still relapse after 10 years, < 5% death or renal failure.

Prognosis is worse for non-responders or those who require maintenance steroids, those with histology other than minimal change, older children or those with high BP.

Acute renal failure

BACKGROUND

ARF is sudden decrease in renal function resulting in retention of wastes and electrolyte imbalance. This definition is not based on urine output since uraemia occurs without oliguria in some drug nephropathies and polyuric ARF may follow relief of obstructive uropathy. However, a minimum urine flow of 300 ml/m² per 24 hours is required to excrete the normal obligate solute load of 500 mosmol/m² per 24 hours. GFR increases with postnatal age to an adult value of 125 ml/min/1.73 m² by 2 years.

See Table 10.7.

DIAGNOSIS

History and examination of the oliguric child may suggest:

1. Nephrotic syndrome and hypovolaemia (see p. 157).
2. Nephritic syndrome — triad of hypertension (may present as encephalopathy), haematuria ('smoky' urine), oedema (periorbital and ankles) suggests glomerulonephritis.
3. HUS — acute nephropathy, microangiopathic haemolysis ± thrombocytopenia and purpura. Prodrome of abdominal pain, vomiting or respiratory tract infection followed in 75% by bloody diarrhoea.

   ARF is rare (0.5/100 000/year) but epidemics occur July–December in preschool children with sporadic cases throughout year.
4. Specific features of the cause, e.g. tonsillitis, HSP, SLE.
5. Drugs.
6. Any ARF can present as hypertension or encephalopathy.

INVESTIGATIONS (Tables 10.8, 10.9 and 10.10)

1. urine — urinalysis, microscopy, culture, U & E, osmolality, hourly output and 24-hour urine collection for protein excretion and creatinine clearance (GFR)
2. throat swab

Table 10.7   Causes of acute renal failure

Pre-renal (renal hypoperfusion)
Dehydration commonest
Haemorrhage
Cardiac failure
Nephrotic syndrome

Renal (established parenchymal damage)	
HUS commonest	
Glomerulonephritis	Mostly due to immune complex deposition (post-streptococcal, post-viral, HSP, SLE, SBE, CSF shunt nephritis)
Acute tubular necrosis	Shock, hypoxia
Interstitial nephritis	Drugs (especially aminoglycosides and cytotoxics) and toxins (e.g. carbon tetrachloride)

Post-renal (obstructive nephropathy or uropathy)
Urethral valves
Calculi
Trauma
Crystal nephropathy (e.g. tumour lysis syndrome)
Haemoglobinuria or myoglobinuria

Any of the above may exacerbate pre-existing renal impairment, i.e. 'acute on chronic'.

3. blood — FBC & film, U & E, creatinine, albumin, HCO_3^- (arterial gases if ill), blood cultures, viral titres, ASOT, ANF, HBsAg
4. renal USS for kidney number, size and to exclude obstruction
5. ECG in hyperkalaemia
6. CXR in fluid overload

MANAGEMENT

In all cases — BP 6-hourly; weight, fluid balance, urinalysis and electrolytes daily

Pre-renal failure

1. Restore circulating volume (see Ch. 2 and 3) with 0.9% saline, or 4% human albumin 15 ml/kg i.v. over 30 min.
2. Then frusemide 1 mg/kg i.v.
3. If the child responds (> 10 ml/kg urine in next 2 hours), continue generous fluid replacement.

In severe cases; urinary catheter, CVP line and dopamine at 'renal' dose (5 μg/kg/min i.v. infusion)

Established renal failure

Conservative management:
1. Fluid restriction to (a) insensible water loss 3 ml/kg/6 hours
   + (b) previous 6 hours' urine output
   + (c) previous 6 hours' Na^+ output

   Frusemide 1 mg/kg i.v. may maintain urine output. *Never* give spironolactone
2. Low protein (1 g/kg per 24 hours), high calorie (400 kcal/m^2 per 24 hours to inhibit protein catabolism), low Na^+ and low K^+ diet
3. Oral penicillin 12.5 mg/kg 6-hourly
4. Hypertension (see Ch. 7, p. 95)
5. Hyperkalaemia > 6.5 mmol/l (see p. 26)
   — calcium gluconate 10% 0.5 ml/kg i.v. over 5 min
   — flush i.v. line

Table 10.8 Biochemistry in pre-renal and acute renal failure

	Pre-renal failure	ARF or partially obstructive renal failure
Urine Na^+ concentration (mmol/l)	< 30	> 30
Urine urea/plasma urea ratio	> 20	< 10
Urine osmolality/plasma osmolality ratio	> 1.15	1.10 approx.

In both pre-renal and acute renal failure there is oliguria (< 300 ml/m^2 per 24 hours or < 0.5 ml/kg/h). Total obstruction leads to anuria (apart from bladder sweat)

Table 10.9 Normal range (mean ±2SD) plasma creatinine

Age (years)	Plasma creatinine (μmol/l)
0	40–90 (reflects maternal creatinine)
0.5	20–50
1	15–40
4	20–45
8	25–60
12	25–70
>12	50–100

Table 10.10 Normal renal function

Age	GFR (ml/min/1.73 m^2)
0	25–60
0.5	40–100
1	50–160
2–12	90–170
>12	90–150

— NaHCO$_3$ 8.4% 2 ml/kg i.v. over 5 min

— calcium resonium 1 g/kg enema 8-hourly

Arrange urgent dialysis, and if these measures are ineffective, start:

— dextrose 25% 2 ml/kg/h i.v. and soluble insulin (e.g. Actapid) 0.1 u/kg/h i.v.

6. Acidosis — if base excess is > –10 mmol/l, give NaHCO$_3$ 8.4% 2 ml/kg and arrange dialysis

Indications for dialysis

1. HUS — refer as soon as the child is oliguric or urea raised as current trend is to dialyse early to reduce neurological complications and to allow transfusion.

For other causes of ARF —

2. Symptomatic uraemia (vomiting, encephalopathy, usually urea > 40 mmol/l) or rapidly rising urea and creatinine
3. Symptomatic fluid overload, especially cardiac failure or pericardial effusion
4. Uncontrollable hypertension
5. Symptomatic electrolyte problems or acidosis
6. Encephalopathy or seizures
7. Prolonged oliguria — conservative regimen controls ARF but causes nutritional failure

Post-renal failure

1. If the bladder is palpable, always catheterise.
2. Ideally, stabilise biochemistry (as for renal failure) before obstruction is relieved surgically.

3. Involve urological surgeon and identify cause/site of obstruction. Nephrostomy may buy time.

PROGNOSIS

Glomerulonephritis. Depends on cause and histology
1. Post-streptococcal — 90% full recovery by 10 years, 5% persistent proteinuria and haematuria.
2. HSP — only 1% develop CRF although 20% have nephropathy (proteinuria > 0.1 g/m^2 per 24 hours or haematuria > 10 red cells/mm^3) at presentation and may develop true nephritic or nephrotic picture. No child with normal urine at presentation suffers nephropathy during a relapse. 0.5% mortality (intussusception, cerebral involvement).

HUS. 75% complete recovery, 10% CRF, 10% neurological deficit, 5% die (usually intracranial haemorrhage).

Chronic renal failure

BACKGROUND

See Table 10.11 for causes. CRF is asymptomatic and urea and creatinine levels within normal range until GFR is 25% of normal (i.e. 20 ml/min/m^2). Thereafter, urea and creatinine levels double as GFR halves. A disproportionate increase in urea over creatinine implies pre-renal exacerbation. Once GFR < 15 ml/min/m^2, acidosis develops and thirst, polyuria and nocturia ensue as dilute urine is excreted. The commonest misconception is that a large urine flow rate is invariably a good sign in CRF. Urine flow rate is not the same as GFR and a large quantity of 'poor quality' urine (i.e. fixed osmolality of 300 mosmol/kg) may be passed despite a falling GFR and hence falling solute excretion.

DIAGNOSIS

Usually anticipated from preceding family history, congenital abnormality, UTI or ARF but may present insidiously as growth failure, anaemia, hypertension, vomiting or unexpected biochemical finding. Measure BP and plot growth on centile chart.

INVESTIGATION

1. Urinalysis and 24-hour urine collection for creatinine clearance.
2. FBC and ferritin; U & E, creatinine, Ca^{2+}, PO_4^{3-} and alkaline phosphatase; albumin.
3. X-ray left wrist for bone age and renal osteodystropy.
4. i.v. isotope (DTPA renogram) is more accurate than creatinine clearance.

Table 10.11 Causes of chronic renal failure

Congenital abnormalities (25%)
Obstructive uropathies (urethral valves, VUJ or PUJ obstruction)
Spina bifida
Dysplastic kidneys

Inherited disorders (8%)
Polycystic kidneys (can present at any age)
Nephronophthisis (check karyotype — phenotypic girl may be XY)
Alport's nephritis (and deafness)
Cystinosis (aminoaciduria, crystalluria ± calculi)

Acquired problems (67%)
Glomerulonephritis
HSP
Reflux nephropathy (recurrent pyelonephritis)
HUS

MANAGEMENT

Conservative treatment

1. Nutrition —
   a. Protein — essential for growth. Therefore, restrict protein only if urea > 20 mmol/l. Never restrict protein to < 5% calorie intake (1.25 g protein/100 kcal) and never to less than 1.5 g/kg per 24 hours if < 2 years or pubertal. Ensure sufficient essential aminoacids and ketoacids.
   b. Calories — minimum requirements per 24 hours are:
      110 kcal/kg for first 10 kg bodyweight
      + 80 kcal/kg for next 10 kg bodyweight
      + 20 kcal/kg thereafter
      Example. A 35 kg child needs 1100 + 800 + 300 = 2200 kcal per 24 hours (1 kcal = 4.2 kjoule)
      CRF causes anorexia and therefore high-calorie supplements or NG feeding may be necessary.
   c. Vitamin supplements, including folate.
2. Renal osteodystrophy — low GFR causes PO_4^{3-} retention, hypocalcaemia and secondary hyperparathyroidism with bone demineralisation.
   a. Dietary PO_4^{3-} maximum 600 mg per 24 hours (dairy products rich in PO_4^{3-})
   b. Calcium carbonate 20–50 mg/kg per 24 hours with meals binds PO_4^{3-} and maintains plasma Ca^{2+}
   c. 1,25-DHCC 20 mg/kg per 24 hours
   Monitor regularly as hypercalcaemia is a risk.
3. Salt and water balance —
   a. Na^+ restriction and diuretics only if clinical fluid overload or hypertension

b. CRF often accompanied by polyuria and renal Na⁺ wasting so Na⁺ supplements are necessary

c. avoid K⁺-containing foods (e.g. bananas, fruit juice)

4. Hypertension — see Ch. 7, p. 95.

5. Anaemia — oral iron only if ferritin is low; transfuse only if symptomatic but do not increase Hb > 9 g/dl. Erythropoeitin may soon be available.

6. Acidosis — oral $NaHCO_3$ up to 4 mmol/kg per 24 hours if plasma HCO_3^- < 15 mmol/l.

7. Do *not* use arm veins for vascular access.

Renal replacement therapy

Dialysis and transplantation are beyond the scope of this book.

Surgical problems

HYPOSPADIAS

Urethral meatus may be ventral glans, penile shaft or perineum. Foreskin appears hooded. Chordee (erect penis not straight) is common.

Circumcision is totally contraindicated; karytotype if meatus is proximal or the scrotum bifid; reconstruction at 1 year.

CRYPTORCHIDISM

Empty scrotum may be due to:

— retractile testis (often palpable at external inguinal ring and can be drawn down)

— undescended testis (1% of term births, more common in preterms; if testes do not spontaneously descend after 1 year, USS may detect a high undescended testis; orchidopexy ideally between 1 and 2 years to optimise fertility)

— ectopic (if ambiguous genitalia, a palpable gonad is almost always a testis)

— absent testis

Undescended and ectopic testes are at increased risk of torsion, trauma or tumour. Seek surgical opinion within 2 hours for every painful testis.

PHIMOSIS

Adherence of the foreskin to the glans is normal up to 5 years. However, ballooning of the foreskin during micturition *is* an indication for surgical separation of adhesions or circumcision, as is recurrent balanitis.

Drug prescribing in renal impairment

1. It may be necessary to reduce the dose or the frequency; since 5 times the drug half-life are required to achieve steady state concentrations, a loading dose (usually the same as for a child with normal renal function) may be indicated for immediate effect.

Table 10.12 Drugs requiring caution in renal disease

Infections	Aminoglycosides, cephalosporins, isoniazid, nalidixic acid, nitrofurantoin, penicillins, trimethoprim
	Amphotericin, flycytosine
	Acyclovir
	Isoniazid
Cardiovascular	Aldosterone antagonists, angiotensin converting enzyme inhibitors, beta-blockers, digoxin, diuretics
Cytotoxics/immunosuppressors	Cisplatin, methotrexate, mercaptopurine, thioguanine, bleomycin, cyclophosphamide, azathioprine, cyclosporin A
Others	Allopurinol, insulin (requirements may fall), non-steroidal anti-inflammatory drugs, including aspirin

2. Avoid nephrotoxic drugs.
3. Check GFR before prescribing known nephrotoxic drugs.
See Table 10.12 for drugs to avoid or adjust dosage in renal impairment.

Enuresis

BACKGROUND

Children are usually dry by day by 2 years and dry by night by 3 years.

Primary enuresis: bladder control is never acquired; secondary enuresis: bladder control is acquired and then lost.

Primary nocturnal enuresis is common and usually due to delayed maturation (10% of 5-year-olds and 5% of 10-year-olds, boys > girls, often family history or socially disadvantaged). Acquisition of control may be delayed by poor toilet training or emotional problems.

Other causes of enuresis include UTI, constipation, diabetes mellitus or diabetes insipidus, structural abnormality of urinary tract (e.g. ectopic ureter, ureterocele or urethral obstruction), neurological abnormality, mental handicap, sexual abuse.

Organic causes are more likely if enuresis is secondary or daytime.

DIAGNOSIS

By history. How was the child toilet trained? Day or night wetting and what time? Parental response? How often? Site and condition of toilet? Related to school term, birth of sibling or bereavement? Symptoms of polydipsia, daytime urgency, polyuria, dysuria, haematuria? Dribbling incontinence is always pathological.

Examination includes abdominal palpation, neurological examination of the lower limbs and observation of the spine, perineal sensation (saddle distribution of loss suggests sacral cord lesion), the external genitalia and urethral meatus, rectal examination and anal tone, BP, height and weight. An older child may be in nappies or plastic pants and show extensive napkin rash.

INVESTIGATION

Initially confined to urinalysis and microscopy and culture of urine.

Management

Must be age-appropriate and rarely indicated before 5–6 years. Success depends as much on the enthusiasm and confidence of the paediatrician, and the parent, as on the method used. Transient success is common, followed by recurrence of the problem.

Basic principles

1. Reassure that there is no abnormality and that the problem is common and treatable.
2. Explain to parents and child, with diagrams, basic anatomy and physiology and that the brain controls these functions even during sleep. Ensure that everyone shares the same vocabulary!
3. Ask the parents to keep a diary.
4. Reward appropriate behaviour and ignore, rather than punish, wetting.
5. Frequent follow-up initially.

Methods

Night lifting and fluid restriction are simple but not of proven efficacy.

1. 'Star' charts: need not just be stars. Select a motif that the particular child values, e.g. picture of a car, ball in pocket of billiard table, etc. Avoid inappropriate rewards such as sweets or money. May work from school age but depends on the intelligence of the child and motivation of the parent. Often fails with the 'streetwise' older child who attaches no value to a gold star.
2. Alarms: child at least 6–7 years old; 80% effective but may

take 3 months. Continue until totally dry for 6 weeks. 10% relapse but will respond to further trial.

3. Drugs: imipramine 25 mg initially is often effective but there is a high relapse rate and risk of side-effects and overdose. Intranasal desmopressin has similar problems. Best reserved for short-term relief during holidays and as a 'crutch' with other methods. Avoid < 6 years.

4. Admission: for interval training by nursing/hospital school staff. Effective in 50%, possibly because children with nocturnal enuresis also pass frequent, small volumes of urine by day.

Endocrine and metabolic problems

Diabetes

DIAGNOSIS

In children diagnosis is made on a raised blood glucose level
(> 11 mmol/l) in the presence of unequivocal symptoms. There is
little place for oral glucose tolerance test in diagnosis. Fasting
normoglycaemia does not exclude diabetes and a raised blood
glucose concentration in an ill child without symptoms is not
diagnostic of diabetes.

DIABETIC KETOACIDOSIS

Definition: clinical rather than biochemical; severe uncontrolled
diabetes with ketosis, requiring emergency treatment with i.v.
fluids and insulin.

**Always consult an experienced paediatric registrar or
consultant if you are unsure of management.**

Basic management plan

Fluid, insulin and K^+ requirements are detailed following this basic
plan:
  1. Admit to a ward equipped to handle diabetic ketoacidosis or
     to ICU.
  2. Weigh and compare with recent weight.
  3. Assess dehydration (often 10–15%); see fluid replacement
     below.
  4. Identify provoking factors, e.g. infection, although these are
     uncommon in childhood.
  5. Initial investigations;
     a. In all cases: blood glucose, HbA_1, Na^+, K^+, urea, creati-
        nine, HCO_3^-, osmolality, FBC; throat swab, urine for
        ketones and culture. Viral titres.
     b. Severe cases: also arterial blood gases, LFT, amylase,
        blood culture and ABO group; save serum.
     c. In newly diagnosed diabetics check islet cell antibodies.
  6. Commence reliable i.v. infusion with 0.9% saline or plasma.
  7. Avoid oral fluid for the first 8–12 hours and consider gastric
     suction (in coma, vomiting or signs of gastric dilatation).

8. Collect urine (but avoid catheterisation unless unconscious) and monitor volume, glycosuria and ketonuria.
9. Connect ECG; monitor lead 2 for K^+-related T wave changes.
10. Careful data collection on flow charts is essential. Ensure continuity from casualty to ward. Document:
    a. clinical status (include coma scale)
    b. biochemical status — measure plasma glucose half-hourly for the first 2 hours and then as below:
       plasma Na^+, K^+ and osmolality at 0, 2 and 6 hours to confirm appropriate increase in Na^+ and that K^+ is in the normal range
    c. fluid given
    d. insulin given

Fluid management in diabetic ketoacidosis

Calculate total volume requirement and plan to replace the deficit over the first 36–48 hours.

The volume required over this time is the deficit + normal maintenance fluids.

Deficit. This may be measured (1 kg weight loss = 1000 ml) or assessed (e.g. if a 20-kg child is estimated to be 10% dehydrated, then the fluid deficit is 2000 ml).

Maintenance fluids. These may be calculated from the standard weight-related formula (see Ch. 3, p. 18).

Procedure.
1. Re-expand the circulating volume urgently (0–1hour): give 0.9% saline or plasma 10–20 ml/kg. Use plasma in severe circulatory failure or when initial saline infusion fails to improve clinical status (difficult cases probably require the additional guidance of CVP measurement).
   Example. For the 20 kg child with 10% dehydration 200–400 ml is given in the first hour.
2. Early rehydration: 0.9% saline + KCl (20–50 mmol/l guided by serial K^+ levels and ECG). The rate is based on providing maintenance and replacing deficit evenly over 36–48 hours; the higher the osmolality the slower the correction. Continue 0.9% saline until either;
   a. blood glucose falls below 14 mmol/l (change to 0.18% saline/4% dextrose + KCl (as directed below) or
   b. plasma Na^+ exceeds 150 mmol/l but blood glucose is still above 14 mmol/l (change to 0.45% saline + KCl, see below).
3. Intermediate/late rehydration: continue 0.18% saline/4% dextrose + KCl until the patient is metabolically stable and able to recommence full oral fluid intake.
Example. For the 20 kg child with 10% dehydration the remain-

ing fluid requirement is 3500 ml–400 ml (given to correct shock) = 3100 ml. This is given over 36–48 hours as described above.

Potassium requirements

Early introduction to fluid regimen is essential. Titrate concentration according to existing guidelines. Check plasma regularly and adjust infusion appropriately:

Plasma K^+ < 2.5 mmol/l: carefully monitor administration of 1 mmol KCl/kg bodyweight by separate infusion over 1 hour.

Plasma K^+ 2.5–3.5 mmol/l: KCl infusion of 3 g/l.

Plasma K^+ 3.6–5.0 mmol/l: KCl infusion 2 g/l.

Plasma K^+ 5–6 mmol/l: KCl infusion 1 g/l.

Plasma K^+ > 6 mmol/l: stop KCl infusion and check plasma level in 2 hours.

Insulin infusion requirements

1. Commence syringe pump infusion of insulin solution (50 units of human soluble insulin per 50 ml 0.9% saline). Connect to the main infusion line and run at 0.05 u/kg/h for children < 10 years. For older children and those younger where the 0.05 u/kg is not decreasing blood glucose at approximately 5 mmol/h, use 0.1 u/kg/h.

2. An initial bolus of insulin should **not** be given.

3. Monitor blood glucose half-hourly for 2 hours and then 1-hourly until the patient is receiving 0.18% saline /4% dextrose and blood glucose is stable or predictable. Aim for a **gradual** blood glucose fall of around 5 mmol/l/h until it reaches 10–15 mmol/l. The frequency of blood glucose measurement may then be reduced to 2-hourly.

4. Convert infusion fluid to 0.18% saline/4% dextrose when blood glucose falls to 14 mmol/l or less, and reduce insulin to 0.05 u/kg/h if on a higher dose. If blood glucose rises above 14 mmol/l increase the infusion rate appropriately (max. 0.1 u/kg/h).

5. Continue insulin infusion until the child is ready to tolerate regular oral snacks and drinks. Then convert to 2 or 3 s.c. insulin injections per 24 hours, or back on to the child's normal insulin regimen. Delay stopping infusion while significant ketonuria persists (Ketostix ≥ 3+).

Plasma sodium

The observed plasma Na^+ levels are usually low at presentation. This depression is caused by an actual deficit due to vomiting and polyuria, and to lipaemia and hyperglycaemia (1 mmol fall in Na^+ for each 2 mmol glucose excess over 5 mmol/l), and transfer of free water from intracellular to extracellular space. A normal or elevated Na^+ at presentation is indicative of osmotic decompensation. Plasma Na^+ should rise during management to partially compensate for the fall in osmolality accompanying correction of hyperglycaemia (and azotaemia).

Bicarbonate

Rarely required unless ketoacidosis is profound (pH<7.1) and there is shock. **Use cautiously if at all**; max. dose:

8.4% NaHCO$_3$ = base deficit × weight in kg × 0.15.
Given via an infusion pump over 1 hour.

Formula for calculating daily subcutaneous insulin requirement

0.75–1.0 u/kg per 24 hours. Divided: 0.5 u/kg per 24 hours as isophane insulin (Protophane); 0.25–0.5 u/kg per 24 hours as soluble insulin (Actrapid).

Example. A 20 kg child. Total dose = 15–20 units insulin.
Trial regimen:

a.m. soluble 4 u and isophane 6 u. Optional extra noon dose of soluble insulin 2–4 units if blood glucose > 12 mmol/l and or ketonuria.

p.m. soluble 4 u and isophane 4 u. Continue to review and be prepared to adjust dosage several times over first few days.

VOMITING IN A DIABETIC CHILD

1. Normal blood glucose and no ketonuria: maintain insulin dose and substitute easily tolerated sugar-containing fluids or foods for usual meals. Check blood glucose 2–4 hourly. Give small supplements (i.e. 2 units) of soluble insulin for hyperglycaemia if needed.
2. Low blood glucose: reduce insulin to half to two-thirds usual dose. Give fluids as above; check 1-hourly until blood glucose rises. Extra short acting insulin may be given during the day if blood glucose values rise.
3. Hyperglycaemia with ketonuria: increase insulin dose by 10%. Give fluids as in 1.
4. Hyperglycaemia + ketonuria: increase insulin dose by 10%. Give supplements of fast acting insulin (2–4 units) if required. Check blood glucose 2–4-hourly and repeat supplement until normoglycaemia and clearing of ketonuria are seen.

NB. If in doubt, the patient needs to be seen and assessed to ensure diabetic ketoacidosis does not occur.

INTERCURRENT ILLNESS IN A DIABETIC CHILD

Intercurrent illness may cause relative insulin resistance leading to hyperglycaemia and possible ketonuria.

Alternatively, diminished food intake may lead to hypoglycaemia. Thus management decisions are based on blood glucose and urinary ketones.

Management

1. Maintain insulin.
2. Give appropriate treatment for the intercurrent illness.
3. Maintain carbohydrate intake as sugar-containing fluids or food. They can be spaced at frequent intervals during the day.
4. Increase insulin in hyperglycaemia; this depends on the level of hyperglycaemia but is often an additional 10% of the normal dose. To prevent hypoglycaemia, decrease the dose to normal as the illness clears.
5. If there is hyperglycaemia and ketonuria, in addition to increasing the baseline intermediate acting insulin an increase in short acting insulin or additional doses are required until ketones are no longer present and the child is normoglycaemic, i.e. > 10 years: 2–4 units soluble insulin; < 10 years: 2 units soluble insulin.

SURGERY

These are suggested guidelines but, as children vary, the approach should be flexible.

Minor elective surgery

1. Admit 1 day prior to surgery and give usual evening insulin.
2. Monitor blood sugar using BM 20/800 strips or Reflomat before main meals and 1 hour after.
3. On the morning of surgery give 50% of the normal dose of both fast acting and intermediate acting insulin.
4. Omit breakfast.
5. Commence 10% dextrose infusion at 08.00 hours giving maintenance fluids.
6. Operate first on the morning list.
7. Give lunch or tea postoperatively and remove the drip after 2–3 hours if well.
8. Give normal evening insulin (increase short acting insulin if glucose > 13 mmol/l).

Major elective surgery

1. Admit 1–2 days prior to surgery or earlier if unstable.
2. Inform the diabetic team and anaesthetist.
3. Adjust insulin to achieve reasonable control with glucose < 13 mmol/l.
4. Monitor blood glucose before meals, 1 hour after and at 10 p.m.
5. On the day of surgery:
   a. no food or s.c. insulin
   b. insert an i.v. line at 08.00 hours, using 10% dextrose (500 ml) with 1 g (13 mmol) KCl added to give maintenance fluids (Table 11.1).
   c. insulin; use human Actrapid, or Velosulin depending on

Table 11.1 Dosage of dextrose and insulin prior to surgery

Bodyweight (kg)	10% dextrose (plus KCl) (infusion rate ml/h)	Actrapid dose (u/h)
10	50	0.5
20	60	1.0
30	70	1.5
40	80	2.0
50	90	2.5
>60	100	3.0

which is usually given. Give via a 50-ml syringe pump. Mix 50 units of insulin in 49 ml normal saline (1 u/ml), so that a flow rate of 1 ml/h delivers 1 u/h insulin.

6. Monitor blood glucose levels 1-hourly (including intra-operatively) whilst the infusion is running so that the rate can be adjusted. Use Reflomat or BM 20/800 strips (lab. results are too slow).

   Adjust as follows:

   a. If glucose < 5 mmol/l: reduce the infusion rate by 50% and check that 10% dextrose infusion is flowing. Re-check 30 min later.

   b. If glucose is > 15 mmol/l: increase the insulin infusion rate by 25% and check 1 hour later.

7. Continue the i.v. regimen postoperatively until oral feeding is recommended. Then, restart the previous insulin regimen.

Emergency surgery

A child admitted for emergency surgery may have a high blood glucose or be in frank ketoacidosis. Surgery should be delayed if possible, as the mortality rate in surgery performed during ketoacidosis is high. Furthermore, diabetic ketoacidosis may mimic an acute abdominal condition. Discussion is needed between the paediatrician, surgeon and anaesthetist.

NB. Infections (especially abscess), steroids, aminophylline, beta blockers and dopamine cause temporary insulin resistance and will increase insulin requirements.

Treatment is as above except:

1. Check urine for glucose and ketones preoperatively.
2. Monitor blood glucose more frequently.
3. Monitor U & E.
4. Give 10% dextrose 0.18% saline (500 ml) with 1 g KCl. Extra fluid may be required for increased insensible losses due to pyrexia.
5. Additional saline may be required if the child is hyponatraemic.
6. Avoid Hartmann's solution which contains lactate.

HYPOGLYCAEMIA IN A DIABETIC CHILD

1. Occasional hypoglycaemic episodes are virtually inevitable. Minimise these while maintaining best possible control of glucose. Family members must be taught to recognise early symptoms and to treat appropriately.
2. Most common causes are bursts of activity without a preceding snack, delayed food or insulin dosage errors.
3. Most episodes can be treated with 10–20 g glucose (as glucose tablets, granulated table sugar, orange or apple juice).
4. If the child is unable to swallow, retain carbohydrate, or unconscious, give Glucagon 0.03 mg/kg, max. dose 1 mg i.m. or s.c. This should raise the blood glucose level within 5–15 min but may be followed by nausea and vomiting. Give oral carbohydrate to prevent further hypoglycaemia.
5. If the child cannot take or retain sugar orally, i.v. glucose at 10 mg/kg/min with frequent blood glucose monitoring is essential.

HYPOGLYCAEMIA BEYOND THE NEONATAL PERIOD (blood glucose < 2.5 mmol/l)

Clinical manifestations

Trembling, nervousness, sweating, pallor, tachycardia, hunger, nausea, vomiting, drowsiness, headache, weakness, inability to concentrate, bizarre behaviour, confusion, coma and seizures.

Emergency management

Hypoglycaemia is an important preventable cause of permanent brain damage, mental retardation and seizures. Therefore the diagnostic evaluation should be performed early and hypoglycaemia treated aggressively.

1. Take blood (the *essential diagnostic sample*) at the time of hypoglycaemia for: glucose, lactate, FFA, β-hydroxybutyrate, alanine, insulin, glucagon, cortisol, GH, NH_3, U&E. (6 ml into lithium–heparin bottle, 5 ml in clotted bottle, 1 ml into fluoride oxalate bottle).
2. Test urine for: ketones, non-glucose reducing substances, organic acids, aminoacids, toxins.
3. A metabolic acidosis on blood gas analysis with high blood NH_4^+ may suggest a metabolic cause.

Acute treatment

a. Symptomatic hypoglycaemia may be treated by an initial bolus of 0.25–0.5 g/kg 25% dextrose.

> **Example.** For a 10-kg child:
> 0.25 g/kg = 10 ml 25% dextrose; 0.5 g/kg = 20 ml 25% dextrose
> For a 30-kg child:

0.25 g/kg = 30 ml 25% dextrose; 0.5 g/kg = 60 ml 25% dextrose.

b. Glucose is then given i.v. at approximately 3–5 mg/kg/min in infants and children and at 5–8 mg/kg/min in newborns.

If the child is asymptomatic omit the initial loading dose.

Example. Acute symptomatic hypoglycaemia in a 10-kg infant:

give 10 ml 25% dextrose as a bolus i.v.

give glucose i.v. at 150% of the usual hepatic glucose production rate (normal rate = 3–5 mg/kg/min; therefore, 150% = 7.5 mg/kg/min)

7.5 mg/kg/min = 108 g per 24 hours. 10% dextrose contains 100 g dextrose in 1 litre.

Therefore, 1080 ml 10% dextrose = 108 g dextrose.

$$\frac{1080}{24} = 45 \text{ ml/h}$$

If 20% dextrose is used the infusion rate = 22.5 ml/h.

If 5% dextrose is used the infusion rate = 90 ml/h.

For hyperinsulinism, 2.5 mg/kg 6-hourly diazoxide should be considered. Discuss with the consultant.

Assessment of hypoglycaemia

Detailed history and examination. In most cases an adequate 'essential diagnostic sample' at the time of hypoglycaemia provides the diagnosis. If hypoglycaemia is suspected or established but no blood collected at this time, admit for:

1. **Formal fasting study.** Aim to establish the degree and frequency of hypoglycaemia by a 24-hour profile under normal conditions in hospital under close supervision.

   a. Draw blood for glucose: fasting (pre-breakfast); 1 hour post-breakfast; pre-lunch; 1 hour post-lunch; pre-dinner.

   b. If hypoglycaemia is detected take the 'essential diagnostic sample' (p. 174) immediately. Send urine for metabolic screen.

   c. Test urine for ketones before breakfast; ketonuria excludes hyperinsulinaemia.

2. **Prolonged 18-hour fast in hospital (day 2).** This stage is most likely to be reached if the suspected diagnosis is ketotic hypoglycaemia. Strict observation in hospital is essential.

   a. Time of starting and length of fast depends on the child's clinical condition (infants < 2 years fast for 6–8 hours; 2–10 years fast for 8–16 hours; > 10 years fast for 16–20 hours). Longer fasts should be commenced at 10 p.m. so hypoglycaemia is more likely to occur during the day.

   b. Insert an i.v. line with a three-way tap.

   c. Check weight.

   d. Collect baseline blood and urine samples for glucose and ketones.

   e. Blood should be drawn for glucose 2–4 hourly or earlier if symptoms occur. Check urine for ketones. Check weight after 6–12 hours' fasting.

f. If hypoglycaemia develops take 'essential diagnostic sample'.

g. At the end of the fast or if hypoglycaemia occurs, glucagon 0.1 mg/kg i.m. (max. 1 mg) should be given and 4 ml blood drawn for glucose and lactate, and the remaining serum used for a possible GH and cortisol level after 5, 15, 30 and 60 min.

3. **Further specific tests.** These are determined by the above findings, e.g. liver biopsy, lactate infusion. Measure C peptide if surreptitious exogenous insulin administration is possible (e.g. Munchausen's syndrome by proxy).

Interpretation (Table 11.2). The prolonged fast is a useful screening procedure. Most children remain normoglycaemic after an appropriate fast. If fasting is too long even normal children become hypoglycaemic. Following the glucagon stimulation test an exaggerated insulin response suggests hyperinsulinism. Absent glycaemic response occurs with disorders of hepatic glycogen metabolism.

Table 11.2 Evaluation of hypoglycaemia

Test	Ketotic hypoglycaemia	Excess insulin	Hormone deficiency*	Enzyme deficiency†
Glucose	Low	Low	Low	Low
Insulin	Normal	++ – ++++	Normal	Normal
GH	Normal	Normal	Low/normal*	Normal
Cortisol	Normal	Normal	Low/normal*	Normal
T₄/TSH	Normal	Normal	Low/normal*	Normal
Lactate	Normal	Normal	Normal	++++
FFA	++++	Low	++ – +++	++++
Ketones‡	++++	Low	++ – +++	++ – ++++
Alanine	Decreased	Normal	Normal	++++

* Deficiency of GH or ACTH may be isolated or associated with deficiency of other pituitary hormones.
† Deficiency of key gluconeogenic enzymes such as glucose 6-phosphatase or fructose 1,6-diphosphatase.
‡ β-hydroxybutyrate and acetoacetate.
Normal = blood level appropriate in relation to the level of blood glucose and duration of fast; ++= mildly elevated; +++ = moderately elevated; ++++ = markedly elevated.

Hypothyroidism

NEONATAL

Laboratory screening (Guthrie test) may suggest hypothyroidism.

Investigations

1. Take a random non-fasting blood sample for TSH, free T_3 and T_4.

2. Knee X-ray for bone age assessment.
3. Perform a ^{123}I-sodium iodide scan (for detection of thyroid tissue).
4. Maternal thyroid function tests.
5. If TSH is low, consider TRH stimulation test.

Treatment

Start replacement therapy with L-thyroxine 10 µg/kg per 24 hours. Adjust on the basis of repeat thyroid function tests. Discuss management with the endocrinology team.

THE OLDER CHILD

Absence of a goitre suggests TSH deficiency or an atopic thyroid gland.

Investigations
1. TSH, free T_3 and T_4.
2. Left wrist X-ray for bone age.
3. Thyroid autoantibodies.
4. Discuss ^{123}I uptake test ± a perchlorate discharge test with the endocrinologist.

Treatment

Treatment is with L-thyroxine. Therapy may be monitored by measuring TSH. The dose should be gradually increased until adequate (initial dose is 2.5 µg/kg per 24 hours).

Hyperthyroidism

NEONATAL

Secondary to maternal hyperthyroidism. Clinical signs include tachycardia, exophthalmus, hyperactivity, wakefulness, irritability, weight loss, goitre.

Treatment
Observe in hospital. If necessary consider:
1. Propranolol 0.7 mg/kg 8-hourly.
2. KI, Lugol's solution 0.2 ml per 24 hours.
3. Carbimazole.
4. Increased nutrition is often needed.
Most patients undergo spontaneous resolution within 6 months, the majority within 2 months.

THE OLDER CHILD

Aetiology

Graves' disease, thyroid adenoma, thyroiditis and, much less commonly, a thyroid carcinoma or TSH-producing tumour may cause raised T_3 and T_4. T_3 thyrotoxicosis is rare.

Investigations

1. Blood for TSH, T_3, free T_3 and T_4.
2. Thyroid auto antibodies.
3. Blood count, ESR.
4. Thyroid scan if nodules are present.

Treatment

1. Severe hyperthyroidism with cardiac decompensation and decreased conscious state (thyroid storm) may occur and is a medical emergency.
   a. Inhibit thyroxine synthesis and release with propylthiouracil 200–400 mg 6-hourly.
   b. KI may be given orally.
   c. Give dexamethasone 1–2 mg 6-hourly to decrease T_3.
   d. If extremely unwell give propranalol i.v. (slow infusion of 0.1 mg/kg).
   e. General support, i.e. rehydration, cooling.
2. Consult a larger text for treatment of hyperthyroidism.

Ambiguous genitalia

Early involvement of the consultant in charge is essential. It is important not to guess the child's sex.

HISTORY

Careful family history is required. Check for history of any maternal drug exposure during pregnancy.

EXAMINATION

The following are particularly useful to the diagnosis:
1. If the testes are present the child is a male pseudohermaphrodite.
2. If the child is hypertensive, this suggests an adrenal problem.
3. Could the external genitalia be fashioned into a functional penis. If not, the child will be reared as a girl.
4. Rectal and USS examination to detect the presence of a uterus. If present then the child is a female pseudohermaphrodite.

INVESTIGATIONS

1. Send a blood sample for urgent chromosomal examination. Buccal smears should also be sent but may be unreliable in the first week of life.
2. Send samples urgently to detect congenital adrenal hyperplasia (see below).

MANAGEMENT

1. If congenital adrenal hyperplasia is confirmed, or if there are symptoms such as mild vomiting and weight loss, give hydrocortisone 20–25 mg/m^2 per 24 hours (approximately 2.5 mg 12-hourly in a term baby). Also give fludrocortisone 0.05–0.1 mg per 24 hours. Salt supplements may be necessary in the initial period (up to 2–4 g per 24 hours). (If the child is unwell treat urgently as below for congenital adrenal hyperplasia.)
2. If congenital adrenal hyperplasia is not confirmed, further tests are indicated to detect underlying conditions; consult a larger text.

Congenital adrenal hyperplasia

Suspect diagnosis in the following situations:
1. Ambiguous genitalia in a newborn.
2. Infant presenting with vomiting and/or collapse, hyponatraemia (Na$^+$ < 130 mmol/l), hyperkalaemia (K$^+$ > 6.5 mmol/l) and often hypoglycaemia.
3. Previous family history or unexplained neonatal death.
4. In the older child, hypertension, virilisation of a girl, and a boy with precocious puberty but small testes.

INVESTIGATIONS

1. Serum for 17-hydroxyprogesterone and 11-deoxycortisol (raised in congenital adrenal hyperplasia).
2. Serum ACTH.
3. Daily plasma and urinary electrolytes to check for salt loss.
4. Daily BP.
5. Plasma renin and angiotensin levels.

MANAGEMENT

1. Correction of salt deficit: **life-threatening circulatory collapse may occur**. Treatment is urgent.

   Plasma volume replacement is given as 10–20 ml/kg of 5% dextrose in normal saline (0.9%) given over 30 min. This may then be replaced with 0.18% or 0.45% saline according to electrolyte status.

2. Fludrocortisone 0.05–0.15 mg p.o. is introduced as soon as the infant tolerates oral preparations.

3. Give 25–50 mg hydrocortisone sta. This dose may be lowered.

Designation of the appropriate sexual identity of the child and longterm supervision should be discussed with the consultant.

Adrenocortical hypofunction

AETIOLOGY

Includes Addison's disease, congenital adrenal hyperplasia, fulminating infections, iatrogenic secondary to prolonged steroid, therapy, unresponsiveness to ACTH.

PRESENTATION

Either as adrenal crisis (vomiting, dehydration, hypotension and hypoglycaemia leading to coma) or insidious (weakness, weight loss and increased pigmentation, areas of vitiligo, anorexia, hypotension, hypoglycaemia).

GI symptoms may be prominent and may be misinterpreted as acute gastroenteritis.

INVESTIGATIONS AND DIAGNOSIS

1. Decreased serum Na^+. Increased serum K^+, hypochloraemic acidosis, hypoglycaemia, increased urinary Na^+ and decreased urinary K^+ may be found. Hypercalcaemia may be present.

2. Check plasma cortisol at 09.00 and 23.00 hours. Low levels point to a lesion in the hypothalamic–pituitary–adrenal axis. Check plasma ACTH at 09.00 hours; levels are usually above 200 pg/ml in primary adrenal failure.

3. ACTH stimulation test:

Short Synacthen test

a. Fasting is not required.

b. Collect blood for plasma cortisol at t = 0 min.

c. Give Synacthen (tetracosactrin) 250 µg i.v. or i.m. (dose for infants = 36 µg/kg).

d. Collect blood at t = 30 and 60 min.

Interpretation. A normal response is a 2–3 fold increase. If the response is subnormal, adrenal insufficiency is present. This is primary if ACTH levels are increased. Response may also be subnormal in secondary adrenal insufficiency.

Prolonged Synacthen test

Indicated if the cortisol response to short ACTH stimulation is inadequate and secondary adrenal insufficiency is suspected.

a. Fasting is not required.
b. Collect plasma cortisol at t = 0 min.
c. Give Synacthen Depot (tetracosactrin) 1 mg per 24 hours i.m. for 3 days.
d. Collect blood for plasma cortisol 4–6 hours after the last Synacthen injection.

Interpretation. An absent response is definitive evidence of primary adrenal insufficiency. There is a response in secondary adrenal insufficiency.

4. AXR for adrenal calcification.
5. Check autoimmune antibodies.

TREATMENT

A. Life threatening circulatory collapse (addisonian crisis)

1. Treat shock with i.v. plasma or normal saline (20 ml/kg).
2. Treat hypoglycaemia (see p. 174).
3. Give hydrocortisone sodium succinate 50 mg stat. i.v. followed by 5 mg/kg per 24 hours given in 6 divided doses.

B. Maintenance

Hydrocortisone replacement (20 mg/m^2 per 24 hours in 2–3 divided doses) and fludrocortisone (0.05–0.15 mg per 24 hours) are required. During periods of stress hydrocortisone dosage should be doubled or trebled. A Medic Alert bracelet must be worn.

Cushing's syndrome

AETIOLOGY

Includes prolonged steroid treatment, adrenal tumour or hyperplasia, and an ACTH-producing pituitary tumour.

CLINICAL FEATURES

Include reduced height and growth, facial and truncal obesity, limb muscle wasting, skin striae, bruising, hypertension, mood changes, and buffalo hump.

In girls, virilism with hirsutism, acne and cliteromegaly; in boys, false precocious puberty (small testes).

INVESTIGATIONS

1. Measure electrolytes.

2. Measure plasma cortisol at 09.00 (normal range 200–700 mmol/l) and 23.00 hours (normal range < 275 nmol/l). A normal rhythm will exclude Cushing's syndrome.
3. Plasma testosterone and androstenedione will be elevated in virilising tumours.
4. Plasma ACTH is always low in adrenal tumours.
5. Elevated 17-oxogenic steroids and free cortisol on a 24-hour urine sample reflect abnormal steroid secretion.
6. Elevated oxogenic steroids and other specific metabolites (pregnanetriol and dehydroepiandrosterone) are suggestive of an adrenal tumour.
7. Dexamethasone suppression tests:

Low dose:

a. Collect 24-hour urine for 17-OHCS and urinary free cortisol:
b. Collect blood samples at 08.00 and 24.00 hours for plasma cortisol (day 1).
c. Give dexamethasone 5 µg/kg 6-hourly for 2 days (days 2 and 3).
d. Collect 24-hour urine for 17-OHCS and free urinary cortisol.
e. Collect blood at 08.00 and 24.00 hours for plasma cortisol (day 4).

Interpretation. Failure to suppress confirms Cushing's syndrome but does not necessarily provide information about the cause.

High dose:

The protocol is the same as outlined above except 2 mg dexamethasone is given orally every 6 hours for 2 days. This will result in suppression of plasma and urinary cortisol in patients with pituitary-dependent Cushing's syndrome but not in those with adrenal adenoma or carcinoma.

8. The high incidence of an adrenal tumour in children justifies imaging studies of the hypothalamo-pituitary region and adrenal glands before completion of endocrine studies, i.e. plain AXR, USS and CT scan.

TREATMENT

Depends on the cause and is beyond the scope of this text.

Metabolic disease

May present at any age. Clinical suspicion must be high so that appropriate investigations and treatment can be initiated immediately.

The possibility should always be considered in an acutely ill child, especially if there are unexplained neonatal deaths or illnesses in siblings.

Consanguinity should increase the index of suspicion.

PRESENTATION

Neonatal

Most babies are normal at birth. Symptoms usually start in the first week and are non-specific, e.g. lethargy, fits, coma, tachypnoea, hepatomegaly, poor feeding, acidosis, hypoglycaemia, hyperammonaemia and sepsis.

Childhood

Suspect in a child with the following signs: recurrent unexplained episodes of illness and lethargy, vomiting, FTT, developmental delay, mental retardation, hepatomegaly or splenomegaly, acidosis, hypoglycaemia and hyperammonaemia.

INVESTIGATIONS

Laboratory facilities and requirements for collection and handling of samples varies from centre to centre. Thus it is essential to discuss investigations with the consultant in charge.

Suggested initial investigations:

1. Screen for sepsis if the child is unwell, i.e. blood and urine cultures, CXR, LP.
2. Urine: check smell and for presence of acetone, reducing substances, ketoacids, dinitrophenylhydrasone, sulphites. Check pH. Send for amino- and organic acid analysis.
3. Serum: FBC, electrolytes (check anion gap), Ca^{2+}, glucose, albumin, blood gases, NH_3, lactic acid, pyruvic acid, 3OH-butyrate, acetoacetate, uric acid, aminoacids.
4. Store at $-20°C$:
   a. urine (as much as possible)
   b. plasma heparinised 5 ml (not whole blood)
   c. CSF 0.5–1.0 ml.
5. Other investigations that may be indicated include EEG, cerebral and cardiac USS.
6. If the child is deteriorating rapidly or dies, a skin biopsy taken under strict aseptic conditions should be placed in transport medium. Post-mortem tissue samples are only suitable if taken within 2 hours of death. Two needle biopsies of tissue suspected as being abnormal (e.g. liver, skeletal muscle) should be taken post mortem, wrapped in aluminium foil and snap frozen in liquid nitrogen. Store deep frozen.

TREATMENT

Treatment should be discussed with a consultant experienced in the care of metabolic illness; if the child is unwell this advice should be sought as a matter of urgency. Sudden metabolic decompensation can be life threatening. While obtaining advice the following initial steps should be undertaken:

1. Stop oral feeds while the child is acutely ill and until a specific diagnosis can be made.
2. Collect samples for investigations above.
3. Sepsis may trigger the metabolic decompensation. If sepsis is possible investigate as above and treat appropriately.
4. Continuous monitoring of conscious state, regular measurement of glucose, electrolytes, NH_3, blood pH and fluid balance.
5. Parenteral glucose infusion should be given to provide energy support and to prevent catabolism. Concentrated glucose solutions may have to be given via a central line (80–100 kcal/kg per 24 hours).
6. Treatment of acidosis: if blood pH is < 7.2 correction with HCO_3^- may be required (see p. 30). Patients with severe acidosis may require up to 1 mmol/kg/h HCO_3^-.
7. If acidosis is refractory to treatment or hyperammonaemia is extreme, peritoneal or haemodialysis should be instituted.
8. Abnormal coagulation is seen in cases of metabolic liver disease. Treatment with FFP may be indicated.
9. Raised ICP should be managed as described on p. 195.
10. Further specific treatment of the acute episode, e.g. administration of pharmacological doses of vitamins to cover the possible vitamin-responsive disorders (e.g. biotin 5–10 mg per 24 hours i.v. and hydroxycobalamin 1 mg per 24 hours i.m.) or carnitine infusion, should be discussed with the consultant in charge.

FURTHER MANAGEMENT

This depends on the specific defect. Discuss with the consultant in charge.

12

Neurology

Seizures

An accurate eye-witness history is 95% of the diagnosis.

FEBRILE CONVULSIONS

A convulsion when febrile and no other cause is found, and there is no past history of convulsions when afebrile.

Background
— 3% of children affected; 30% will have more than one
— unusual < 6 months and > 5 years

Diagnosis
Most commonly associated with viral URTI. Meningitis and UTI are the two commonest serious infections causing febrile convulsions.

Investigation
Perform LP and collect urine (see Ch. 10) in:
1. all children in whom no source for the fever is found on examination
2. all infants < 12 months even if there are signs of URTI

Treatment

A. Emergency treatment of a convulsion
1. O_2 by mask
2. 5mg diazepam stezolid p.r.
3. Insert i.v. catheter — if still fitting, 0.25 mg/kg diazepam (Diazemuls) i.v. dilute 10 mg in 10 ml saline and give dose over 3 min until effective — apnoea a risk.

B. Further treatment. Treat meningitis (see below) and UTI (see Ch. 10), otitis media or tonsillitis (see Ch. 16) as appropriate

C. Antipyretic measures
1. 10 mg/kg paracetamol *every* 4 hours or 5 mg/kg ibuprofen *every* 6 hours irrespective of temperature

2. undress, tepid sponge, fan in the room but *not on* the child

Follow-up

1. No follow-up or EEG unless frequent febrile convulsions
2. Only valproate and phenobarbitone demonstrated to decrease recurrence

Table 12.1 Differential diagnosis of 'funny turns'

Convulsions	
Non-epileptic	*Epileptic*
Febrile	Major motor seizure
Hypoglycaemia	— may be precipitated by TV or
Hypocalcaemia	flashing lights
Hysterical pseudoseizures	— may be tonic, clonic or tonic-
Hypoxia (including	clonic
Munchausen's by proxy)	— may be tongue-biting and urinary
	incontinence
Jerks or spasms	
Non-epileptic	*Epileptic*
Infantile colic	Infantile spasms
Tics	Simple partial seizure
Dystonia (especially in children	Myoclonic seizures
with cerebral palsy)	
Oculogyric crises	
(metoclopramide induced)	
Sudden loss of consciousness	
Non-epileptic	*Epileptic*
Breath holding	Tonic seizures
Reflex anoxic seizure	Myoclonic seizures
Cardiac syncope (arrhythmia	(thrown to the ground or
or outflow obstruction)	akinetic 'drop attack')
Faint (vasovagal attacks)	
Basilar migraine (headache	
not a feature of epileptic	
seizure)	
Trances	
Non-epileptic	*Epileptic*
Hypoglycaemia	Minor motor seizures
Masturbation	Minor status
Poor concentration	Complex partial seizures
Glue sniffing or drugs	
Vertigo	
Non-epileptic	*Epileptic*
Labrynthitis	Complex partial seizures
Benign paroxysmal vertigo of	
infancy	
Basilar migraine	
Odd behaviour	
Non-epileptic	*Epileptic*
Tantrums and pseudoseizures	Complex partial seizures
Nightmares and sleepwalking	
Hypoglycaemia	
Drugs	

rate — consider after > 5 febrile convulsions and continue for 2 years. The subsequent risk of epilepsy is unaltered.

3. Risk factors for recurrence and epilepsy (3%)
   a. onset < 15 months
   b. prolonged (> 30 mins)
   c. focal
   d. developmental or neurological abnormalities
   e. sib or parent with epilepsy

Advise parents

1. antipyretic measures (as above)
2. supply of rectal diazepam
3. call GP/take to hospital if it lasts > 15 min
4. no immunisation is absolutely contraindicated. Prescribe 10 days' 4-hourly paracetamol following MMR immunisation.

AFEBRILE SEIZURES

Background

— $\frac{1}{3}$ of children with an afebrile seizure never have another one
— 10% will progress to chronic epilepsy

Diagnosis

From the history. The differential is shown in Table 12.1

1. 'Blue episodes': common in babies < 1 year. May be associated with feeds of choking. Cause is rarely identified.
2. Breath-holding: toddlers. Always preceded by anger/emotion and often a cry; cyanosis follows and a major motor seizure may result from hypoxia.
3. Reflex-anoxic seizures: precipitated by pain (often a fall or bump to the head); pallor follows, then pulselessness and loss of consciousness.
4. Stokes–Adams attack: no warning. Abrupt loss of consciousness with pallor. Heartbeat may be present throughout (but inadequate output) and peripheral pulse may be absent briefly. A true major motor seizure may follow anoxia.
5. Faint: rare < 10 years. Warning with feeling warm, sick, vertigo. Collapse and pallor but no abnormal movements or cyanosis.
6. Hyperventilation: deliberate prior to diving or involuntary with emotion in a teenager. Peripheral paraesthesia and tetany are common but loss of consciousness may occur.
7. Hysterical pseudoseizures: usually start gradually and resolve quickly (opposite of true epilepsy).
8. Migraine: flashing lights may be followed by hemiparesis or dysphasia but never by clonic movements. Basilar migraine may cause loss of consciousness.

Immediate treatment

1. If the fit has stopped, place in the recovery position with oral airway if necessary.
2. If the child is still fitting, see Table 12.2.

Investigations

A. For every child, every time
1. Full examination but especially
   a. head circumference (see Tables 12.7 and 12.8), skull shape, sutures, dysmorphic features
   b. fundi and pupils
   c. BP
      post-ictal drowsiness, Todd's paresis (hypotonic) and up-going plantars may persist for several hours
2. Developmental assessment once fully conscious (see Ch. 6).

B. For the first afebrile fit only (unless otherwise indicated)
1. Blood glucose, U & E, Ca^{2+}.
2. If there are features of meningism or encephalopathy
   a. LP (unless raised ICP suspected in which case urgent CT scan or cranial USS is indicated)
   b. no EEG after a single afebrile fit since $\frac{1}{3}$ of children never have another.

C. Two or more afebrile fits
1. UV light examination for ash-leaf depigmentation (tuberose sclerosis)
2. EEG: type of epilepsy determines choice of drug (see below)

Table 12.2 Management of status epilepticus

Supportive therapy
Secure airway. Place in recovery position. Do not restrain.
Give facial/nasal O_2 with a high flow rate.
Dipstick test for capillary glucose determination (see Ch. 11 for hypoglycaemia).
Take blood for U & E, Ca^{2+}, lab. glucose and save 2 ml in heparin tube for toxicology
Obtain i.v. access
Blood gas/acid–base analysis if fits have continued for > 20 min
Measure BP
Seizure control

0 min	diazepam (i.v. titrate up to 1.0 mg/kg (max 10 mg < 3 years; max 15 mg > 3 years). Avoid diazepam in head injury or raised ICP diazepam (rectal) 5 mg 6 months–3yr; 10 mg > 3 years
5 min	paraldehyde i.m. 1 ml/year age plus 1 ml (max 10 ml; 5 ml at each site) or paraldehyde p.r. 0.3 ml/kg in equal volume of arachis oil
15 min	phenobarbitone i.v. 20 mg/kg (max 750 mg) over 10 min
20 min	phenytoin i.v. 20 mg/kg (max 1 g at 2 mg/kg per min rate = 10 min infusion). Monitor ECG and BP
30 min	chlormethiazole i.v. 0.8% solution 2 ml/kg over 10 min; if successful maintain for > 2 hours at 1–4 ml/kg/h. Ventilation may be necessary
40 min	thiopentone (general anaesthesia), maintain for > 2 hr at 5 mg/kg/hr i.v. maximum. Ventilation always necessary.

Proceed stepwise if treatment unsuccessful.
Apnoea may follow diazepam. Flumazenil i.v. 10 µg/kg is antagonist.

---

3. ECG, CXR, 24-hour tape if cause may be cardiac
4. Cranial USS (if anterior fontanelle is open) or CT scan if focal fits or raised ICP (3% of childhood seizures are due to brain tumour)

Further management

1. No follow-up of single afebrile fit if above investigations are normal.
2. EEG after 2 fits: a normal EEG does *not* exclude epilepsy and an abnormal EEG does *not* automatically indicate anticonvulsants.
3. Anticonvulsants must be 'earned' and starting them depends on fit frequency and views of the parents and child. Two fits per year may be preferable to daily anticonvulsants for some families. Once started, continue for 2 years minimum and taper off over 2 months. Within 2 years of stopping treatment, 50% will have a fit:

   a. major motor — first choice < 1 year, oral phenobarbitone 20 mg/kg loading dose and 6 mg/kg per 24 hours maintenance
      — 1st choice > 1 year, oral sodium valproate initially 10 mg/kg per 24 hours and increase gradually up to 30 mg/kg per 24 hours. Check FBC and LFT before starting treatment and after 3 months.

   b. minor motor — oral ethosuximide 15–50 mg/kg per 24 hours

   c. infantile spasms — oral clonazepam 0.1 mg/kg per 24 hours (ACTH injections for 6 weeks initially)

   d. simple or complex partial — oral carbamazepine start at 5 mg/kg per 24 hours and increase gradually up to 20 mg/kg per 24 hours

4. Increase dose gradually until seizure control is adequate *or* maximum recommended dose is reached (Table 12.3) *or* side-effects occur. Monitoring drug levels is useful if non-compliance is suspected. Avoid polypharmacy.
5. Advise parents

   a. no cycling in traffic, no climbing sports
   b. adult present at bath time and when swimming
   c. 2 years fit-free for a driving licence
   d. no relationship to IQ
6. Write to school

Prognosis

70% are seizure-free and off treatment after 15 years.

Headaches

BACKGROUND

1. Majority have no underlying organic problem.

Table 12.3 'Therapeutic levels' of common anticonvulsants

1.	Lower limits *not* given; if a low dose of anticonvulsant is effective in preventing seizures, the blood concentration is irrelevant.
2.	All anticonvulsants share common toxic side-effects — ataxia, dysarthria, nystagmus, drowsiness — which may be seen even within the recommended limits.
3	The levels below are based on trough plasma samples. There is some variation between labs.

Anticonvulsant	Max. recommended plasma concentration (mg/l = µg/ml)
Carbamazepine	10
Ethosuximide	100
Phenobarbitone	45
Phenytoin	20
Sodium valproate	100

2. Chronic headache:
   a. systemic hypertension, including coarctation and pharochromocytoma
   b. intracranial hypertension — benign
      — space occupying lesion
   c. other 'things' in the head — sinusitis
      — toothache or malocclusion
      — earache
      — refractive errors
   d. depression
3. Acute, severe or focal headache:
   a. trauma
   b. migraine
   c. meningitis or encephalitis
   d. intracerebral haemorrhage

DIAGNOSIS

95% on the history. Examination must *always* include:
1. fundi and full neurological examination
2. BP
3. femoral pulses
4. cranial bruits
5. teeth and ENT
6. head circumference

INVESTIGATION

For the majority of children, no tests are required. Investigate only:
1. A sinister history (frequent, severe headache or neurological symptoms)
2. Combination of headache with fits
3. Complex migraine (i.e. focal deficits during an attack)

4. Any abnormal physical signs

Only 3% of skull X-rays performed for headache are abnormal.

MANAGEMENT

Any treatment has a placebo effect in 40% of children with headaches.

1. Explain to parents that headaches are common in children, a cause is rarely found, and 95% are symptom-free within 6 months of referral. The majority of children require no treatment or investigation.
2. If the child is an inpatient and the headache is severe, 3–5 mg/kg per 24 hours p.o. codeine phosphate (in 4 divided doses).
3. If a positive diagnosis of migraine is clear, give (early in the attack) one of:
   a. paracetamol 10 mg/kg 4-hourly regularly
   b. Migraleve (buclisine, paracetamol and codeine). For a child > 10 years, 1 pink tablet at onset and 1 yellow tablet 4-hourly (max. of 3 in 24 hours).
   c. domperidone 0.2–0.4 mg/kg orally or 1 mg/kg p.r. Metoclopramide 2.5 mg orally or i.m. also relieves the nausea but extrapyramidal side-effects may occur.

Remember — a child with continuous headaches does *not* have migraine

Central nervous system tumours in childhood

BACKGROUND

A. Brain tumours
1. 75% are infratentorial
   — cerebellar and posterior fossa signs are common and early
   — headaches and papilloedema are late features
2. 25% supratentorial
   — 50% are craniopharyngiomas — short stature
   — visual field defects
   — 50% are cerebral hemisphere tumours — focal neurological deficits
   — seizures
B. Spinal cord tumours
   — usually benign
   — *but* cause damage early by compression
   — focal neurological deficits in the limbs, or altered gait, impaired sphincter control, raised ICP if spinal blockage, back pain (*back pain is very rarely a functional symptom in childhood*)

CNS tumours in children are usually primary but leukaemia and neuroblastoma may occur in the cord or brain.

INVESTIGATION AND MANAGEMENT

Depend on the presentation, the tumour and the site, and should be undertaken in a specialist centre. See p. 191 for the acute management of headache (p. 190), raised ICP (p. 195), seizures (p. 187). LP is contraindicated before a CT scan.

Coma

BACKGROUND

Coma is graded by the Glasgow Coma (GC) Scale (see Table 2.9). A low GC score is very worrying.

CAUSES

1. *Head injury.*
2. *Hypoxia–ischaemia*: cardiac arrest, respiratory arrest or failure, 'near-miss' SIDS, suffocation, severe hypotension.
3. *Infection*: meningitis, encephalitis, cerebral abscess, generalised septicaemia.
4. *Epileptic*: see pp 188 and 195.
5. *Vascular*: haemorrhage (intracerebral and subarachnoid are usually spontaneous; subdural or extradural may follow NAI or skull fracture), stroke, hypertensive encephalopathy.
6. *Metabolic*: hypoglycaemia, diabetic ketoacidosis, renal failure, adrenal failure, liver failure, Reye's syndrome, hypernatraemia or hyponatyraemia.
7. *Toxic*: accidental (< 5 years) or deliberate (> 10 years) ingestion of salicylates, paracetamol, iron or lead; tricyclics or travel sickness pills (dilated but reactive pupils); opiates or lomotil (small pupils); anti-convulsants (nystagmus); alcohol, glue, toluene.
8. *Raised ICP*: results from
   a. cerebral oedema (can occur secondary to any of 1. to 7. above)
   b. hydrocephalus (may be acute or chronic)
   c. space-occupying lesion (tumour or abscess)

DIAGNOSIS

Have a system for dealing with the child with altered consciousness level:
1. Airway, breathing, circulation (see Ch. 2). If decerebrate posturing or fixed dilated pupils, intubate and hyperventilate immediately.
2. Assess GC score. Heel-prick for BMstix to exclude hypoglycaemia.
3. Look for external signs of trauma to the head, neck, spine, chest (think of pneumothorax), abdomen (ruptured viscus,

haemoperitoneum, floating bladder). Note external injuries such as bruises and burns.

Features which suggest cervical injury

a. cervical abrasion or upper spine tenderness
b. afebrile meningism
c. diving injury or fall from tree or horse
d. Down's syndrome
e. paraplegia or absent sensation below the neck

Features which suggest a basal skull fracture

a. bilateral periorbital haemorrhage ('racoon eyes')
b. bruising behind the ear
c. CSF otorrhoea or rhinorrhoea (CSF is positive for glucose on BMstix, mucus is not)

4. Insert i.v. cannula and replace fluids based on 1. and 3. above (see Ch. 2). Control fits (see pp 188 and 195) and treat hypoglycaemia (see Ch. 11).
5. Rapid neurological examination of the unconscious child:
    a. pupillary size, symmetry and reflexes
    b. conjugate gaze, nystagmus, doll's eyes reflex (provided no neck injury — if the eyes fix when the head is rotated, doll's eyes reflex is positive and prognosis is better than if the eyes move with the head).
    c. fundoscopy
    d. presence of gag reflex, corneal reflexes
    e. tone and reflexes in all four limbs and plantar responses
    f. signs of meningism. For signs of meningism or petechial rash, give i.v. or i.m. antibiotics (see p. 197) immediately — do *not* defer until LP is completed.

6. Take blood for:
    a. blood glucose
    b. U & E
    c. Ca^{2+}
    d. arterial blood gas (breathing air if possible)
    e. save 5 ml lithium heparin sample for LFTs, NH_3, toxicology
    f. crossmatch if signs of trauma

    Once the child is stable, transfer to ICU.

FURTHER INVESTIGATION

1. If there are no signs of raised ICP, and no cause for coma is apparent, do LP *and measure pressure*. Blood staining which does not clear serially suggests subarachnoid haemorrhage.
2. If there are signs of raised ICP, urgent neurosurgical referral and CT scan, are needed.

3. Skull X-rays (see below, head injuries), cervical spine X-rays and CXR as appropriate.

FURTHER MANAGEMENT

Monitor:
1. Colour (or pulse oximetry)
2. Pulse, respiratory rate, hourly BP, temperature
3. Pupils
4. GC score
5. Fluid balance

Give eye and mouth care, and regular turning.

Specific treatment depends on the cause — the basic management of some common CNS causes of coma is given below (see Ch. 2 for hypotension, Ch. 7 for hypertension, p. 188 for status epilepticus, Ch. 11 for hypoglycaemia, DKA, electrolyte disorders, and Ch. 15 for poisoning).

Head injury

1. Take a full history from an eye-witness. Was the child unconscious at any time and, if so, for how long?
2. Full general and neurological examination. Mild pallor, irritability or sleepiness, and vomiting are all common and not necessarily signs of raised ICP.
3. Cervical spine X-ray (see p. 193).
4. Skull X-ray required if:
   a. unconscious > 5 min
   b. unconscious < 5 min but (i) high velocity object
                              (ii) bruising or scalp laceration
                              (iii) < 1 year
   c. not unconscious but (i) retrograde amnesia > 5 min
                          (ii) persistent vomiting
                          (iii) scalp haematoma or injury by sharp object
                          (iv) suspected NAI — full skeletal survey
5. Admit if:
   a. definite period of loss of consciousness, irrespective of duration
   b. any memory loss
   c. any convulsions or abnormal neurological examination (including GC score < 15)
   d. persistent vomiting or severe headache
   e. parents unlikely to recognise deterioration
6. Post-traumatic convulsions:
   Diazepam is absolutely contraindicated.

< 5 years: phenobarbitone 10 mg/kg i.v. then 6 mg/kg per 24 hours as 8-hourly divided doses. The loading dose may be repeated once.

> 5 years: phenytoin up to 15 mg/kg i.v. (at 1 mg/kg/min) with ECG monitoring; then 5 mg/kg per 24 hours as 8-hourly divided doses.

7. Seek a neurosurgical opinion if:
   a. GC score is < 10 *or* if it is > 10 but fluctuating rapidly
   b. focal neurological signs or focal fits
   c. open head injury, depressed or basal skull fracture
   d. signs of raised ICP (see below)
8. If GC score is ≤ 8, admit to ICU for ICP monitoring.
9. Observations after admission
   a. Child is alert and orientated: record pulse, BP, respiratory rate and GC score on admission, at 1 hour and then 4-hourly. Record when urine is first passed.
   b. Child is drowsy: monitor above observations every 30 min until he is no longer drowsy.
10. Fluids:
    a. free oral fluids if taken
    b. if vomiting, start i.v. fluids after 6 hours. Give $\frac{2}{3}$ of maintenance requirements only
11. Home the day after admission if:
    (a) all observations are normal
    (b) no vomiting after a full meal
    (c) full discharge examination
    (d) advise the parents of warning signs (drowsiness, vomiting, severe headache, unsteady gait)

Raised intracranial pressure (ICP)

BACKGROUND

May present acutely or chronically (Table 12.4). Hydrocephalus is the commonest cause in children < 1 year.

DIAGNOSIS

Symptoms

These are non-specific, especially the younger the child: vomiting, early morning headache, diplopia or visual loss, irritability or drowsiness, 'off feeds'.

Signs

OFC crossing centile lines, bulging fontanelle (closes 12–18 months), wide sutures, 'sun-setting' (cornea visible *above* iris), papilloedema, III or VI nerve palsies.

Table 12.4 Causes of raised intracranial pressure

Acute onset (hours–days)

Cerebral oedema	Trauma, anoxia, meningitis, encephalitis, Reye's syndrome, lead intoxication, hypertensive encephalopathy, aggressive rehydration (especially if hypernatraemic initially and in diabetic ketoacidosis), liver or renal failure
Vascular	Extradural, subarachnoid or intracerebral haemorrhage (trauma or AV malformation) or venous thrombosis
CSF	Acute hydrocephalus (especially blocked ventricular shunt)

Slow onset (days–weeks) See also Table 12.7
CNS tumour (brain or cord)
Cerebral abscess
Subdural collection (usually traumatic — consider NAI)
Hydrocephalus from any cause
'Benign' intracranial hypertension (associated with hypo- or hypercalcaemia, withdrawal of steroids and venous sinus thrombosis)

Look for skull trauma. Measure BP. Rising BP, falling pulse and depressed respiration are signs of imminent 'coning'.

INVESTIGATION

1. Do not perform LP if raised ICP is possible.
    If an LP is done and the child is lying on his side and not crying, a pressure > 15 cmH$_2$O suggests raised ICP.
2. Urinalysis ('shunt' nephritis associated with microscopic haematuria).
3. U & E, Ca^{2+} and blood sugar.

Depending on the presentation, consider:

4. Blood cultures and acute viral serology.
5. Blood NH$_3$ and LFT.
6. Skull X-ray and CT scan.

Benign intracranial hypertension is a diagnosis of exclusion.

Optic neuritis is a differential. Papilloedema is often asymmetrical, as is visual loss, and no other symptoms or signs of raised ICP. If CT scan excludes space-occupying lesion, perform LP to measure pressure and examine CSF. Treat optic neuritis with 2 mg/kg prednisolone for 1 week and taper off dose over the following week.

MANAGEMENT

1. Observations are as for significant head injury (see p. 194).
2. Treat the cause.
3. Correct metabolic abnormalities slowly.
4. Measures to reduce ICP:

a. head up position (35°) and avoid constriction of neck veins

b. mannitol 20% (1 g/kg i.v. over 20 min) for the rapidly deteriorating child to buy time for other measures

c. dexamethasone (0.5 mg/kg i.v. or p.o. every 6 hours) is useful if the cause is a tumour or 'benign' intracranial hypertension (monitor visual fields as this 'benign' disorder may cause permanent visual failure)

d. fluid intake $\frac{2}{3}$ of maintenance. Inappropriate ADH syndrome may occur

e. treat convulsions (pp 188 and 195)

f. if raised ICP persists, consider:

   (i) elective ETT and artificial hyperventilation to a $PaCO_2$ of 3–3.5 kPa

   (ii) surface cooling to induce hypothermia of 32°C
   We would recommend these measures in:
   — severe head injury with GC score of ≤ 8
   — following craniotomy to evacuate haematoma
   — Reye's syndrome or other acute encephalopathy (viral, burns, lead, hepatic) if GC score is ≤ 8
   — raised ICP of any cause sufficient to cause focal neurological signs; flaccidity or decerebrate posturing; apnoea
   These measures should be accompanied by:

   (iii) sedation and paralysis: morphine 10–30 µg/kg/h i.v.
   midazolam 0.06–0.24 mg/kg/h i.v.
   and
   atracurium 0.3–1.2 mg/kg/h i.v.

   (iv) ICP monitoring using a subarachnoid screw. Aim to maintain a cerebral perfusion pressure (mean arterial BP–mean ICP) of 50–90 mmHg.

Meningitis

BACKGROUND

1. In any child who presents with fever, altered behaviour, vomiting or seizures, an LP must be considered. Threshold is lower if antibiotics are already given.

2. The most likely organism is:

   a. neonate: *E. coli*, group B *Streptococcus*, *Listeria monocytogenes*

   b. preschool child: *Haemophilus influenzae* type B is the commonest but also *Meningococcus* and *Pneumococcus*

   c. older children: *Neisseria meningitidis* and *Str. pneumoniae*

   d. child with a ventricular shunt: *Staph. aureus* and *Staph. epidermidis*

   e. child recently abroad: consider *Mycobacterium tuberculosis*

   f. recurrent meningitis: *E. coli* if sacral sinus, *Str. milariae* if spread from sinusitis

DIAGNOSIS

Symptoms
Very non-specific in the younger child (irritability or lethargy, poor feeding or vomiting, seizures).

Signs
Meningism is usually present in the older child (headache, photophobia, neck stiffness and positive Kernig's sign). Purpuric rash may accompany meningococcaemia or *Haemophilus* septicaemia.

IMMEDIATE TREATMENT

1. If a rash is present, give parenteral cefotaxime 50 mg/kg immediately — *DO NOT DEFER UNTIL LP*.
2. Treat seizures (see Table 12.2).
3. Start i.v. infusion and give plasma 15 ml/kg over 30 min if the child is shocked.

INVESTIGATIONS

1. Take blood for FBC, U & E, blood cultures, acute viral titres and blood glucose.
2. Perform LP — measure opening pressure, request CSF glucose and protein, microscopy and gram stain (Tables 12.5 and 12.6). Specify Ziehl–Nielsen stain if TB is at all possible.
   Do not perform LP if:
   a. there are signs of raised ICP, deep coma, protracted seizures, unequal or dilated pupils, focal neurological signs
   b. the child is shocked with purpuric rash
   Under these circumstances, defer LP (but not antibiotics) until raised ICP is treated and the child is stable.

TREATMENT

1. CSF may be normal in very early infection. Therefore, if meningitis is strongly suspected clinically, treat irrespective of CSF.
2. Always start treatment if any polymorphs are present. Do not try to distinguish bacterial and viral meningitis on the basis of clinical or CSF findings. If the CSF shows abnormal numbers of WBCs, even if they are lymphocytes and no organisms are seen on gram stain, treat with i.v. antibiotics for 48 hours until 'culture negative'.
3. *Antibiotics*
   Prior to a definitive positive culture, our 'blind' therapy, irrespective of age, is:
   i.v. cefotaxime 50 mg/kg 6-hourly

Table 12.5 Normal CSF

	Neonate	Infant < 1 year	Child > 1 year
Appearance	May be yellow (if jaundiced, or xanthochromic after traumatic delivery)	Gin clear	Gin clear
Cells (per mm³ = per μl = × 10⁶ per litre)			
Polymorphs	0	0	0
Lymphocytes	0–15	0–10	0–5
Erythrocytes	0–500	0	0
	Up to 50 RBCs may be found following an apparently atraumatic tap and need no further investigation		
Protein (g/l)	0.3–2.0	0.2–1.0	0.15–0.45
Glucose (mmol/l)	Not less than 60% of a simultaneous blood glucose		

Table 12.6 Abnormal CSF

	Bacterial meningitis	Bacterial meningitis but already on antibiotics	Viral meningitis	Tuberculous meningitis
Appearance	Turbid	May be clear	Usually clear	Hazy
Cells (per mm³)				
Polymorphs	10–50 000	10–1000	May be 50% of lymphocyte count in early stages	10–1000
Lymphocytes	A few	10–1000	10–1000	10–1000
Erythrocytes	If a traumatic tap, allow 1 WBC for 800 RBCs in CSF *or* compute ratio from peripheral FBC. If in doubt, treat as bacterial meningitis. If CSF is xanthochromic, presence of RBCs suggests recent haemorrhage			
Gram stain	Organisms often seen	May be no organisms (and sterile culture)	No organisms	May be organisms on ZN
Protein (g/l)	0.8–4.0	0.8–2.0	0–1.5	0.6–6.0
Glucose	< 60% of blood	Normal or low	≥ 60% of blood	Very low

If a cerebral abscess is present, CSF usually shows elevated protein and excess of lymphocytes

ZN = Ziehl–Nielsen stain

4. *N. meningitidis*: i.v. benzyl penicillin 50 mg/kg 4-hourly for 7 days.
   Str. pneumoniae: i.v. benzyl penicillin 50 mg/kg 4-hourly for 10 days.
   Haem. influenzae: i.v. cefotaxime 50 mg/kg 6-hourly for 10 days.

5. *Supportive measures*
   $\frac{2}{3}$ maintenance fluids.
   Neurological observations as for head injury (p. 195).
   Serial head circumference measurements in infant.
6. *Prophylaxis*
   Rifampicin 10 mg/kg 12-hourly orally to all household members and all 'kissing' contacts within the previous 10 days and also to the index child once oral intake is tolerated.
   Neisseria meningitidis: continue for 2 days
   Haemophilus influenzae: continue for 4 days
7. *Isolate* all possible meningitis cases until culture is negative or Rifampicin regimen completed.
8. *Tuberculous meningitis* (see p. 213)

PROGNOSIS AND FOLLOW-UP

Sensorineural deafness is the commonest serious sequel of viral meningitis. Mortality is 5–10% in bacterial meningitis. A quarter have major neurological sequelae (e.g. seizures, deafness, blindness, cerebral palsy, developmental delay). *All* children should have hearing formally tested 3 months after viral or bacterial meningitis.

Viral encephalitis

BACKGROUND

Three forms are recognised:
1. Acute viral meningoencephalitis, e.g. herpes simplex type I (HSE), CMV, rabies.
2. Postinfectious encephalitis causes damage by demyelination, e.g. following chickenpox, rubella, mumps, measles. Many present with ataxia because of cerebellar involvement.
3. Subacute sclerosing panencephalitis.

DIAGNOSIS

Symptoms
Headache, vomiting, altered behaviour or consciousness level, seizures (often focal).

Signs
Impaired consciousness, meningism, cranial nerve palsies and other focal neurological signs, papilloedema, fever.

INVESTIGATIONS

1. LP (if no contraindications — see p. 198). CSF usually contains cells, which may be polymorphs if very early (e.g. in-

creased cell count in 97% of HSE *but* acellular CSF does *not* exclude the diagnosis, e.g. rabies).
2. Acute and convalescent viral serology.
3. Virus isolation from CSF, stool, urine.
4. In HSE, EEG may show focal or unilateral temporal lobe changes accompanied by corresponding CT scan changes.

TREATMENT

1. General management and observation of the unconscious child (mouth and eye care, frequent turning, urinary catheter, enteral or parenteral alimentation after 5 days).
2. Treat raised ICP.
3. Acyclovir i.v. 10 mg/kg 8-hourly improves the prognosis in HSE.

Reye's syndrome

BACKGROUND

An acute encephalopathy which follows a prodromal illness and is accompanied by hepatocellular liver failure due to fatty infiltration. Known associations:
1. Therapeutic doses of aspirin
2. Chicken pox or influenza
3. Defects of fatty acid oxiation enzymes, urea cycle enzymes and organic acidaemias.

DIAGNOSIS

Usually follows a mild respiratory illness or viral exanthema with vomiting. This is followed by altered consciousness, convulsions, tachypnoea (or apnoea — a 'near-miss' SIDS) and hepatomegaly.

INVESTIGATIONS

1. Blood $NH_3 > 80$ μmol/l
2. Transaminases > 100 iu/l
3. Prolonged PT (prothrombin ratio > 1.5)
4. Glucose, electrolytes and arterial gases as baseline
5. Reye's is associated with raised ICP — therefore avoid LP
6. EEG is unhelpful as it shows only non-specific encephalo-pathic changes
7. Exclude other causes of acute encephalopathy:
   a. blood cultures
   b. acute and convalescent viral serology
   c. blood salicylate, paracetamol and lead levels

    d.   save plasma and urine for analysis for fatty acid and organic acid disorders.

MANAGEMENT

1. Admit to ICU; neurological observation as for severe head injury (see p. 195)
2. Invasive monitoring of ICP and aggressive treatment improves prognosis (see p. 196)
3. Treat liver failure (see Ch. 9), although this does not improve encephalopathy since there is primary cerebral oedema. Pass NG tube and give:

   lactulose 1 ml/kg
   neomycin 50 mg/kg   }   per 24 hours in 3 divided doses
   cimetidine 30 mg/kg

4. Treat seizures   < 5 years: phenobarbitone i.v.
                  > 5 years: phenytoin i.v.
5. Obsessional attention to fluid balance:
   Operational goals are (a) high/normal blood glucose (8–10 mmol/l)
                                  (b) normal electrolytes and plasma osmolarity (280–320 mosmol/kg)
                                  (c) urine output ≥ 0.5 ml/kg/h
                                  (d) normal BP
                                  (e) maintain CVP 2–4 cmH$_2$O above midaxillary line
6. Treat coagulopathy with i.v. vitamin K and FFP 10 ml/kg i.v. as indicated

PROGNOSIS

Overall mortality is approx. 45%

Permanent neurological sequelae in up to 50% of survivors

Prognosis is worse if: (a) the child is very young
                     (b) GC score is < 8
                     (c) plasma NH$_3$ > 300 μmol/l
                     (d) CPK > 500 iu/l
                     (e) plasma free fatty acids > 0.85 mmol/l

Recurrence is more likely if an enzyme defect is demonstrated.

Child with abnormal head size

LARGE HEAD (Table 12.7)

1. Look for signs of raised ICP. If present, admit and refer urgently to the neurosurgeon.
2. If ICP is clinically normal and there are no headaches, measure OFC serially as an outpatient. Measure parents' OFC. If OFC

Table 12.7 Causes of macrocephaly (i.e. > 97 th centile) or an enlarging head (i.e. crossing centiles)

Normal intracranial pressure
Large brain
    normal variant — always measure the parents' OFC
    cerebral gigantism (Soto's syndrome)
    storage diseases
Thickened skull
    thalassaemia
    osteopetrosis
Raised intracranial pressure
Hydrocephalus
    communicating (e.g. post-meningitis)
    non-communicating (e.g. posterior fossa tumour or associated with spina bifida)
Chronic subdural effusion
    birth trauma
    NAI
    following meningitis

grows parallel to centiles, probably a normal variant. If there is progressive macrocephaly, arrange cranial CT scan (or USS if anterior fontanelle is open).

SMALL HEAD (Table 12.8)

Investigation is rarely rewarding:
1. measure parents' OFC and child's height and weight.
2. SXR to exclude craniosynostosis.
3. Maternal phenylalanine level.
4. Screen for congenital infection and look for intracranial calcification on SXR.
5. Karyotype.
6. Cranial USS.

The unsteady child

BACKGROUND

Ataxia may be acute or chronic (Table 12.9) and may present in casualty or outpatients.

DIAGNOSIS

Clinically, in addition to the wide-based unsteady gait, there may be other features of cerebellar dysfunction.

Ask about atypical seizures and medicines in the home. Look for signs of recent viral infection, raised ICP, focal neurological signs and telangiectasia of the sclera.

Table 12.8 Causes of microcephaly (< 3rd centile) or head growth falling away from the centiles

Normal variant	The child is proportionately small for height and weight also
Dwarfism (e.g. Russell–Silver syndrome)	OFC, height and weight are in proportion but all are > 3 SD below the mean
Familial	The parents have small heads Height and weight may be normal
Primary microcephaly	No obvious underlying cause but sometimes autosomal recessive pedigree Usually mentally retarded and backward sloping forehead
Secondary microcephaly	A known congenital or acquired cause Usually mentally retarded congenital infection fetal alcohol syndrome maternal phenylketonuria perinatal haemorrhage or infarct meningitis or encephalitis specific, rare syndromes, e.g. Smith–Lemli–Opitz syndrome chromosomal syndromes, e.g. Down's syndrome, 18 deletion premature fusion of skull sutures, e.g. Apert's syndrome

INVESTIGATION

Depends on presentation but consider:

1. Blood and urine for toxicology and aminoacid chromatography
2. Acute and convalescent viral titres and blood cultures
3. LP (CSF protein shows an elevated protein in Guillain–Barré syndrome; xanthochromia and RBCs reflect haemorrhage; LP is absolutely contraindicated if abscess is suspected)

Further detailed investigations for rarer causes include:

4. Blood film for acanthocytes, blood vitamin E levels, cholesterol, jejunal biopsy (abetalipoproteinaemia)
5. EEG (minor status or encephalopathy)
6. CT or USS scan (abscess, tumour hydrocephalus)
7. ECG and echocardiogram (Friedrich's ataxia)
8. Motor nerve conduction studies (peroneal muscular atrophy)
9. Muscle biopsy (mitochondrial cytopathy)

The child with weakness

May present as focal or generalised weakness (see Table 12.10) or spasticity or hypotonia (see Table 12.11).

Table 12.9 Causes of ataxia

Acute ataxia
'Toxic' ataxia
    Alcohol or solvent abuse
    Anticonvulsants
    Sedatives
    Lead
    Intermittent maple syrup urine disease
Following viral infection
    Acute cerebellar ataxia 7–10 days later, especially after chicken pox but
    also rubella, measles, enteroviruses and infectious mononucleosis
    Ataxia may accompany postinfection polyneuritis (Guillain–Barré
    syndrome)
Posterior fossa space occupying lesion
    Bacterial abscess
    Haemorrhage
Epilepsy
    e.g. minor status
Chronic ataxia
Ataxic cerebral palsy
Posterior fossa space occupying lesion
    Tumour (including neuroblastoma — 'dancing eyes' syndrome)
    Obstruction of fourth ventricle outlet and hydrocephalus
Progressive ataxias of childhood
    Friedrich's ataxia
    Ataxia telangiectasia
    Abetalipoproteinaemia
    Refsum's disease
    Metachromatic leucodystrophy
    Mitochondrial cytopathy
    Early onset hereditary cerebellar ataxia

SPINAL CORD COMPRESSION (Table 12.10)

A neurological emergency.

Symptoms
Back pain, paraesthesia in the legs, leg weakness, altered urinary
function, constipation.

Signs
Thoracic lesions associated with upper motor neurone signs in the
legs (although toes may be downgoing and reflexes reduced in
early phase) whereas lumbar cord abnormalities usually show
lower motor neurone signs in the legs. Test for sensory level.

Management
1. Do *not* perform LP.
2. Dexamethasone 0.25 mg/kg i.v. (max. 10 mg) and refer to a
   neurosurgeon. At myelography, take CSF to look for infection
   or transverse myelitis.

Table 12.10 Causes of weakness

Remember that power may be limited by pain or lack of cooperation.

Confusingly, lesions in the brain may produce classic upper motor neurone weakness (spastic CP) or 'central hypotonia' (e.g. early CP, Down's syndrome, acute hemiplegia of childhood, Todd's paresis following a seizure)

Spinal cord problem (back ache is very rare as a functional symptom in childhood)
    trauma or atlanto-axia dislocation
    bony abnormalities in Down's, achondroplasia and Morquio's syndrome
    syringomyelia
    tumour (e.g. dermoids, teratomas, gliomas, neuroblastomas, neurofibromas)
    abscess
    postinfectious transverse myelitis

Anterior horn cell problem
    spinal muscular atrophy (Werdnig–Hoffmann disease)
    poliomyelitis

Motor nerve problem
    Focal neuropathy
        Bell's palsy
        brachial plexus injury at birth (Erb's palsy)
        local trauma
    Generalised motor neuropathy
        Guillain–Barré syndrome (postinfection polyneuritis)
        lead poisoning
        acute intermittent porphyria
        drugs, e.g. vincristine

Neuromuscular junction problem
    myasesthenia gravis (neonatal presentation if the mother is affected)

Myopathy
    muscular dystrophy
    dermatomyositis
    mitochondrial myopathy
    inherited metabolic myopathies

Table 12.11 The floppy infant

In addition to the causes of hypotonia associated with nerve or muscle weakness (see Table 12.10), hypotonia is also associated with:
Mental handicap of any cause
CP
Prematurity
Drugs or severe systemic illness
Malnutrition
Down's syndrome
Prader–Willi syndrome
Ehlers–Danlos syndrome
Hypothyroidism
Rare storage diseases and other inborn errors of metabolism

3. Check for primary tumour sites (e.g. abdominal examination, CXR, FBC) and for the café-au-lait spots of neurofibromatosis.

BELL'S PALSY

Background

An acute, isolated lower motor neurone palsy of the facial nerve. Probably post-viral and recurrence is not uncommon. A small proportion is related to trauma, Guillain–Barré syndrome, hypertension, geniculate herpes zoster, suppurative otitis media or Melkersson's syndrome.

Diagnosis

Ptosis is never a feature. The child may have difficulty blinking or closing his eye and the forehead is also affected. Onset may be sudden or gradual and may be preceded by post-auricular pain.

Prognosis

Over 80% make a complete recovery but this may take 3 months. A painless, incomplete palsy suggests good outcome. Pain, hyperacusis and diminished taste may indicate worse prognosis, and if such a child is seen within 4 days, consider prednisolone 2 mg/kg for 4 days (tapered off over another 4 days).

MYASTHENIA GRAVIS

Background

1. True myasthenia can present at any age.
2. Transient neonatal myasthenia may also occur for 2–4 weeks if the mother has myasthenia. If no signs develop by 3 days of age, they will not do so and the infant can be discharged.

Presentation

Ptosis and diplopia are the commonest. Crises may occur during intercurrent infection or minor surgery. In the newborn, hypotonia, poor suck and feeble respiration.

Diagnosis

Confirmed by marked response to anticholinesterase, e.g. neostigmine 0.1 mg/kg i.m. or edrophonium chloride (Tensilon) 0.2 mg/kg i.v.

Management

Supportive therapy (pharyngeal suction, ventilation) until optimal control is achieved with oral anticholinesterases. Dosage is titrated against parasympathetic side-effects (salivation, abdominal cramps, bradycardia).

13

Infectious diseases

Many infectious diseases are covered in other chapters; consult the index.

Pyrexia of unknown origin

Early discussion with the consultant in charge is indicated.

HISTORY

Must be detailed; include timing and progression of symptoms, contact with recent illness, recent travel abroad and contact with travellers, recent drugs and immunisations, contact with pets, past medical history, occupation of parents, place of abode, ethnic group of the child.

EXAMINATION

Meticulous; check for bone and joint infection, skin lesions, enlarged glands, dehydration and intra-abdominal sepsis (diagnosis of appendicitis can be difficult in young children).

INVESTIGATIONS

In an ill child without an obvious focus, the following investigations are suggested:
1. Take blood for FBC + film and differential, LFT, blood cultures, baseline serum for viral titres, CRP and monospot.
2. Stool and urine cultures; urine microscopy.
3. CXR.
4. Mantoux test.
5. LP may be indicated clinically.
   NB. Typical signs of meningitis may be absent in children < 18 months.
6. If the child has recently returned from abroad, malaria, enteric infections, TB and hepatitis must be excluded.

PROLONGED FEVER

The major causes of a prolonged fever are infections, connective tissue disease and malignant disease (see Table 13.1).

A. Infections

If fever persists, repeat FBC and differential, blood cultures and CXR. Send agglutination tests for typhoid, paratyphoid, brucella and leptospirosis. Repeat viral antibodies at 10 days, including EB virus, CMV, toxoplasmosis. Examination and/or history may indicate search for pyogenic abscess or exclusion of low-grade osteomyelitis by isotope bone scan. Subacute bacterial endocarditis may also cause PUO.

B. Connective tissue or autoimmune disease

Indications of such a disorder include:
1. Persistently high ESR
2. Low leukocyte alkaline phosphatase level
3. Hypergammaglobulinaemia
4. Autoantibodies in the serum (e.g. thyroid, liver) and ANA

C. Malignant disease

Investigations such as repeated FBC and film, bone marrow aspiration and radiological examination may be indicated.

TREATMENT

Depends on the underlying cause. A child presenting with fever

Table 13.1 Causes of prolonged fever

Bacterial diseases	**Viral diseases**
Abscesses; dental, liver, pelvic, perinephric, subdiaphragmatic	Cytomegalovirus
	Hepatitis
Bacterial endocarditis	Infectious mononucleosis
Osteomyelitis	
Brucellosis	
Leptospirosis	**Fungal diseases**
Salmonellosis	Histoplasmosis
Sinusitis	Candidiasis (systemic)
Tuberculosis	Blastomycosis
Parasitic diseases	**Collagen diseases**
Malaria	Juvenile rheumatoid arthritis
Toxoplasmosis	Polyarteritis
Visceral lava migrans	SLE
Others	
Drug fever	
	Periodic fever
Colitis	Kawasaki's disease
Pancreatitis	Familial dysautonomia
Thyrotoxicosis	Serum sickness
	Malignancy

alone and who is not very ill does not usually warrant antibiotics 'on spec' without appropriate examination and investigation.

Osteomyelitis

SIGNS

Fever, malaise, pain, erythema, swelling and tenderness of the affected bone.
NB. In neonates local signs may be absent.

INVESTIGATIONS

1. FBC + blood film, CRP and blood cultures.
2. X-rays may show soft tissue swelling initially but bone changes may be absent for up to 10 days.
3. The need for radionuclide bone scans and needle aspiration should be discussed with the orthopaedic surgeon. In acute osteomyelitis, surgical drainage is required if there are signs of an abscess.
4. Full examination for other foci of infection.

TREATMENT

1. Give i.v. flucloxacillin until clinical improvement is seen (4–6 days) then orally for 4 weeks. If an organism other than *Staph. aureus* is suspected (e.g. *Haem. influenzae*) give a second antibiotic such as chloramphenicol. Give neonates i.v. gentamicin in addition to flucloxacillin.
2. Pain relief by splinting and immobilising the affected limb with analgesia as required.
3. Obtain orthopaedic opinion.

Septic arthritis

Usual pathogens: *Staph. aureus, Haem. influenzae* and *Str. pneumoniae*.

SIGNS

Fever, malaise, joint inflammation, limp or pseudoparalysis.

INVESTIGATIONS

1. FBC and blood film, CRP, blood cultures.

2. X-ray of the joint and surrounding bones.
3. Orthopaedic referral for arthrocentesis. Send joint fluid for gram stain and culture, WBC and differential and total protein.

TREATMENT

1. Urgent orthopaedic opinion as to the need for drainage of the joint.
2. Antibiotics: in children < 5 years, i.v. chloramphenicol until symptoms improve, then orally; > 5 years, i.v. flucloxacillin plus i.v. ampicillin until symptoms improve.

   Oral therapy must follow for 3 weeks and is based on in vitro sensitivities, e.g. oral flucloxacillin for *Staph. aureus* infection, amoxycillin for sensitive *Haem. influenzae*, or cefaclor if the cause is unknown or if oral flucloxacillin cannot be tolerated.
3. Analgesia as required. Initial immobilisation helps to relieve pain.

Compound fracture

In addition to appropriate surgical management, antibiotic therapy is indicated as the risk of infection is high. Give flucloxacillin plus gentamicin, both i.v. for 48 hours. Antibiotic therapy should be continued or modified if signs of infection develop. Cultures from the wound and blood may aid the decision.

Bites

HUMAN

May cause serious infection.

Management

1. Wash the wound carefully with normal saline (0.9%); ensure appropriate surgical management (debride and exclude other structural damage, e.g. to tendons). Because of the risk of infection wounds are not usually sutured. If in doubt or if the bite may cause cosmetic problems (e.g. facial) discuss with the plastic surgeon.
2. Determine tetanus status (see p. 228).
3. Prophylactic antibiotics (oral Augmentin or erythromycin).
4. Frequent follow-up to check for infection.

ANIMAL

Management

1. Most wounds can be sutured after cleansing and debridement. Avoid suturing small wounds on the hand or puncture wounds as the risk of infection is high.
2. Check tetanus status.
3. Antibiotics; give for bites to the hands, face or for puncture wounds (e.g. oral Augmentin or erythromycin).

Tuberculosis

Aetiology: *Mycobacterium tuberculosis* infection.
Clinical manifestations may include:
 1. persistent cough
 2. pleural effusion
 3. cervical lymphadenopathy
 4. meningitis
 5. PUO
 6. FTT
 7. hepatosplenomegaly
 8. aseptic pyuria
 9. monoarticular arthritis
10. back pain

SCREENING

When TB is suspected, enquiry into contacts with active TB, a Mantoux test and CXR are needed.

Mantoux test

0.1 ml of tuberculin PPD dilution 100 u/ml (10 iu) is injected intradermally into the skin of the upper flexor part of the forearm so that a bleb is produced, typically 7 mm in diameter. The results should be read 48–72 hours later. Reactions up to 4 mm of induration are considered negative. Reactions of over 10 mm induration are positive. Generally, induration of 5–9 mm indicates *M. tuberculosis* infection though interpretation varies between countries. In the presence of a history of previous BCG vaccination, induration of 15 mm or more may be regarded as evidence of infection and should be managed as if BCG had not been given.

For Mantoux tests in patients in whom TB is suspected or who are known to be hypersensitive to tuberculin, a dilution of 10 iu/ml should be used. If negative, repeat using the strength above.

If Mantoux test and CXR are positive collect:
1. Three early morning urine collections and gastric aspirates; also sputum if possible.

2. LFT.
3. If an effusion is present, pleural biopsy may aid diagnosis. Send fluid for examination and for culture of acid-fast bacilli.
4. If miliary disease is suspected, a biopsy of bone marrow may help with diagnosis.
5. Lethargy or abnormal neurological findings suggest the need for CSF examination, including culture and examination for acid-fast bacilli. Infants < 6 months should all have CSF examination.
6. With proven TB, skin tests and CXR of contacts are needed. The culture for acid-fast bacilli may not be positive for up to 6 weeks. A presumptive diagnosis based on clinical presentation, CXR and positive Mantoux test indicate need for treatment. Demonstration of acid-fast bacilli confirms the diagnosis.

TREATMENT

Treatment should only be carried out with the supervision of medical staff experienced in the management of tuberculous infection as this may vary from region to region.
1. Positive skin test, negative CXR and asymptomatic child: give isoniazid 10 mg/kg p.o. (max. 300 mg) once per 24 hours for 1 year). CXR at 6 and 12 months. Serious TB will almost never develop in a child with primary TB who receives isoniazid treatment for 1 year.
2. Primary tuberculosis and cervical adenitis, meningitis, miliary or progressive lung TB: give rifampicin 20 mg/kg once per 24 hours (max. 600 mg per 24 hours) + isoniazid 20 mg/kg once per 24 hours (max. 400 mg per 24 hours) for 12 months. Also give pyrazinamide 30 mg/kg once per 24 hours with pyridoxine 10 mg once per 24 hours for 2 months.

Contacts

1. Household contacts of active TB require CXR and Mantoux test. Give isoniazid 10 mg/kg per 24 hours. If still Mantoux-negative at 3 months and contact is treated, discontinue and give BCG.
2. Newborn of a mother with active TB: give isoniazid for 8 weeks or until mother's sputum is culture-negative (which ever is longer) and then perform Mantoux test. If negative, stop isoniazid and give BCG. Follow up.

Steroids

Consider in pleurisy, pericarditis, meningitis or stridor due to lymph node obstruction.

NB. Patients should be monitored clinically for adverse drug reactions (consult BNF or MIMS) during treatment and be seen at least monthly. Fortunately drug side-effects are rare in childhood.

Immunodeficiency

Persistent or recurrent infections should raise the suspicion of underlying immunodeficiency.

Immunodeficiency may be:

1. Primary (e.g. a deficiency in the humoral, T lymphocyte, complement or phagocytic system), or
2. Secondary (e.g. viral infections, metabolic disorders, immuno-suppressive agents, prematurity, Down's syndrome, etc.)

SYMPTOMS SUGGESTIVE OF A POSSIBLE IMMUNE DISORDER

Recurrent lower respiratory tract infections, chronic otitis media, bronchiectasis, recurrent or chronic skin sepsis, FTT associated with recurrent infections and chronic diarrhoea; chronic or recurrent candidal infection; recurrent conjunctivitis; unusual or opportunistic organisms causing infections.

Table 13.2 Investigations for suspected immunodeficiency (venous blood)

Immune component	Quantitative	Functional
Immunoglobulin and antibody formation	Immunoglobulin and subclass concentrations Specific antibody titres	Opsonisation Agglutination Neutralisation
Lymphocytes	Lymphocyte count Cell surface antigens	Proliferative responses (e.g. mitogens) Regulatory function: suppressor and helper assays, lymphokine production Skin testing, mumps, ppd
Complement	Individual components	CH_{50}/CH_{100} Opsonisation
Phagocytic	Neutrophil and eosinophil numbers	Chemotaxis Phagocytosis NBT reduction O_2 consumption Superoxide production Iodination Bacterial killing

INVESTIGATIONS

1. General: FBC + film and differential, blood cultures and X-rays relevant to the infection.
2. Consider non-immunological tests, e.g. sweat test, HIV status.
3. Immunological tests: before performing complex investigations (Table 13.2) discuss the case with an immunologist. A simple initial approach is to determine total lymphocyte and neutrophil numbers from peripheral blood, measure IgG, IgA and IgM, and IgG subclass concentrations and to assess lymphocyte responses to the mitogen phytohaemagglutinin (approximately 1 ml of blood is needed). If normal, the majority of primary immunodeficiency disorders will be excluded. (Further tests, see Table 13.2).

MANAGEMENT

Aggressive treatment of infections is indicated. Specific treatment of the immune defect will depend on the abnormality discovered (e.g. gammaglobulin replacement therapy in children with hypogammaglobulinaemia). Liaise with the consultant, immunologist and microbiologist.

NB. Avoid live vaccines. Irradiate blood products given to all patients suspected of immunodeficiency to avoid GVHD.

Kawasaki's disease

Aetiology is unknown.

DIAGNOSIS

Made when an acute illness occurs and five out of six of the following are present:
1. fever
2. rash
3. acute cervical lymphadenopathy
4. conjunctivitis
5. mucosal change, e.g. strawberry tongue, erythema and fissured lips
6. periungual desquamation, erythema of palms and soles, oedema of hands and feet

INVESTIGATIONS

No diagnostic test is available. High ESR, leukocytosis and thrombocytosis. Untreated, 15% develop coronary artery aneurysm.

TREATMENT

Discuss with the consultant.

1. Gammaglobulin 400 mg/kg per 24 hours i.v. for 4 days markedly reduces the incidence of coronary artery changes.
2. Aspirin may be indicated; discuss with the consultant.

Viral infections

MEASLES

Prodromal phase may include fever, cough, koplik spots, pharyngitis and conjunctivitis. After 2–4 days, a maculopapular rash develops. Duration of the illness is 14 days. Incubation period is up to 14 days.

Infectivity. Infectivity is from the beginning of the prodromal phase to 7 days from the date of the appearance of the rash.

Complications. Laryngitis, bronchitis, otitis media and pneumonia may develop. Encephalitis (rare) may develop several days after the rash.

Treatment. Paracetamol as required. Antibiotics as indicated for secondary infections such as otitis media and pneumonia.

Immunocompromised child. Specific groups are listed under contraindications to immunisation to live vaccines (see p. 225). If such children come into contact with measles, human normal immunoglobulin should be given as soon as possible after exposure. To prevent an attack give: < 1 year 250 mg; 1–2 years 500 mg; > 3 years 750 mg.

MUMPS

Swollen and tender parotid and salivary glands. Fever and malaise. Illness lasts 7–10 days. Incubation period is 12–21 days.

Infectivity. From 3 days before onset of the illness to 9 days after onset of parotid and salivary gland swellings.

Complications. Meningo-encephalitis. VIII nerve damage. Orchitis is rare.

Treatment. Paracetamol as required.

CHICKEN POX (varicella)

Maculopapular lesions evolving into vesicles. Fever, itching. Incubation period is 14–21 days.

Infectivity. Pre-illness is 5 days. The child should be isolated until 6 days after the last crop of vesicles. Duration of the illness is 5–10 days.

Complications. Meningo-encephalitis, ataxia, pneumonia. Secondary bacterial infection of chicken pox lesions.

Treatment. Paracetamol and antipruritics (e.g. calamine lotion). Antibiotics for secondary bacterial infection.

Immunosuppressed children who have not had chicken pox should receive varicella zoster immunoglobulin (VZIG) (0.2 ml/kg) if there is *any* concern of contact with chicken pox.

Control of infection. See below.

HERPES ZOSTER (Shingles)

Due to reactivation of varicella zoster virus at any time after chicken pox. Spreads to appropriate cutaneous dermatome causing a maculopapular rash evolving into vesicles. Herpes simplex virus can also cause a rash limited to a dermatome. Viral culture will confirm the diagnosis of herpes zoster.

Treatment. Acyclovir should be given to the immunosuppressed person. Immunosuppressed children who have not had chicken pox should receive zoster immune globulin (0.2 ml/kg) following exposure to herpes zoster.

Treat bacterial superinfection, e.g. with augmentin. Neutropenic patients should also receive broad spectrum antibiotics.

Oral corticosteroids are not indicated as post-herpetic neuralgia is rare.

With V cranial nerve involvement, refer to the ophthalmologist due to the possibility of keratoconjunctivitis or uveitis.

Analgesia for pain: initially paracetamol.

RUBELLA (German measles)

Cervical and occipital lymphadenopathy with a generalised macular rash. Illness lasts for 2–5 days. Incubation period is 14–21 days.

Isolate the infected person for 7 days from the onset of rash. Warn parents to advise any pregnant contacts of the child to visit their GP irrespective of previous vaccination.

Treatment. Symptomatic.

Complications. Arthralgia, encephalitis, thrombocytopenia, congenital rubella.

HAND, FOOT AND MOUTH DISEASE

Fever followed by vesicles on the hands, feet and mouth. Incubation period is 1–2 days.

Treatment. Antiseptic mouth toilet may be given.

EPSTEIN–BARR VIRUS (infectious mononucleosis, glandular fever)

Clinical features may include sore throat (often with exudate on tonsils), malaise, fever, lymphadenopathy, splenomegaly, hepatomegaly and jaundice. A maculopapular rash may occur, especially following amoxycillin.

Investigations. FBC and film shows lymphocytosis with atypical lymphocytes. Monospot test is positive after the second week of the illness. Monospot may be negative if < 5 years but patients will have positive serology for EBV.

Treatment. Symptomatic. Illness usually lasts 5–20 days and a prolonged convalescence may be required. Prednisolone is recommended for marked splenomegaly or airway obstruction. Amoxycillin (and ampicillin) is contraindicated.

CYTOMEGALOVIRUS

History and physical findings are similar to EBV infection. Diagnosis is by observing a rise in antibody to CMV or by culture of virus.

Treatment is supportive. (An antiviral agent is available but discuss with the virologist prior to use.)

AIDS

Paediatric HIV infections usually occur in babies born to infected mothers. Such infants have a 30–50% chance of acquiring the infection. HIV infection should be considered in infants of i.v. drug abusers, prostitutes or if the father is a haemophiliac or bisexual. Apart from gammaglobulin, previous receipt of any blood products may have put a child at risk for AIDS. Haemophiliacs treated with factor VIII may be antibody-positive to HIV.

Clinical features

Weight loss, malaise, diarrhoea, persistent oral *Candida*, PUO, lymphadenopathy, splenomegaly, unusual infections and progressive neurological disease are seen. The most common presentation is pneumonia caused by *Pneumocystis carinii*. Unique features of AIDS to the paediatric population include persistent parotitis, lymphoid interstitial pneumonitis and recurrent serious bacterial infections. Kaposi's sarcoma is unusual in childhood.

Diagnosis

Serological testing is required. In children < 15 months it is necessary to repeat any positive antibody tests to eliminate false positive results due to passively acquired maternal antibody. Viral culture and antigen detection may have a role in early diagnosis.

Treatment

There is no definite therapy available for HIV infection at present. Management includes treatment of AIDS associated infection and general support.

Pneumocystis pneumonia is treated with co-trimoxazole or pentamidine. Prophylactic therapy with co-trimoxazole is advised to prevent *Pneumocystis* pneumonia. Because of poor tolerance to co-trimoxazole in some children aerosolised pentamidine (shown to be efficacious in preventing pneumocystic pneumonia in adults) should be considered. Discuss with the consultant.

After exposure to chicken pox or shingles, varicella zoster immunoglobulin should be given. Clinical varicella and herpes may be treated with acyclovir.

The MMR vaccine is currently recommended for HIV-infected children. Use of DPT, *Haem. influenzae*, pneumococcal, inactivated polio and influenza vaccines may be beneficial to HIV-positive children. Breast feeding by HIV positive mothers is inadvisable. Other live vaccines such as oral polio should be avoided.

Fungal infections

Serious localised or systemic fungal infection is most likely to occur in patients who are immunocompromised or who have a serious underlying disease. Treatment with broad spectrum antibiotics and the presence of an indwelling catheter for venous access also predispose to fungal infections.

EXAMINATION

Include inspection of skin and fundi. Cardiac USS may be indicated to exclude endocarditis.

INVESTIGATIONS

If serious fungal infection is suspected, the advice of an infectious disease consultant should be sought.
1. Blood cultures: preferably arterial blood and not via an indwelling catheter.

2. Urine for microscopy and culture; presence of a positive culture and yeasts and hyphae in aspirated bladder urine, in the absence of a urinary catheter or other foreign body, suggest systemic candidiasis.
3. LP; in systemic candidiasis and *Cryptococcus neoformans* infection there is a high incidence of CNS infection.
4. Tissue biopsy; detection of fungi in intestinal or respiratory secretions is common and only indicates mucosal contamination. Biopsy of an intestinal or oesophageal lesion or lung for histological examination and culture is preferred for diagnosis. Mucormycosis is diagnosed by histological examination and culture of affected tissue following biopsy.

TREATMENT

Discuss with the microbiologist and consultant in charge.
1. Almost all systemic fungal infections are susceptible to amphotericin B. If the fungus is sensitive to 5-fluorocytosine (never use alone), this should be used, allowing lower doses of amphotericin B to be used.

     For the amphotericin test dose and infusion doses, see p. 351. Serious hypokalaemia and renal impairment may occur. Monitor serum K^+, creatinine and AST levels regularly. Reduced dose may be required if hypokalaemia, renal or hepatic toxicity occurs.
2. If candidal infection is restricted to the bladder, it may respond to continuous bladder irrigation with amphotericin B.
3. Chronic mucocutaneous candidiasis may be treated with oral ketoconazole. Discuss with the consultant.

Parasitic infections

NB. Infestation with several worms at one time is common.

Eosinophilia. Protozoa do not cause an eosinophilia. Eosinophilia is often the first clue that a helminth infection is present.

   Anaemia is a non-specific finding in parasitic infections and is inconsistent.

Examination for parasites. Helminth ova and protozoal cysts may be identified in old specimens of faeces but warm, fresh specimens are necessary for identification of living forms.

   The presence of erythrocytes in the stool may suggest an amoebic colitis while leukocytes suggest bacterial infection or inflammatory bowel disease and not a parasitic cause.

Serological tests. May be especially helpful with amoebiasis and toxoplasmosis.

PROTOZOAN INFECTIONS

Malaria

Four types of species of *Plasmodium* may infect man by a mosquito bite: *P. falciparum, P. vivax, P. ovale* and *P. malariae.* Diagnosis should be considered in any sick child who may have been exposed.

Clinical features. These are non-specific and include fever, rigors, lethargy, malaise, headaches, muscle and joint ache with or without splenomegaly. In younger children pallor or jaundice may be seen. GI complaints may be prominent. Fever may become periodic once infection is established. The child may appear well between fevers.

Treatment. It is essential to detect malaria caused by *P. falciparum* and treat immediately in hospital until well.

Severely ill patients usually have *P. falciparum* infection and require supportive treatment as needed for complications such as anaemia, convulsions, pulmonary oedema, shock, hyperglycaemia, DIC and renal failure.

Other forms of malaria may be treated as an outpatient. Discuss treatment with microbiologists.

Drug therapy.
1. For all types of malaria, except chloroquine-resistant *P. falciparum*, give chloroquine orally (see p. 353), followed by primaquine for 14 days (0.1 mg/kg 8-hourly), given after chloroquine.
2. For chloroquine-resistant *P. falciparum* or if sensitivity is uncertain; give quinine (see p. 360) for 7 days, followed by Fansidar 1 tablet/20 kg bodyweight once only plus primaquine as above.

NB. Measure blood glucose during quinine therapy as hypoglycaemia may occur. Perform daily parasite counts in severe malaria or if resistance is suspected. Do not use steroids for cerebral malaria.

Prophylaxis. Detailed information may be obtained from Liverpool (051-708 9393), London (071-636 8636), and East Birmingham (021-772 4311), Schools of Tropical Medicine.

Entamoeba histolytica (amoebiasis)

Mild colonic infection may cause diarrhoea alternating with constipation. Amoebic dysentery usually presents with bloody diarrhoea, mild fever, abdominal tenderness and malaise. Appendicitis may occasionally be incorrectly diagnosed. It may affect the liver causing tender enlargement with a filling defect on scan. LFT may show minimal derangement.

Diagnosis. Fresh stool microscopy to demonstrate motile protozoa and minimal leukocytes with erythrocytes. With liver involvement alone, serological tests are very helpful.

Treatment. Metronidazole (see p. 357).

Giardia lamblia (giardiasis)

May cause chronic or recurrent diarrhoea, offensive smelling stools and malabsorption. There may be no symptoms.

Diagnosis. Made by examining fresh, warm stools and duodenal juice.

Treatment. Metronidazole (see p. 357).

Toxoplasma (toxoplasmosis)

Usually asymptomatic. Infection may be congenital or acquired. Neonatal hepatitis, uveitis, retinitis, microcephaly, hydrocephalus, chorio retinitis and mental retardation may result from the former. The latter causes glandular fever-type illness or meningo-encephalitis.

Diagnosis. Check for rising antibody titres. Newborn infections may be diagnosed by demonstration of IgM *Toxoplasma* antibodies or persistence of antibodies beyond 3–4 months.

Treatment. Discuss with an infectious disease specialist.

HELMINTH INFECTIONS

Ascaris lumbricoides (round worms)

Transient lung migration may cause pneumonia with cough, bloody sputum, pulmonary infiltrates and fever (Loeffler's syndrome). Occasionally vague abdominal discomfort and rarely intestinal obstruction and appendicitis seen.

Diagnosis. Larvae may be seen in the sputum and ova in the faeces by direct examination. Eosinophilia is present.

Treatment. Mebendazole; for children > 2 years, see p. 357.

Enterobius vermicularis (thread worm, pin worm)

Very common; perianal itching and vaginitis.

Diagnosis. The worms may be seen in the perianal area or on the surface of faeces. Adhesive tape on the perianal area to collect ova should be done first thing in the morning and repeated up to five times if negative.

Treatment. Mebendazole; see p. 357. Treat the whole household. A therapeutic trial may be indicated if diagnosis is suspected but thread worms are not found.

Ancylostoma duodenale, Necator americanus (hook worm)

Penetration of the skin may cause a papulovesicular eruption. Mild pneumonitis with eosinophilia may develop. Larvae may be found in the sputum. Abdominal cramps and diarrhoea may occur.

Diagnosis. Detection of ova in stools.

Treatment. Mebendazole for children > 2 years; piperazine for children < 2 years; see p. 357.

Trichuris trichiura (whip worm)

Usually asymptomatic; diarrhoea (occasionally bloody) and abdominal pain may occur.

Diagnosis. Demonstration of ova in faeces. Eosinophilia is not present.

Treatment. Mebendazole; see p. 357.

Toxocara canis and toxocara cati (toxocariasis)

History of close contact with dogs or pica. Symptoms may include fever, transient pneumonia, hepatosplenomegaly. Blurred vision with retinal granuloma may occur.

Diagnosis. Fluorescent antibody tests and ELISA. The parasite is rarely demonstrated. Eosinophilia, leukocytosis. Hypergammaglobulinaemia.

Treatment. When required for inpatients with ocular involvement, give thiabendazole (see p. 361); max. 3 g per 24 hours. Ophthalmological opinion is required. Anti-inflammatory agents such as corticosteroids may be needed.

Strongyloides stercoralis

May be asymptomatic or cause diarrhoea and abdominal pain.

Diagnosis. Larvae found in fresh faeces or duodenal aspirate.

Treatment. Thiabendazole; see p. 361.

Trichinella spiralis (trichinosis)

Usually a history of eating pork. Fever, facial and periorbital oedema, headaches, photophobia and conjunctivitis and myalgia may suggest the diagnosis. Signs of encephalitis may occur.

Diagnosis. Marked eosinophilia (after 3 weeks). Serological tests (positive from the third week). Muscle biopsy may show characteristic larvae. Negative biopsy does not rule out diagnosis.

Treatment. Thiabendazole for 5 days; see p. 361.

Beef tape worm

These patients are asymptomatic; segments of tape worm are found in stools.

Treatment. Niclosamide, single dose; see p. 358.

Pork tape worm

Caused by ingestion of pork. Symptoms are rare. Diagnosis is by passage of segments in stools; treatment is as for beef tape worm.

Echinococcus granulosus (hydatid)

Often a history of contact with dogs and sheep. Slow growing and usually asymptomatic but cysts may occur. Serological tests are usually positive. Casoni test is usually positive.

Treatment. Accessible cysts are removed surgically. If surgery is contra-indicated or if cysts spill during surgery mebendazole should be given.

Immunisation (Table 13.3)

No child should be denied immunisation without serious consideration. If in doubt consult 'Immunisation against Infectious Disease' issued by the Department of Health or a local specialist.

Obtain consent and enquire about the child's fitness and suitability before each immunisation. Warn parents of possible side-effects (p. 227) and advise parents on fever control.

NB. Ensure knowledge and facilities are available to deal with anaphylactic shock (see p. 227).

NOTES ON IMMUNISATIONS

1. Give intradermal injections into the site of deltoid insertion. Deep s.c. and i.m. injections should be given into the anterolateral aspect of the thigh or deltoid muscle.
2. Immunise premature babies at 2 months from birth irrespective of prematurity.
3. No opportunity should be missed to immunise children even if they are older than the recommended age. If the course of immunisation is interrupted it should be resumed and completed as soon as possible but not repeated.
4. If more than one live vaccine is needed at the same time, give either simultaneously in different sites (unless a combined preparation is used) or give 3 weeks apart.
5. If immunising children >10 years old against diphtheria, use special adult vaccine.
6. Consider giving pertussis course to unimmunised children < 6 years if in close contact with younger children to whom they may pass the disease.

Table 13.3 UK recommended immunisation schedule

Age	Vaccine	Route	Dose	Notes
Birth	BCG	Intradermal	0.05 ml	For children at high risk of TB, i.e. Asian/ African and those with history of TB in a relative
	Hepatitis B course	Deep s.c. or i.m.	1 ml	For children of Hepatitis B carriers
2 months (1st dose) 3 months (2nd dose) 4 months (3rd dose)	Diphtheria + pertussis + tetanus (DPT) + Hib	Deep s.c.. or i.m.	0.5 ml	Primary immunisation course Diff. limb
12–18 months	Polio	Oral	3 drops	
	Measles + Mumps + Rubella (MMR) + Hib	Deep s.c. or i.m.	0.5 ml	Can be given at any age after 12 months even with a history of measles, mumps or rubella
4–5 years	Diphtheria & + Tetanus	Deep s.c. or i.m.	0.5 ml	Booster doses
	Polio	Oral	3 drops	
10–14 years	Rubella	Deep s.c.	0.3 ml	Girls only unless documented evidence of MMR
	BCG	Intradermal	0.1 ml	Not within 3 weeks of live vaccine Need prior tuberculin skin test
15–18 years	Tetanus	Deep s.c. or i.m.	0.5 ml	Booster
	Polio	Oral	3 drops	

CONTRAINDICATIONS

General

1. Acute febrile illness. A minor infection, e.g. snuffles without fever or systemic upsets, is not a contraindication.
2. Do not give live vaccines (measles, mumps, rubella, oral polio and BCG) to children who:

a.   are on high-dose steroids (> 2 mg/kg per 24 hours for more than 1 week). Postpone until at least 3 months after treatment has stopped.

b.   are on immunosuppressive treatment, e.g. chemotherapy. Do not give until at least 6 months after treatment has stopped.

c.   have malignant disease.

d.   have impaired immunological function, e.g. hypogamma-globulinaemia.

These children should be given injection of immunoglobulin if exposed to chicken pox or measles.

Siblings of such children should have the MMR vaccination, but not oral polio (use inactivated polio instead).

3.   Live vaccines should not be given for 3 months after or 3 weeks before immunoglobulin injection or to pregnant girls.

4.   For HIV patients, seek specialist advice.

Specific

1.   Pertussis:

a.   Absolute contraindications are severe local or general reaction to the preceding dose defined as:

Local: extensive area of redness/swelling which becomes indurated and involves most of the anterolateral surface of the thigh or major part of circumference of the upper arm.

General: fever > 39.5°C within 48 hours, anaphylaxis, broncho-spasm, laryngeal oedema, generalised collapse, prolonged unre-sponsiveness, prolonged inconsolable screaming, convulsions occurring within 72 hours.

b.   The following are not absolute contraindications to immunisation and should be discussed with a consultant so immunisations are not omitted: children with cerebral damage in the neonatal period, personal history of convulsions, family history of idiopathic epilepsy.

2.   Polio:

a.   Vomiting or diarrhoea.

b.   Do not give if the child is in contact with an immunosuppressed child; give inactivated polio vaccine instead.

3.   Measles:

a.   Severe egg allergy (may cause anaphylaxis).

b.   Allergy to neomycin or kanamycin.

4.   Rubella:

a.   Pregnancy.

b.   Allergy to neomycin/polymyxin.

5.   BCG:

a.   Positive tuberculin skin test. Refer all for further investigation and supervision (see p. 212).

b.   Generalised septic skin conditions.

6.   Tetanus:

Severe reaction to a previous dose (defined as for pertussis).

ADVERSE REACTIONS

Diphtheria/pertussis/tetanus

Pain, redness and swelling around the injection site, mild malaise and pyrexia lasting 1–2 days after injection. Persistent nodules can occur if injection is not given deeply enough.

There is no conclusive evidence that pertussis vaccine can cause permanent brain damage.

Polio

One recipient and one contact case of paralytic polio in 2 million doses of the vaccine. Advise strict personal hygiene for contacts of recent vaccines, particularly for washing their hands after changing napkins.

Measles

Malaise, fever and/or rash 7 days after injection lasting 2–3 days. Febrile convulsions in 1/1000 children (much lower rate than that accompanying naturally acquired illness).

Mumps

Parotid swelling in 1% 21 days after injection. Mumps meningoencephalitis in 1/400 000 doses.

Rubella

Mild rubella-like illness and arthralgia 1–3 weeks after vaccination. Self limiting thrombocytopenia.

ANAPHYLAXIS

Recipients of vaccine should remain under observation until they have been seen to recover from the procedure. It is not possible to specify an exact length of time.

Symptoms

1. Pallor, limpness and apnoea.
2. Upper airway obstruction: hoarseness and stridor as a result of angio-oedema involving hypopharynx, epiglottis and larynx.
3. Lower airway obstruction: dyspnoea and wheeze.
4. Cardiovascular: sinus tachycardia, profound hypotension in association with tachycardia, severe bradycardia.
5. Skin: characteristic rapid development of urticarial lesions.

Management

1. Lie in the left lateral position. If unconscious, insert airway.
2. Give 1/1000 adrenaline by deep i.m. injection. (< 1 year 0.05 ml; 1 year 0.1 ml; 2 years 0.2 ml; 3–4 years 0.3 ml; 5 years 0.4 ml; 6–10 years 0.5 ml) unless the patient's condition is good and there is a strong central pulse.

3. O_2 by facemask.
4. Send for help; never leave the patient alone.
5. If appropriate, begin cardiopulmonary resuscitation.
6. Chlorpheniramine maleate (Piriton) 2.5–5 mg and hydro-cortisone 100 mg may be given i.v.
7. If there is no improvement in the patient's condition in 10 min repeat the dose of adrenaline up to a max. of 3 doses.
8. All cases should be admitted to hospital for observation.

Treatment of patients with tetanus-prone wounds

The following are considered tetanus-prone wounds:
1. A wound or burn sustained more than 6 hours before surgical treatment.
2. Any wound or burn that shows any of the following: puncture-type wound, clinical evidence of sepsis, contact with soil or manure, devitalised tissue.

NB. Thorough surgical toilet of the wound is essential whatever the tetanus immunisation history of the patient.

SPECIFIC ANTI-TETANUS TREATMENT

1. If the last of the three-dose course of tetanus vaccine or rein-forcing dose was within the last 10 years:
   a. if the wound is clean, no treatment;
   b. if the wound is tetanus-prone, a dose of absorbed vaccine may be given if risk of infection is especially high; otherwise, no treatment.
2. If the last of the three-dose course of tetanus vaccine or reinforcing dose was more than 10 years previously:
   a. if the wound is clean, give a reinforcing dose of adsorbed vaccine;
   b. if the wound is tetanus-prone, give a reinforcing dose of adsorbed vaccine plus a dose of human tetanus immunoglobulin.
3. If not immunised or immunisation status is not known with certainty:
   a. give a full three-dose course of adsorbed vaccine if the wound is clean;
   b. if the wound is tetanus-prone give a full three-dose course of vaccine plus a dose of human tetanus immunoglobulin in a different site.

NB. Patients with impaired immunity who suffer a tetanus-prone wound may not respond to vaccine and may require anti-tetanus immunoglobulin in addition.

Dose of anti-tetanus immunoglobin. Prevention: 250 iu, or 500 iu i.m. if more than 24 hours have elapsed since the injury, if contamination is heavy and for burns.

14

Haematology and oncology

See Table A.2 (p. 363) for normal values. Hb reaches its lowest level at 3 months and 'physiological' hypochromia and microcytosis are seen at 1 year.

History
1. Overt blood loss — epistaxis, haematemesis, haematuria, blood in stools
2. Dietary assessment
3. Steatorrhoea, previous surgery or recent GI infection which might explain malabsorption
4. Chronic infection or inflammation
5. Drugs — especially cytotoxics, antibiotics, antimalarial, anticonvulsants, analgesics
6. Symptoms of anaemia — lethargy, tiredness, shortage of breath on exertion

Examination
1. Conjunctivae for pallor. Always measure Hb.
2. Stomatitis and koilonychia are rare in childhood.
3. Jaundice.
4. Bruising or petechiae.
5. Hepatosplenomegaly.
6. Signs of cardiac failure.
7. Signs of malabsorption/FTT.

HYPOCHROMIC ANAEMIA

See Table 14.1 for causes. Remember, MCV and iron indices are age-dependent (see Tables A.2 (p. 363) and 14.2)

Iron deficiency anaemia

Background. The commonest cause of anaemia in childhood. Causes are:
1. Dietary deficiency — commonest cause, particularly in families of lower socioeconomic class. Also, infants

Table 14.1 Causes of hypochromic anaemia

Disorder	MCV	Serum iron	Serum ferritin	TIBC	Hb electrophoresis
Iron deficiency	↓	↓	↓	↑	N
Beta thalassaemia major	↓	↑	↑	N	↑ HbF (> 90%) and HbA₂ (> 3.5%)
Beta thalassaemia minor (trait)	↓	N	N	N	↑ HbA₂ (> 3.5%) and half have increased HbF (> 1% after 6 months of age)
Anaemia of chronic disorder	↓/N	↓	↑/N	↓	N
Sideroblastic anaemia	↑/↓ or dimorphic	↑	↑	N	N

Note 1. In addition to sideroblastic anaemia, other causes of a dimorphic blood film are:
   a.   recent blood transfusion
   b.   mixed iron and folate/vitamin B₁₂ deficiency
   c.   chronic haemolysis and secondary folate deficiency
2.   Coexistent iron deficiency and beta thalassaemia trait may result in a normal HbA₂ (2–3.5%). If in doubt, treat with iron for 3 months and repeat Hb electrophoresis. Correct diagnosis is important to avoid unnecessary iron treatment and for genetic counselling.

weaned after 6 months, toddlers who dislike meat and vegetables, and ethnic minorities.

Iron deficiency itself leads to anorexia.

2.   Increased demand — prematurity, multiple birth, adolescence.

3.   Blood loss — neonatal: antepartum haemorrhage, twin-to-twin transfusion, fetomaternal haemorrhage.

   — Older child: usually GI, including reflux oesophagitis.

4.   Malabsorption — coeliac disease, cow's milk intolerance, inflammatory bowel disease, post-gastroenteritis. The latter three may also involve blood loss.

Table 14.2 Normal iron indices for various ages

Age	Serum iron (μmol/l) Mean (range)	Serum ferritin (μg/l) Mean (range)	TIBC (μmol/l) Mean (range)
1 month	22 (10–30)	250 (150–350)	36 (28–44)
6 months	15 (5–25)	30 (14–200)	58 (48–66)
1 year	14 (5–25)	30 (12–250)	64 (56–70)
5 years	22 (11–34)	40 (18–250)	64 (56–70)

Note: Serum ferritin is proportional to amounts of storage iron and less vulnerable than serum iron to daily fluctuation and the influence of concurrent illness.

Management

1. Blood for Hb, iron studies (Table 14.2) and blood film. Often there is associated thrombocytosis. Screen non-white children for haemoglobinopathy at same time (see p. 237).
2. If iron deficiency anaemia is confirmed, give 2 mg/kg elemental iron per 24 hours in 3 divided doses for 3 months. Warn that the stools will appear dark.
3. Check Hb, iron, reticulocytes and film after 1 month (to confirm compliance and response) but do not expect complete resolution until 3 months' iron therapy is completed. Temper and appetite often improve with treatment. Continue iron for another 3 months after normal Hb levels are achieved.
4. Transfusion is only rarely necessary (see p. 240).
5. If response to iron is poor, either poor compliance (iron may cause constipation or diarrhoea) or the cause is not dietary deficiency. Consider the following investigations:
   a. urinalysis
   b. ESR
   c. faecal occult blood
   d. barium swallow and meal
   e. jejunal biopsy
   f. bone marrow examination

   and see pp 232–240 for the possibility of another anaemia coexisting with iron deficiency.

Prophylaxis. In all premature infants, start Sytron 10 drops per 24 hours at 1 month of age until weaned onto solids.

HAEMOLYTIC ANAEMIA

Background

Aetiology — *physiological*: in the newborn, haemolysis of cells containing HbF.

— *pathological* (Table 14.3): isoimmune is commonest in the newborn and viral-induced autoimmune is commonest in older children.

Diagnosis

Family history, drug history and ethnic origin are important.
   Splenomegaly is found in association with haemolysis in:
      spherocytosis
      early in sickle cell disease (later splenic atrophy)
      thalassaemias
      malaria
      glandular fever
and hypersplenism of any cause (e.g. malignancy, portal hypertension).

   Laboratory investigations are necessary for accurate diagnosis. Consider the following scheme:

Table 14.3   Classification of haemolytic anaemias

Intrinsic red cell defects
Abnormal membrane
    spherocytosis (autosomal dominant)
    elliptocytosis
Abnormal haemoglobin
    sickle cell disease
    thalassaemias
Enzyme deficiency
    G6PD (X-linked)
    pyruvate kinase

Extrinsic problems
Immune (DCT usually positive)
    Isoimmune: maternal antibodies affect fetal and neonatal red cells
                    ABO incompatibility
                    Rhesus incompatibility
                    other rare atypical antibodies

    Autoimmune: *warm antibody type* — mostly IgG
                    idiopathic
                    drugs (e.g. penicillin)
                    autoimmune diseases (e.g. SLE, chronic active
                    hepatitis, inflammatory bowel disease)
                    lymphoma
            cold antibody type — mostly IgM
                    idiopathic
                    infectious (infectious mononucleosis,
                    mycoplasma, CMV, rubella)
                    paroxysmal cold haemoglobinuria
                    lymphoma
Malaria
Microangiopathic
    HUS
    DIC
Hypersplenism

Investigations

1. Is there increased red cell destruction?
    a.   FBC — low Hb
    b.   elevated unconjugated bilirubin
    c.   elevated urinary urobilinogen
    d.   reduced plasma haptoglobins
2. Is there increased red cell production?
    FBC — polychromasia, macrocytosis due to retulocytosis (> 4%)
3. Is the haemolysis mainly intravascular?
    a.   free plasma Hb
    b.   haemoglobinuria or haemosiderin in urine (if chronic)
    c.   schistocytes, burr cells or helmet cells suggesting micro-angiopathy. U & E for HUS
    d.   thrombocytopenia and abnormal clotting suggests DIC

    e.   pancytopenia suggests hypersplenism

4. Why are the RBCs being destroyed?

    a.   genetic cause:

        (i) RBC morphology — spherocytes, elliptocytes. Although spherocytosis is autosomal dominant, family history may be negative because of variable expressions. The osmotic fragility test may be normal in the newborn and spherocytes may not be present. Therefore, repeat at 3 months

        (ii) haemoglobinopathy (see Table 14.7)

        (iii) enzymopathy — red cell pyruvate kinase assay, G6PD deficiency screen. Both may cause neonatal jaundice. In G6PD deficiency (X-linked), drugs may precipitate haemolysis (Table 14.4) and very rarely a girl may be homozygous.

    b.   acquired:

        (i) immune— positive DCT (although may be negative in ABO incompatibility). Determine blood groups and rhesus status of mother and infant.

        (ii) infection — bacterial cultures, viral serology, mycoplasma antibodies, monospot, thick film malarial parasites.

        (iii) paroxysmal nocturnal haemoglobinuria — Ham's acid lysis test.

Treatment

See Ch. 19 for phototherapy and exchange transfusion.

Outside the newborn period, treat the cause and transfuse only if Hb is < 7 g/dl or in cardiac failure.

MACROCYTIC ANAEMIAS

Background

The causes are shown in Table 14.5.

Table 14.4 Precipitants of haemolysis in G6PD deficiency

Drugs or toxins
    Aspirin
    Chloramphenicol
    Chloroquine
    Dapsone
    Fava beans
    Nalidixic acid
    Nitrofurantoin
    Primaquine
    Quinine
    Sulphonamides (including co-trimoxazole)
    Vitamins C and K
Most bacterial and viral infections

Folate deficiency may occur by the age of 3 months whereas congenital vitamin B_{12} malabsorption may not present until 3 years. Acquired vitamin B_{12} malabsorption ('juvenile pernicious anaemia') occurs after 8 years of age.

Diagnosis

Enquire about diet, past medical history and family history. Examine for enlargement of liver, spleen or thyroid. Neurological signs are rarely found in childhood vitamin B_{12} deficiency.

Consider the following:

Investigations

1. FBC for white cell and platelet count.
2. Film for appearance of polymorphs and reticulocyte count.
3. Unconjugated bilirubin — haemolysis is associated with vitamin B_{12} deficiency and causes a reticulocytosis.
4. Serum vitamin B_{12} level (normal 150–1000 ng/l). Schilling test assesses radioactive vitamin B_{12} absorption (with and without intrinsic factor) by measuring urinary excretion following an oral dose.

Table 14.5 Causes of macrocytic anaemia

Cause	Other features
Vitamin B_{12} deficiency	Often hypersegmented neutrophils.
	May be leukopenia or thrombocytopenia
Congenital malabsorption	Autosomal recessive
	No intrinsic factor antibodies
	May be associated immunodeficiency
Juvenile pernicious anaemia	Intrinsic factor antibodies
	May be other autoimmune disease
Disease of terminal ileum	Congenital short gut
	Surgery
	Crohn's disease
	Rarely coeliac disease
Deficient dietary intake	Often vegetarian, or a diet deficient in protein, fruit and vegetables
Folic acid deficiency	Usually poor diet deficient in protein, folate and vitamin C
	Trimethoprim may interfere with folate metabolism in premature infants
	Also anticonvulsants
Liver disease	Target cells on blood film
Hypothyroidism	Target cells on blood film
Reticulocytosis	Polychromasia and other evidence of haemolysis on blood film (reticulocytes are larger cells)
Aplastic anaemia	Associated leukopenia and thrombocytopenia
Rare metabolic disorders	Lesch–Nyhan syndrome, orotic aciduria (urea cycle disorder)

Remember that MCV is age-dependent (Table A.2, p. 363)

5. Intrinsic factor autoantibodies.
6. Serum (normal 3–20 ng/ml) and red cell folate levels (normal 100–650 ng/ml).
7. Tests for generalised malabsorption if ileal disease is suspected.

Treatment

Improved diet. Congenital and acquired pernicious anaemia require lifelong treatment with monthly i.m. vitamin B_{12} injections (weekly initially until Hb is normal). Folic acid should *not* be given.

NORMOCYTIC ANAEMIAS

Up to 20% of iron deficiency anaemias are accompanied by a normal blood film. The majority of normocytic anaemias are secondary to another disease (Table 14.6) and the reticulocyte count is usually low. The picture may be more complicated because of associated iron deficiency, either because of poor dietary intake (chronic diseases often associated with anorexia or malabsorption) or chronic blood loss (e.g. varices in liver disease, inflammatory

Table 14.6   Causes of normocytic anaemia

Acute haemorrhage
Renal disease
Liver disease
Hypothyroidism
Chronic infection (osteomyelitis, CSF shunt infection, TB, SBE)
Chronic inflammation (JRA, SLE, inflammatory bowel disease)
Marrow failure
    Aplasia or hypoplasia. May affect white cell and platelet precursors also.
        Congenital — Blackfan–Diamond syndrome
                  — Fanconi's anaemia
        Acquired — idiopathic (commonest)
              — radiation
              — drugs (cytotoxics, chloramphenicol, carbimazole, phenytoin, sulphonamides)
              — toxins (benzenes, carbon tetrachloride, glue sniffing)
              — during or after infections (parvovirus, severe bacterial or viral infection)
              — autoimmune
    Malignant infiltration. The commonest are:
        leukaemia
        lymphoma
        neuroblastoma
    Storage diseases
        cystinosis
        Gaucher's disease
        Niemann–Pick disease
        osteopetrosis (marble bone disease)

bowel disease — thrombocytosis $> 450 \times 10^9/l$ with iron deficiency suggests chronic blood loss).

ESR is often raised. Other causes of a very high ESR (> 50 mm/h) are:

chronic infection (especially osteomyelitis and SBE)

chronic inflammation (especially JRA, SLE, polyarteritis nodosa)

malignancy

OTHER RED CELL APPEARANCES

In addition to hypochromic, haemolytic, macrocytic and normocytic blood films, rare abnormalities are:

1. Target cells — severe iron deficiency
    — sickle disease
    — thalassaemia
    — liver disease
    — post-splenectomy or asplenia syndrome
2. Heinz bodies (intracellular globin precipitate). This results in increased RBC rigidity and decreased RBC survival
    — G6PD deficiency
    — haemoglobinopathies
    — post-splenectomy or asplenia syndrome
3. Howell–Jolly bodies (intracellular DNA fragments)
    — haemoglobinopathies
    — post-splenectomy or asplenia syndrome
    — leukaemia
    — cytotoxic drugs
    — severe vitamin B_{12} or folate deficiency
4. Reticulocytosis (see Table A.2 (p. 363) for age dependence). Implies an active marrow
    — haemolytic anaemia
    — chronic bleeding (often accompanied by thrombocytosis)
    — response to iron, vitamin B_{12} or folate treatment

HAEMOGLOBINOPATHIES

Sickle cell disease

Background. Heterozygotes have 'sickle trait'; homozygotes have 'sickle disease'. Sickle disease does not cause problems in the newborn because HbF does not contain beta chains. Occurs in children whose families originate from Africa or the West Indies.

Diagnosis

1. Clinically suspected because of pallor, hepatomegaly and/or splenomegaly (only if detected before 8 years) and/or jaundice or one of the crises (see management). Usually present between 3 months and 6 years.

2. Screen before surgery, all Afro-Caribbean children with anaemia, or those whose parents have the disease or trait.
   Screening tests include:
   a. Prenatal diagnosis possible from fetal red cells or liquor fibroblasts.
   b. Neonatal diagnosis by Hb electrophoresis. Repeated at 6 months.
   c. Older child (i) RBCs become sickle shaped under low O_2 tension, e.g. thiocyanate test.
   (ii) 'Solubility test': RBCs sickle following addition of sodium metabisulphite.
   These 'sickling tests' are positive in both trait and disease.
   (iii) Hb electrophoresis distinguishes trait from disease.

Clinical diagnosis

'Sickle trait'. Hb may be 10–12 g/dl, sickling test is positive but film is normal.

Hb electrophoresis shows HbA and HbS. Asymptomatic unless hypoxic (e.g. altitude, anaesthesia). Examination normal. Do *not* treat with iron.

'Sickle disease'. Hb 5–9 g/dl, reticulocytes > 10%, sickled cells, target cells, Howell-Jolly bodies on blood film, positive sickling test, Hb electrophoresis shows HbS but no HbA with variable HbF (the more, the milder the disease).

1. *Pneumococcal infection* — susceptible because of 'autosplenectomy' (recurrent infarction). Should receive pneumococcal vaccine and prophylactic penicillin until adulthood. Also at risk of *Salmonella* osteomyelitis.
2. *Painful crisis* — infarction of bone, joint, spleen or lung. May be precipitated by infection. Papillary necrosis of the kidneys may occur with haematuria and renal failure.
3. *Aplastic crisis* — marrow failure usually secondary to infection, often parvovirus. Anaemia but no reticulocytosis.
4. *Haemolytic crisis* — acute or chronic haemolysis with jaundice, anaemia and reticulocytosis.
5. *Megaloblastic crisis* — folate deficiency complicating chronic haemolysis.
6. *Hepatic crisis* — pigment stones/inspissation causes obstructive jaundice.
7. *Sequestration crisis* — Hb falls because of pooling in spleen rather than marrow failure or haemolysis. The child may be shocked. There is splenomegaly and reticulocytosis.

Management

Prevention: avoid hypoxia, chilling, dehydration
             seek early treatment of infection

regular folate 1 mg/day

pneumococcal vaccine and prophylactic penicillin.

Not regular blood transfusions.

Acute crises: many are precipitated by infection and exacerbated by dehydration.

broad spectrum antibiotics after blood cultures

i.v. fluids; avoid hypotension

keep warm and give analgesia

correct hypoxia and acidosis

transfuse only if dangerous fall in Hb, or shocked in sequestration crisis, with *warmed, fresh blood* until Hb 7 g/dl.

Estimate size of spleen, Hb, reticulocytes daily.

The sickle gene may occur in association with other haemoglobinopathies (Table 14.7) but still only in Afro-Caribbean families.

BETA THALASSAEMIA

Background

Heterozygotes need no treatment (and should not receive iron) but

Table 14.7 The haemoglobinopathies

Haemoglobinopathy	Hb electrophoresis	HbF (%)	HbA$_2$(%)
Normal	HbA predominates	< 2	< 3
Sickle disease (homozygote)	HbS predominates HbA absent	5–20	< 3
Sickle trait (heterozygote)	HbA present HbS present	< 2	< 3
Sickle/C disease	HbC present HbS present	< 2	< 3
S beta thalassaemia	HbS predominates HbA absent	2–30	< 3
Beta thalassaemia major (homozygote)	HbF predominates HbA absent or diminished	10–90	< 8
Beta thalassaemia minor (heterozygote)	HbA predominates	< 8	< 10
Alpha thalassaemia 4-gene deletion	Hb Barts (tetramer of gamma chains) Usually lethal in utero		
3-gene deletion	HbH (tetramer of beta chains) Severe haemolytic anaemia		
1- or 2-gene deletion	HbA predominates 10% Hb Barts at birth Microcytic, hypochromic film	< 2	< 3

homozygotes are transfusion dependent. Occurs in children from the Mediterranean, the Indian subcontinent. Is *not* a cause of neonatal jaundice but homozygotes usually present by 1 year.

Diagnosis

1. Clinically, thalassaemia major shows severe anaemia, jaundice, gross hepatosplenomegaly and even cardiac failure. Later, stunted growth and frontal bossing.
2. Screening of at-risk racial groups with anaemia, FTT or prior to surgery (see Table 14.7).
    In thalassaemia minor, the film may be hypochromic microcytic; in thalassaemia major, this is accompanied by reticulocytosis.

Management of thalassaemia major

1. Regular transfusion to keep Hb 8–10 g/dl.
2. Desferrioxamine 400 mg i.v. at the end of each transfusion to delay iron overload.
        Consider daily s.c. maintenance desferrioxamine.
3. Folic acid supplements but *not* iron.
4. Splenectomy if hypersplenism is causing pancytopenia.
    Give pneumococcal vaccine 0.5 ml *before* splenectomy.

The other haemoglobinopathies in Table 14.7 are all rare in the UK but the alpha thalassaemias may cause neonatal haemolytic jaundice, unlike the beta thalassaemias and sickle disease.

Blood transfusion

INDICATIONS

Acute haemorrhage (see Ch. 2)

Whether to transfuse, and the rate and volume, depend on pulse and BP *not* the Hb concentration which will be normal initially. Take blood for FBC and crossmatch, and give *fresh O negative CMV-negative* uncrossmatched blood if there is life-threatening haemorrhage.

Anaemia (see Table A.2 (p. 363) for age dependence)

Transfuse if:

1. cardiac failure is attributed to anaemia — give packed cells more slowly (see below) with frusemide 0.5 mg/kg i.v. midway through transfusion.
2. Hb < 6 g/dl in chronic iron deficiency.
3. Hb < 8 g/dl in marrow failure, recent cytotoxic therapy or thalassaemia major, as Hb is likely to fall further.
4. PCV < 40% and O_2 or ventilator dependent.

5. Hb < 9 g/dl and surgery is urgently indicated. Do not transfuse if surgery is elective — defer operation and find and treat the cause.

Transfusion should be considered at higher Hb values if there are ongoing losses which are likely to continue, e.g. GI bleeding. Do *not* transfuse for chronic anaemias if another treatment is available, even if it takes longer to work.

RATE AND VOLUME OF TRANSFUSION (see above)

For elective transfusion:
1. volume of packed cells required (ml) = weight (kg) × 3 × desired rise in Hb (g/dl)
2. if whole blood is used (ml) = weight (kg) × 5 × desired rise in Hb (g/dl)
   In both cases, rate = 3 ml/kg/h

Circulating blood volume is approx. 80 ml/kg body weight.
   Transfusions of more than 25 ml/kg are rarely indicated except in acute haemorrhage.

COMPLICATIONS

1. Haemolytic transfusion reactions — due to antigen/antibody incompatibility. Fever, rigors, haemoglobinuria. Stop the transfusion and given generous i.v. fluids to avoid renal failure.
2. Febrile non-haemolytic reactions — fever, rigors, urticarial rash, particularly following repeated transfusions, and especially with white cell or platelet transfusions. Stop the transfusion and give 2 mg/kg hydrocortisone i.v. (may cause intense perineal itching) and 0.2 mg/kg chlorpheniramine i.v. In some children, this complication cannot be avoided (but try leukocyte-poor blood or use blood or platelet filter) and the transfusion must be continued.
3. Massive transfusion — hyperkalaemia, hypocalcaemia, acidosis, hypothermia and DIC are all risks.
4. Transmission of infection — now probably the most serious hazard of trivial transfusion.
   a. HIV screening of donor blood generally tests for antibody positivity and there is a variable latent period between viral infection in the donor and seroconversion. HIV antibody tests have a false negative rate of up to 2% (i.e. blood is infected but the test is negative). Blood products (e.g. FFP) may be pooled from thousands of donors, increasing the risk further.
   b. Hepatitis B is screened for but not non-A, non-B.
   c. CMV can be transmitted by transfusion and cause life-

threatening illness in the immunosuppressed. Therefore, use only CMV-negative blood for:

(i) neonates

(ii) children with malignancies

(iii) children receiving immunosuppressive drugs

(iv) children with congenital or acquired immuno-deficiency

(v) children awaiting transplantation

If blood transfusion is *vital* and no CMV-negative blood is immediately available, use a white cell filter.

d. Bacterial contamination can occur, or gain entry via the vascular access, and malaria can also be transmitted.

5. Circulatory overload and pulmonary oedema — slow the rate of transfusion, give frusemide 1mg/kg i.v., increase PEEP if on IPPV.

Always ask yourself
1. Is this transfusion necessary?
2. Is there an alternative? e.g. waiting for oral haematinics to work or using a synthetic colloid of human albumin (which has a lower risk of infection or reaction than blood) solution to expand intravascular volume; although obviously this does not alter O_2 carrying capacity, it may dramatically improve O_2 delivery to tissues by improving perfusion.

Polycythaemia

BACKGROUND

The causes are listed in Table 14.8.

See Table A.2 (p. 363) for age dependency. The danger of a high Hb is that hyperviscosity is associated with poor perfusion and cerebral, renal or inferior vena cava thrombosis.

CLINICAL DIAGNOSIS

1. Plethora may be confused with cyanosis and true cyanosis may be detectable with a normal PaO_2 if Hb is very high. There may be cyanosis because of CHD.

2. In the newborn, cerebral irritability, PFC and jaundice may be present.

Table 14.8 Causes of polycythaemia

In the newborn
> Delayed cord clamping
> SGA infant
> Macrosomic infant of diabetic mother
> Twin-to-twin transfusion
> Maternofetal transfusion

In the older child
> Cyanotic CHD
> Chronic hypoxia of any other cause, including living at altitude and chronic obstructive sleep apnoea
> Associated with malignancies, including phaeochromocytoma and cerebellar haemangioblastoma
> Following renal transplant and occasionally with other renal abnormalities

MANAGEMENT

Newborn

Measure the PCV on an arterial sample which has been centrifuged at 3000 rpm for 10 min. If PCV > 72% (or > 65% if symptomatic), perform partial exchange transfusion (infuse 20 ml/kg plasma or normal saline via a peripheral vein whilst removing 20 ml/kg blood from a peripheral arterial line; perform over 30 min; infuse 10 ml before beginning withdrawal).

Older child

Look for the cause. Correct concurrent iron deficiency.

Platelets and coagulation

BRUISING AND BLEEDING

Background

Causes of abnormal bleeding are given in Table 14.9. The commonest cause of bruising is trauma.

Diagnosis

In the neonatal period, the commonest causes are:
1. Trauma — especially very immature or breech
2. Thrombocytopenia
    a. passive transfer of maternal antibody — ITP, ATP, SLE
    b. sepsis — with or without DIC; thrombocytopenia associated with low grade bacteraemia from indwelling catheters
    c. congenital infection
    d. rare syndromes and inherited thrombocytopenias

Table 14.9 Causes of abnormal bleeding

A. *Abnormality of the platelets*
1. Thrombocytopenia
   (a) Decreased production — generalised bone marrow failure (see Table 14.6)
   — specific megakaryocyte failure, usually following viral infection (including congenital) but also inherited forms or associated with syndromes
   (b) Increased destruction — immunological (ITP or ATP)
   — DIC (including HUS)
   — Kasabach–Merritt syndrome (giant haemangioma)
   — hypersplenism
   — Wiskott–Aldrich syndrome (eczema and prone to infection)
2. Normal platelet count
   Abnormal platelet function — Von Willebrand's disease

B. *Abnormality of clotting factors*
1. Decreased or abnormal production — vitamin K deficiency, malabsorption, liver disease and warfarin all deplete factors II, VII, IX, X
   — haemophilia A and Von Willebrand's disease (factor VIII)
   — haemophilia B (factor IX), i.e. Christmas disease
2. Antagonism — heparin
3. Consumption — DIC (including HUS)

C. *Abnormality of vascular endothelium*
1. HSP
2. Infections, especially meningococcaemia (may be DIC also)

---

3. Clotting problem
   a. haemorrhagic disease of the newborn (vitamin K deficiency, usually breastfed)
   b. haemophilia (only rarely presents in the neonatal period)

In the older child, all causes in Table 14.9 are possible.

History
1. Blood loss currently or after dentistry, circumcision, tonsillectomy
2. Bruising and degree of trauma
3. Diet
4. Steatorrhoea
5. Drugs (especially cytotoxics)
6. Recent viral infection (may precipitate ITP or HSP)

Table 14.10   Interpretation of common coagulation tests

	PT	PTT	TT
Vitamin K deficiency Liver disease Warfarin	Prolonged	Normal	Normal
Haemophilia A Haemophilia B Von Willebrand's disease	Normal	Prolonged	Normal
Heparin (reptilase time normal) DIC (raised FDPs, thrombocytopenia)	Prolonged Prolonged	Very prolonged Prolonged	Prolonged Prolonged

Examination

1. Coincident anaemia or infection
2. Characteristic extensor and lower limb pattern of HSP, often with arthropathy
3. Signs of meningitis, liver disease, splenomegaly
4. Pattern of bleeding
   a. abnormality of platelets — spontaneous petechiae or purpura, epistaxis, GI or GU tract, fundi and intracranial bleeding
   b. abnormality of clotting factors — larger skin bruises following trivial trauma, bleeding into muscles or joints
   c. vasculitis — the purpura is *palpable*

Investigation

Summarised in Fig. 14.1 and Table 14.10. Labs use their own controls or normal ranges. Most clotting times are longer in premature and even healthy neonates.

Bleeding time.   Useful but rarely performed as requires coopera-

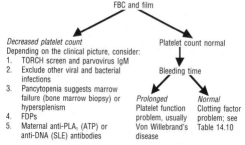

Fig. 14.1   Investigation of bleeding problem

tion. Normally ≤ 8 min. Prolonged in thrombocytopenia and Von Willebrand's disease. In the latter, family history may be negative but diagnosis is confirmed by low factor VIII activity, low factor VIII antigen level, decreased platelet aggregation.

Prothrombin time (PT). Principally assesses *extrinsic path* and prolonged by deficiencies of factors II, V, VII, X, fibrinogen.

Partial thromboplastin time (PTT). Principally assesses *intrinsic path* and prolonged by heparin and deficiencies of factors II, V, VIII, IX, X, XI, XII.

Thrombin time (TT). Assesses final common pathway and prolonged principally by abnormalities in the amount or activity of fibrinogen, i.e. heparin, FDPs, hypofibrinogenaemia. The TT with reptilase is usually normal in the presence of heparin but much higher in DIC than the TT without reptilase. The TT with reptilase is usually normal in the presence of heparin but much higher in DIC than the TT without reptilase.

Management

Often controversial and depends on the cause but the following are important guides:

Thrombocytopenia

1. Platelet transfusion is of more value in decreased production rather than increased consumption. One unit should raise the count by 20×10^9/l/m^2 in the former and the incremental count 30 min after the end of transfusion is helpful in diagnosing rapid consumption.
2. Platelet transfusion is indicated in any thrombocytopenic disorder if there is active bleeding, or prior to surgery (but not bone marrow biopsy); or if the platelet count is $< 10 \times 10^9$/l (unless ITP) or $< 20 \times 10^9$/l in the febrile neutropenic child. Platelets are not crossmatched but a donor from the same ABO group is used.
3. No treatment has been shown convincingly to alter morbidity or mortality in ITP although several transiently increase the platelet count:
    a. platelet transfusion — very transient response. Not recommended unless there is active bleeding
    b. oral prednisolone 2 mg/kg per 24 hours for 5 days
    c. human immunoglobulin ('Sandoglobulin') 0.4 g/kg per 24 hours by iv. infusion for 5 days

The latter two are usually only considered if platelets $< 5 \times 10^9$/l and after bone marrow examination has excluded leukaemia (extremely rare as a cause of isolated thrombocytopenia).
4. In neonatal ATP, maternal platelets can be given.

Abnormality of clotting factors

1. If vitamin K deficiency is possibly contributory, give i.v. vitamin K (300 µg/kg/day slowly to max. 10 mg).

2. If there is active bleeding and the exact diagnosis is unclear, give FFP 10ml/kg i.v. over 30 min.

3. DIC implies a triad of thrombocytopenia, abnormal clotting times and elevated FDPs. There is simultaneous overactivity of thombosis and fibrinolysis with consumption of platelets and clotting factors, abnormal bleeding and sometimes an associated microangiopathic haemolytic anaemia.

   Treatment of DIC remains controversial. Platelets and FFP should be given as sparingly as possible. If haemorrhage is significant, give 15 ml/kg FFP i.v., 4 u/m^2 platelets and cryoprecipitate i.v. if fibrinogen concentration < 100 mg/dl. Sepsis or profound shock are the commonest causes of DIC.

4. In haemophilia A, factor VIII concentrate is currently preferred to cryoprecipitate because of the lower risk of HIV. Level of factor VIII in the affected child's blood is < 20% but does not require treatment unless there is clinical bleeding.

> Units of factor VIII required = weight (kg) × % rise in factor
> VIII desired

Aim for level of 15% in superficial bleeding or haemarthroses and 100% in head injuries (even if no clinical sign of bleeding). Always admit head injuries. Factor VIII half-life = 12 hours. Counsel parents that there will be, on average, 35 bleeding episodes/year and arrange hepatitis B vaccination.

Vasculitis. There is no treatment for HSP except adequate analgesia. Haematuria and arthropathy are not indications for admission necessarily but abdominal pain is.

THROMBOCYTOSIS

The causes are:
1. Increased production — infection
   — haemorrhage
   — Kawasaki's disease
   — bone marrow malignancy
2. Decreased destruction — after splenectomy

Platelet counts $> 1000 \times 10^9/l$ may cause bleeding or thrombosis. Thrombocytosis in Kawasaki's disease is one of the few remaining paediatric indications for aspirin.

Oncology

Background

Commonest childhood cancers are leukaemias 35% (mostly ALL), lymphomas 10%, CNS tumours 25%, neuroblastoma 5%, Wilms' tumour 5%. Only leukaemias and lymphomas are dealt with in this chapter (see relevant chapters for tumours at other sites) and the only information given is that which a non-specialist junior doctor would require. The comments on cytotoxic drugs, immunosuppression and infection apply to all cancers.

Diagnosis

Commonest presentations of haematological malignancy are:

1. Symptoms and signs of anaemia
2. Abnormal bleeding
3. Recurrent or overwhelming infection
4. Enlargement of liver, spleen or lymph nodes
5. Mediastinal mass (stridor, SVC obstruction, widened mediastinum on CXR), pleural or pericardial effusion
6. Incidental finding on FBC (see Tables 14.3, 14.6, 14.8, 14.9, 14.11 and p. 363)

Diagnosis and type of *leukaemia* are usually confirmed by FBC (WBC may be high or low but peripheral blast cells are usually present) and bone marrow biopsy. Diagnosis and type of *lymphoma* are confirmed by biopsy of lymph node or at laparotomy.

Pretreatment investigations

1. Height and weight (see surface area nomogram)
2. FBC and film
3. U & E and creatinine
4. Ca^{2+} and PO_4^{3-} and serum alkaline phosphatase
5. LFT and albumin
6. Clotting screen
7. Uric acid
8. Immunoglobulins
9. Viral antibodies
10. Save 5 ml blood for frozen storage
11. Blood culture
12. Karyotype

Table 14.11 Abnormalities of white cell count

Causes of raised white cell count
Infection
Inflammation
'Stress', including recent seizure or burns or diabetic ketoacidosis
Corticosteroid treatment
Leukaemia

Causes of low white cell count
Bone marrow failure, including leukaemia, cytotoxic drugs and radiotherapy
Hypersplenism (including lymphoma)
Sepsis, especially neonatal and overwhelming septicaemia but also typhoid, brucellosis and yellow fever
SLE

13. Urine culture and CMV excretion
14. CXR
15. LP for routine microscopy and culture of CSF and request 'cytospin' to look for blast cells implying CNS involvement. Platelet cover required if count $< 20 \times 10^9$/l
16. Bone marrow aspiration *and* trephine biopsy for histochemical staining, chromosome anomalies, monoclonal antibody studies of B and T cell markers (null cell carries best prognosis), and marrow architecture. Platelet cover is rarely necessary.

LP and bone marrow biopsy should be coordinated during a single general anaesthetic, often with the insertion of an indwelling central venous catheter ('Hickman' line).

In addition, abdominal USS, CT scan, lymphangiography, skeletal survey and isotope bone scan may be indicated depending on the presentation, the diagnosis and the need for staging.

Investigations during treatment

1. FBC before each pulse of treatment.
   If PMN $< 1 \times 10^9$/l or platelets $< 100 \times 10^9$/l, doses may require reduction but treatment should not be delayed.
2. LFT and creatinine every 2 months or before each treatment with platinum or methotrexate.
3. If cisplatin is used: measure plasma Mg^{2+} before each treatment, GFR every 3 months and audiometry every 6 months.
4. If doxorubicin or daunorubicin is used: ECG before treatment and when accumulative dose reaches 100 mg/m², 200 mg/m² and 300 mg/m² and at each treatment thereafter.

Management

Common problems are dealt with below. Specific treatments are not dealt with because they are complex, tumour-specific and rapidly changing as new protocols are devised.

TUMOUR LYSIS SYNDROME

Rapid cell death within hours of initiation of chemotherapy can lead to the following metabolic problems and ARF (urate nephropathy) which may exacerbate these problems:

1. Hyperkalaemia — especially if initial WBC is high. Measure plasma K^+ 4-hourly for the first 12 hours of treatment and then 12-hourly, aiming for $K^+ = 3.5$–6.0 mmol/l. ECG changes are a late sign.
2. Hyperphosphataemia — usually accompanied by hypocalcaemia.

3. Hypercalcaemia — rare unless there is massive bony involvement.
4. Lactic acidosis — suspect if increased anion gap in the absence of ketonuria or renal failure.
5. Hyperuricaemia — vomiting, coma or renal failure may occur but arthropathy is rare.

Prevention

These complications can be minimised by use of the regimen described below (although hyponatraemia and hypokalaemia can occur with such large volumes of i.v. fluids), started 12 hours before chemotherapy.

1. i.v. fluids at twice maintenance (i.e. 3 l/m^2 per 24 hours given as 500 ml 0.9% saline to every 1000 ml 0.18% saline/4% dextrose).
2. i.v. allopurinol 5 mg/kg 8-hourly.
3. i.v. NaHCO$_3$ 3 mmol/kg per 24 hours (1 ml of 8.4% NaHCO$_3$ = 1 mmol) initially, adjusted to keep urine pH > 6.5.
4. For the 12 hours 'prehydration', add 20 mmol KCl (13.5 g) to alternate 500-ml bags of fluid. Once chemotherapy starts, withhold further i.v. KCl until plasma K$^+$ is measured after 4 hours and then give i.v. supplements to maintain K$^+$ = 3.5–6.0 mmol/l.

This regimen presumes normal renal function at diagnosis. Weigh the child daily, measure urine output and use frusemide 0.5 mg/kg i.v. if there is either excessive positive fluid balance or oliguria.

PROBLEMS WITH CYTOTOXIC DRUGS AND RADIOTHERAPY

1. Do not mix cytotoxics in the same syringe and flush cannula with 0.9% saline between drugs.
   Side-effects:
   GI tract — mouth ulceration, anorexia, nausea, vomiting, diarrhoea

   Bone marrow — pancytopenia, immunocompromise
   Lymphoreticular system — immunocompromise
   Hair follicles — alopecia

   Many drugs also cause skin rashes and abnormality of liver or renal function. Doses may have to be modified in view of the latter. Any drug may cause an anaphylactic reaction. More specific drug side-effects are given in Table 14.12 and particular problems are dealt with below.

   Radiotherapy also produces most of the above side-effects acutely (i.e. within 6 weeks of treatment) and, in addition, late complications (after 6 months) include radiation pneumonitis and hepatitis, short stature, hyperpigmentation, hypothyroidism and GH deficiency, learning defects.

Table 14.12 Side-effects of commoner cytotoxic drugs

Drug	Side-effects
Alkylating agents	
Cyclophosphamide	Haemorrhagic cystitis, fever, pneumonitis
Ifosfamide	Haemorrhagic cystitis
Busulphan	Pneumonitis, gynaecomastia, hyperpigmentation, cataracts
Antimetabolites	
Methotrexate	Hepatotoxicity, nephrotoxicity, skin rash, pneumonitis, peripheral neuropathy, encephalopathy. Headache, fever and convulsions after intrathecal methotrexate.
Purine analogues (6-mercaptopurine and thioguanine)	Hepatotoxicity and jaundice, skin rash, hyperpigmentation
Pyrimidine analogues (cytarabine)	Hepatotoxicity, GI haemorrhage, neuritis, conjunctivitis, 'flu'-like illness with arthralgia, skin rashes
Plant alkaloids	
Vincristine, vinblastine and vindesine	Neurotoxicity (muscle weakness, cramps, areflexia, cranial nerve palsies, jaw pain) including autonomic neuropathy (constipation common — give prophylactic lactulose), hepatotoxicity, skin rash, SIADH
Antibiotics	
Doxorubicin, daunorubicin and epirubicin	Orange urine, cardiotoxicity (transient ECG changes or irreversible cardiomyopathy and cardiac failure — risk related to cumulative dose)
Actinomycin D	Glossitis
Bleomycin	Acute hypotension and fever, erythema of fingers, pulmonary fibrosis
Amsacrine	Oesophagitis, haematuria cardiotoxicity, abnormal LFT
Miscellaneous	
Asparaginase	Pancreatitis, coagulopathy, abnormal LFT, hyperglycaemia
Platinum compounds (cisplatin and carboplatin)	Nephrotoxicity, flushing, burning or pruritus, facial swelling and bronchospasm, ototoxicity
Mitozantrone	Abnormal LFT, elevated creatinine, cardiotoxicity
Etoposide (VP16)	Acute hypotension, bronchospasm

2. Vincristine, doxorubicin, daunorubicin and actinomycin are very irritant.
   If extravasation occurs:
   a. stop the infusion

   b. give i.v. dexamethasone 4mg and remove the cannula
   c. use a 22G needle to infiltrate intradermally around the extravasation site a further 4mg dexamethasone and 1500 u (1 ampoule dissolved in 1 ml water) hyaluronidase.
       DO NOT GIVE HYALURONIDASE INTRAVE-NOUSLY.
   d. if doxorubicin is extravasated, infiltrate 4 ml of 4.2% $NaHCO_3$ widely also.

3. Intrathecal methotrexate — use only the intrathecal preparation
    — remove CSF for microscopy before giving methotrexate
    — only give methotrexate if there is free flow of CSF and stop immediately if any resistance is felt

4. Folinic acid rescue — a lethal dose of methotrexate is given i.v. and the normal tissue rescued by i.v. folinic acid 15 mg 6-hourly for 48 hours. Methotrexate level is measured 48 hours after start of treatment (Table 14.13)

5. Haemorrhagic cystitis — is a common side-effect of cyclophosphamide and ifosfamide. This can be prevented by:
   a. prehydration as described above
   b. twice maintenance fluids for 6 hours following each dose
   c. Mesna (which binds the damaging agent in the urine) 500 mg/m^2 i.v. at first dose of cytotoxics, and 4 and 8 hours later

ANTI-EMESIS

Background
Nausea and vomiting are common side-effects of cytotoxic drugs (through

Table 14.13 Folinic acid rescue following methotrexate

Plasma methotrexate concentration at 48 hours	Action
<0.1 μmol/l	Discontinue folinic acid
0.1–0.4 μmol/l	Continue folinic acid 15 mg 6-hourly for another 48 hours
0.4–0.9 μmol/l	Increase folinic acid to 30 mg 6-hourly for the next 48 hours. Repeat levels and follow as above
> 0.9 μmol/l	Increase folinic acid to 100 mg/m^2 6-hourly until methotrexate level < 0.4 μmol/l. Then as above

both CNS and GI effects) but always consider whether vomiting is due to:
1. systemic, urinary or GI infection
2. intestinal obstruction
3. raised ICP
4. fear ('anticipatory' vomiting which may be helped by diazepam 0.25 mg/kg orally the night before and on the morning of treatment)

Management

Two non-interacting drugs can be given alternately to reduce the interval between anti-emetic doses. Try, in the following order:

1. Domperidone
   0.2–0.4 mg/kg 4-hourly p.o.
   or 1 mg/kg 6-hourly p.r.
   or 0.7 mg/kg 4-hourly i.v.
2. Metoclopramide
   0.2 mg/kg 4-hourly i.v./p.o.
   Dystonic reactions are commonest in older girls and treated with procyclidine 5 mg i.v. or benztropine 1 mg i.v. Both doses can be repeated after 20 min if symptoms reappear.
3. Prochlorperazine
   0.25 mg/kg 6-hourly i.v./p.o./p.r.
4. Chlorpromazine
   0.5 mg/kg 4-hourly p.o./i.v./p.r.
   Unpopular with children > 5 years as very sedating
5. Nabilone (start 12 hours before treatment and continue 24 hours after)
   < 18 kg: 0.5 mg 12-hourly p.o.
   18-36 kg: 1 mg 12-hourly p.o.
   > 36 kg: 1 mg 8-hourly p.o.
6. Dexamethasone
   0–4 years: 2 mg 8-hourly p.o./i.v.
   4–14 years: 4 mg 8-hourly p.o./i.v.
7. Ondansitron
   Very expensive so reserved for children receiving platinum drugs. Dose is based on the child's surface area:

	Treatment (i.v.) 8-hourly	Post-treatment (p.o.) 8-hourly
< 0.6 m²	5 mg/m²	2 mg/m² for 3–5 days
0.6–1.2 m²	5 mg/m²	4 mg/m² for 3–5 days
> 1.2 m²	8 mg/m²	8 mg/m² for 3–5 days

Diazepam, nabilone, domperidone, rectal prochlorperazine and dexamethasone should all be started the night before cytotoxics.

PAIN RELIEF

Background

1. Regular pain relief is superior to 'as required'.

2. The oral route is kinder but nausea, vomiting or the need for rapid analgesia indicate the i.v. route. Avoid i.m. if possible as this is painful and haematoma is likely if platelets < 20 × 10⁹/l.

3. Give enough analgesia to control pain. Strong analgesia should *not* be withheld because the child is not terminally ill.

4. Once pain control has been achieved, it may be possible to reduce the dose (rather than the frequency).

Management

1. Mild pain — *paracetamol* 15 mg/kg 4-hourly p.o./p.r. For mouth ulcers apply 1% hydrocortisone in glycerine paste 2-hourly and antiseptic mouthwash 2-hourly alternately each hour.

2. Moderate pain — *dihydrocodeine* 1 mg/kg 4-hourly p.o. This is less constipating than codein but start prophylactic lactulose 0.25 ml/kg 12-hourly p.o.

3. Severe pain — *diamorphine* 0.2 mg/kg 4-hourly p.o.
    or 0.1 mg/kg 4-hourly i.v.
    or 0.025 mg/kg/h by i.v. infusion
    Start prophylactic lactulose 0.25 ml/kg 12-hourly p.o.
    Addiction is rare but tolerance is common; therefore the dose may need to be increased but will not cause respiratory depression. Slow release morphine (MST Continus) 0.2 mg/kg 12-hourly p.o. may be more appropriate for chronic pain.

USE OF CENTRAL VENOUS CATHETERS

Background

CXR should show the tip in the SVC or right atrium. The commonest complications are:

1. Infection — usually *Staph. epidermidis*. If blood cultures taken through the line and from a peripheral vein are positive with the same organism, the line is probably infected and should be removed.
    Tricuspid valve vegetations and endocartitis may also occur and can be detected by echocardiography. Local skin infection at the site of insertion may also occur.

2. Clotting — give 5000 u streptokinase into the line and leave for 30 min. Repeat dose once if still unable to withdraw blood. Is there a clamp or clip closed on the line?

Using a Hickman or Broviac line

1. All procedures are sterile (including giving drugs and changing bags) and require the use of sterile towels and gloves.

2. An assistant must spray line and connectors with methylated spirits. Clean the bung with an alcohol swab and allow to dry before inserting the needle.

3. Change giving sets every 48 hours.

4. Use only Luer locks.

5. 'Break' into the line as infrequently as possible and rationalise drug charts so that drugs are given at same times.
6. Always withdraw 5 ml 'dead space' before taking blood samples. Do not use for gentamicin levels.
7. No routine flushing of Hickman catheters is required; only flush after treatment. Use 5 ml normal saline containing 1 u/ml heparin. Flush double-lumen Hickman lines weekly. Flush Broviac catheters twice weekly.

INFECTION IN THE IMMUNOSUPPRESSED CHILD

Background

Infection is the cause of death in 75% of leukaemics and may be acute and overwhelming or insidious and atypical. Potentiating factors are:

1. Bone marrow involvement impairs WBC production.
2. Lymphomas particularly impair T cell function (hence TB, fungi, Listeria).
3. Corticosteroids and cytotoxic drugs impair B cells and humoral immunity (hence bacterial infection, Pneumocystis).
4. Indwelling venous lines.
5. GI ulceration, anal fissures.
6. Poor nutrition.

'Neutropenic'

The child is at greatest risk when PMN $< 1 \times 10^9$/l and the risk is greatest from his own organisms, especially the gut.

Diagnosis of infection

Apart from the usual symptoms and signs in any child, some empirical rules are necessary for the neutropenic child in which fever may herald a life-threatening emergency:

1. Start treatment if temperature is $> 39°C$.
2. Start treatment if temperature is $> 38.5°C$ on two occasions, at least 4 hours apart.
3. Start treatment if infection is suspected, even in the absence of fever.
4. Do not give paracetamol or other antipyretics until treatment is started.

Examine carefully for a source of fever daily, especially the mouth, throat, ears and perineum.

Pretreatment investigations

Before starting antibiotics always:

1. FBC and film, U & E + creatinine
2. Peripheral and central line blood cultures
3. Throat swab
4. Swab any skin lesion, including fissure-in-ano
5. CRP

6. CXR
7. Urine and stools for microscopy and bacterial and viral culture but do not defer antibiotic treatment while awaiting these specimens.

Only perform an LP if clinically indicated.

Empirical treatment

Until a positive culture is obtained:

1. Azlocillin 75 mg/kg 8-hourly i.v.
2. Gentamicin (or tobramycin at the same dose if known renal impairment) 2.5 mg/kg 8-hourly i.v. Check trough (pre-dose) and peak (30 min post i.v. dose) gentamicin levels around the third dose.
3. Nystatin 100 000 u 4-hourly p.o.
4. Treat fever with paracetamol 15 mg/kg 4-hourly p.o.
5. If culture-negative after 72 hours and well and afebrile, stop treatment.
6. If culture-negative after 72 hours but still febrile, add cefotaxime 50 mg/kg 6-hourly i.v.
7. If still febrile after 5 days and culture-negative, consider amphotericin, starting at 0.25 mg/kg daily i.v. (side-effects are anaphylaxis and commonly hypokalaemia).
8. If culture-positive, ensure that the organism is sensitive to the current treatment regimen. Treat for a minimum of 10 days and until PMN $> 1 \times 10^9$/l. Consider stopping cytotoxic drugs.
9. Treat clinical herpes, chicken pox or shingles with acyclovir 10 mg/kg 8-hourly i.v. for 1 week. Stop chemotherapy.

Prevention of infection

1. Oral antiseptic mouth care and *gentle* but regular brushing of teeth.
2. Avoid constipation, rectal examination and rectal temperatures.
3. Avoid shop-washed salads, paté, cream cheese and cheese-cake.
4. Avoid contact with other infected inpatients or family members.
5. Regular Septrin prophylaxis against *Pneumocystis*.
6. If in contact with measles, even if only suspected, give human immunoglobulin 1 g/m² (max. dose 1 g) i.m.
7. If in contact with chicken pox or shingles, give zoster immune globulin 1 g/m² (max. dose 1 g) i.m.
8. If zoster immune globulin is unobtainable, give acyclovir 200 mg p.o. 5 times per 24 hours for 1 week.
9. Live vaccinations (polio, MMR, BCG) must not be given to the child or other siblings.
10. Advice to parents — watch for tiredness, paleness, breathlessness, cough, diarrhoea, tummy ache, headache, rash, fever — if worried, do not give paracetamol but telephone ward immediately.

THROMBOCYTOPENIA

See p. 246 but indications are different in the child with cancer.
Give 4 u/m^2 of platelets (ABO compatible) if:

1. Platelet count $< 20 \times 10^9$/l and overt bleeding.
2. Platelet count $< 20 \times 10^9$/l and fever $> 38.5°C$.
3. Platelet count $< 20 \times 10^9$/l and requiring blood transfusion.

Platelet transfusions may be required twice daily to meet these criteria.

15

POISONING

Always suspect poisoning in children with symptoms that cannot otherwise be explained, e.g. unusual behaviour, tachypnoea, tachycardia, drowsiness or coma.

Self administration of a poison in a child > 7 years may be an attempt at suicide.

Initial management

1. Detailed history; include parents', relatives' and friends' medications as necessary.
2. Accept the largest estimated amount that may have been ingested when determining management.
3. General medical examination will often reveal supporting evidence for a particular ingestion. Document neurological and respiratory status well to allow later comparison.
4. Confirm the specific poison by qualitative and, if possible, quantitative measurement on blood, urine or gastric samples. Discuss with the lab. to check they are able to identify the agent concerned.

Investigations

Urine 25 ml for toxicology screen; blood 5–10 ml for quantification of substances picked up on urine testing and for detection of agents such as alcohol, methanol and acetone.

Management of the unstable or unconscious patient following ingestion

1. Nurse in ICU. Monitor conscious state, BP and blood glucose.
2. Assess the need for mechanical ventilation on clinical and blood gas observations.

3. Maintain circulation — consider plasma expansion and a pressor agent (e.g. dopamine).
4. Give 5% i.v. dextrose infusion at $\frac{2}{3}$ maintenance.
5. Paraldehyde (p.r.) or i.v. diazepam may be given to control seizures (diazepam may induce further respiratory depression requiring ventilation).
6. Antibiotics are only indicated for bacterial superinfection and are not required prophylactically.
7. Check U & E, Hb and WBC. Save specimens as above.
8. Consider the differential diagnosis. Give appropriate antidote or therapy.

Removal of poison

It is good practice to consult poison centres concerning specific poisons. **Poison centres are open 24 hours a day, every day, for advice**.

Telephone: Belfast 0232-420503
Birmingham 021-554 3801
Dublin 0001-745588
Edinburgh 031-229 2477
London 071-635 9191 or 071-407 7600

Treatment of some specific agents are mentioned in this chapter but if there is any doubt consult one of the above numbers.

METHODS

1. Ipecacuanha paediatric syrup followed by a large drink

a. 6–12 months: give 10 ml once only under medical supervision followed by clear fluids.
b. 1–10 years: give 10–15 ml followed by clear fluids. If vomiting does not occur within 20–30 min, repeat the same dose once.
c. > 10 years: give 30 ml of ipecacuanha syrup followed by clear fluids (200 ml).

Contraindications. Following the ingestion of caustic agents, hydrocarbons, detergents and in comatose or fitting children. Beware of administration to children who have ingested substances that may cause rapid coma or convulsions. Gastric lavage with a cuffed ETT may be indicated instead.

NB. NEVER use salt water as an emetic. Salt poisoning may occur.

2. Gastric lavage

This is unpleasant.

a. If the child is comatose or convulsing or may rapidly become so, a cuffed ETT must be placed in situ to prevent aspiration of gastric contents into the lung.
b. Wrap the child in a sheet for restraint and place on his left side.
c. Insert a large-bore tube (at least 28FG) using KY jelly to facilitate the procedure.
d. Measure the distance to the stomach. Ensure entrance to the stomach by injecting air and auscultating over the stomach. Always aspirate for stomach contents prior to lavage.
e. Lavage with 0.45% saline in 10–20-ml aliquots. Continue until clear.
f. Charcoal may be left in the stomach if indicated (see below).
g. Occlude the end of the tube on removal to prevent aspiration.

3. Activated charcoal

Check with a poison centre before use. Activated charcoal forms a stable complex with some ingested toxins, preventing their ab- sorption.

Do not give before ipecacuanah as it will bind to it and make it ineffective. The dose is 1 g/kg p.o. in infancy and 15–30 g for children. It may be given following vomiting or via an NGT after gastric lavage. It is not effective against acids, alkalis and many alcohols and metals.

4. Methods to improve excretion

These should only be used in serious poisoning, after consultation with a poison centre. Most cases can be handled conservatively, allowing the child to metabolise or excrete the poison.

Excretion may be enhanced by a fluid diuresis, an ionised diuresis and an osmotic diuresis. A diuretic diuresis may very occasionally be used.

Dialysis is rarely needed for emergency management of poisons. Haemoperfusion and haemodialysis tend to be more effective than peritoneal dialysis. In the young child who cannot undergo these procedures, an exchange transfusion may be required.

Cathartics may hasten passage through the GI tract and in some cases may reduce absorption (e.g. $MgSO_4$ 0.25–0.5 g/kg: max. 15 g/dose).

Specific poisons

IRON POISONING

Toxicity is likely following ingestion of 60 mg/kg elemental iron; 20–60 mg/kg is possibly toxic.

Phase 1: symptoms usually occur 30 min to 2 hours after ingestion and include abdominal cramps, vomiting, drowsiness and bloody diarrhoea.

Phase 2: period of apparent recovery, intensive observations must continue.

Phase 3: 6–24 hours after ingestion there may be fever, shock, metabolic acidosis, convulsions, coma and liver impairment.

Phase 4: 3–4 weeks after ingestion, stricture of the GI tract may occur. Hepatotoxicity is possible.

Investigations

Include: FBC, blood glucose, U & E, blood group and save/crossmatch, serum iron, TIBC. AXR for radio-opaque tablets. Repeat serum iron 3–4 hours postingestion.

Treatment

1. Give ipecacuanah.
2. Oral 'complexation' (i.e. $NaHCO_3$ with desferrioxamine) is of questionable value.
3. Treat hypotension: i.v. fluids, including plasma, as required to correct fluid loss and acidosis. $NaHCO_3$ may be required. If the child is unresponsive to these measures, administer dopamine (5 µg/kg/min) and titrate as needed to the desired response (max. 15 µg/kg/min). Administer a cathartic (magnesium citrate 4 ml/kg up to 300 ml/dose).
4. Desferrioxamine is a specific antidote and should be given if: the serum iron exceeds the TIBC (if obtained); peak serum iron is > 350 µg/dl (62.5 µmol/l); the patient becomes symptomatic and serum iron result is not readily available.
   Beware an anaphylactic reaction
   Dose: administer up to 15 mg/kg/h i.v. Faster rates may cause hypotension. Do not exceed 80 mg/kg per 24 hours.
   Indications for stopping desferrioxamine include improvement in the patient's clinical condition, serum iron within the normal range, disappearance of the red urinary colour.
5. Dialysis is only used in the presence of oliguria or anuria and is only effective when iron is bound to desferrioxamine.
6. Consider exchange transfusion in severely symptomatic patients.

PARACETAMOL

The most serious effect is liver damage which does not become apparent for 2–7 days and may be fatal.

Treatment

1. Give ipecacuanha.
2. Take blood 4 hours after paracetamol ingestion for paracetamol levels, baseline LFT and PT.

3. Plot plasma paracetamol level on the nomogram contained in the literature accompanying the N-acetylcysteine (Parvolex). If hepatic toxicity is probable and ingestion was < 15 hours ago, give N-acetylcysteine by an i.v. infusion: 150 mg/kg in the first 15 min, 50 mg/kg for the next 4 hours, 100 mg/kg over the next 16 hours (total dose 300 mg/kg). Dilute in 5% dextrose. Beware anaphylaxis.

   N-acetylcysteine may be harmful if given > 15 hours after ingestion.

   Bronchoconstriction may occur in asthmatic patients.
4. Avoid forcing fluids and enzyme inducing drugs.
5. If poisoning is severe, seek advice from a specialist centre with regards to transfer for future management.

ANTICHOLINERGIC POISONING

Atropine-like agents, e.g. hyoscine (travel sickness tablets), atropine and ipratropium bromide in excess, and some berries.

Effects include flushed hot skin, dilated pupils, tachycardia, hyperpyrexia, urinary retention, diminished bowel sounds, hallucinations and coma.

Laboratory levels of drugs/plants producing anticholinergic effects are not useful.

Treatment
1. Emesis; give ipecacuanha syrup unless the child could rapidly become comatose or convulse.
2. Administer charcoal slurry (1–2 g/kg in infants, 15–30 g in children) and one dose of cathartic.
3. Monitor BP and temperature.
4. Discuss with a poison centre.

TRICYCLIC ANTIDEPRESSANTS

Doses over 10 mg/kg are increasingly dangerous.

The most harmful effects are cardiac arrhythmias, AV block and tachycardias. Other effects include agitation, drowsiness, ataxia, hallucinations, vomiting, convulsions, coma and hypo/hypertension.

Treatment
1. Emesis is now contraindicated as rapid neurological deterioration is known to occur.
2. Administer charcoal slurry (1–2 g/kg in infants, 15–30 g in children) and one dose of cathartic.
3. Gastric lavage with a cuffed ETT in situ may be indicated if performed up to 12 hours after ingestion, or in patients who are comatose or at risk of convulsing.
4. Monitor ECG for 48 hours if symptomatic.

5. Insert an i.v. line.
6. Treat convulsions with diazepam (0.25–0.4 mg/kg/dose, max. 10 mg/dose). If seizures cannot be controlled or they recur administer phenytoin.
7. **Ventricular arrhythmias:** treat conduction defects with phenytoin 15 mg/kg by i.v. infusion over 30 min. Beware of the negative inotropic effects of phenytoin.

    Administer $NaHCO_3$ 1 mmol/kg initially and as needed to achieve blood pH of 7.45–7.55. Check serum K^+ levels and maintain at 4–5 mmol/l. Unresponsive arrhythmias may respond to lignocaine (1 mg/kg).

    NB. Dysopyramide, quinidine, procainamide are contraindicated. Pacing may be required. Treat ventricular fibrillation with defibrillation (3–5 J/kg) and with phenytoin.

    SVT does not warrant treatment unless it is causing hypotension or cardiac failure. Treat by cardioversion.

    NB. If cardiac arrest occurs continue resuscitation for at least 2 hours as the effects may be reversible.

PHENOTHIAZINES

Symptoms: in general, hypotension, miosis, hypothermia, CNS depression, quinidine-like effects on the myocardium, urinary symptoms and seizures.

Extrapyramidal effects (oculogyric crisis, stiff neck, torticollis, protruding tongue, and trismus) may even occur following therapeutic doses.

Treatment

1. Emesis with ipecacuanha in recent large ingestions unless the child could rapidly become comatose or convulse.
2. Administer activated charcoal slurry (1–2 g/kg infants, 15–30 g in children) and one dose of cathartic.
3. Hypotension: administer plasma i.v. If unresponsive give dopamine (5 µg/kg/min).
4. Seizures: give i.v. diazepam (0.25–0.4 mg/kg/dose, max. 10 mg/dose). If not controlled give phenytoin.
5. Monitor ECG: serious conduction defects may be treated with phenytoin (15 mg/kg i.v. over 30 min).
6. **Dystonic reactions** (see extrapyramidal signs above): give either
    a. procyclidine (< 2 years 0.5–2 mg, > 2 years 2–5 mg, > 12 years 5 mg), or
    b. diphenhydramine 1–2 mg/kg (max. 50 mg) i.m. or i.v. over 2 min, or

    c. benztropine mesylate (Cogentin) (if > 3 years) 1–2 mg i.v. followed by maintenance for 2 days.

7. Hypothermia: manage with external warming.

CENTRAL NERVOUS SYSTEM DEPRESSANTS

Narcotics (morphine and dihydromorphine), benzodiazepines, alcohol, sedatives and barbiturates.

— History of ingestion is often denied in older patients.
— All induce CNS and cardiorespiratory depression in acute overdosage.
— Pupils are often constricted following morphine or dihydromorphine.
— Hypoglycaemia is common in children after alcohol ingestion.

Treatment

1. If comatose, give naloxone 0.01 mg/kg i.v. If no response is seen, repeat the dose 1 min later giving 0.1 mg/kg i.v. If no response is seen, then narcotic overdose is unlikely.
2. Removal of substances from the GI tract: care has to be taken because of CNS depression. Ipecacuanha and gastric lavage without a cuffed ETT in situ may be dangerous.
3. Give 10% dextrose i.v. following alcohol ingestion in children accompanied by very regular blood glucose estimations as profound hypoglycaemia may occur several hours after ingestion.
4. Consider haemodialysis for patients with severe alcohol intoxication.
5. Patients may need respiratory support in the form of ventilation.
6. Seizures: treat with diazepam (0.25–0.4 mg/kg/dose, max. 10 mg/dose) but beware of respiratory depression. If unresponsive, treat with phenytoin.

SOLVENT INHALATION AND ABUSE

Clinical presentation may be with acute intoxication or chronic abuse with withdrawal.

Acute intoxication

Onset of effect is usually within minutes with resolution over several hours. Symptoms vary according to the substance inhaled but there is often initial excitation with euphoria, often with sneezing, coughing, salivation, nausea and vomiting. This may lead to CNS depression with confusion, disorientation, disinhibition, hallucinations and aggression. This may be followed by depressed reflexes and ataxia leading to stupor, seizures and cardiorespiratory arrest. Death may occur from asphyxia, arrhythmias, respiratory arrest, liver failure or trauma.

Chronic abuse

May be associated with CNS manifestations, hepatotoxicity, nephrotoxicity, and bone marrow depression.

Withdrawal symptoms include tremulousness, tachycardia, disorientation, hallucinations, agitation and seizures.

Investigations

High index of suspicion is needed. Save blood for toxin analysis. Heparinise refrigerated sample and save urine for drug screen. Discuss suspicions with laboratory staff.

Treatment

Admit for observation and supportive care. Withdrawal symptoms usually respond to a long acting sedative such as diazepam given in a sufficient dose to produce a calm, seizure-free state.

SALICYLATE POISONING

Ingestion of 150 mg/kg will cause symptoms which include hyperventilation leading to an initial respiratory alkalosis. This is often quickly followed by a metabolic acidosis. Ketosis may occur and rarely hypoglycaemia. Vomiting, diarrhoea, sweating, fever, dehydration, tinnitus, vertigo, restlessness, confusion, convulsions, coma and circulatory collapse may be seen.

Peak serum levels may occur 2 hours after ingestion.

Investigations

FBC, electrolytes, blood gases, serum ketones, blood glucose, PT and serum salicylate level.

Treatment

1. If there is any doubt about symptoms or if the salicylate level is above 2.9 mmol/l (40 mg/100 ml) then hospital admission is necessary.
2. Give ipecacuanha syrup.
3. Give activated charcoal and administer one dose of cathartic.
4. Intravenous fluids in the form of dextrose/saline should be given to replace losses and maintain normoglycaemia.
5. Vitamin K i.m. may be given to correct hypoprothrombinaemia.
6. Severe bleeding may require FFP, clotting factors and whole blood.
7. Check salicylate level, electrolytes, pH, and CO_2 at least 3- hourly if unwell.
8. Our policy is to use forced alkaline diuresis if the blood salicylate level at 4–6 hours is > 200 mg/l in children < 18 months; > 400 mg/l in children 18 months–12 years; > 600 mg/l in children > 12 years. If > 1000 mg/l, refer for haemodialysis. Check details with the poison centre.

For forced alkaline diuresis take baseline blood gases, U & E and osmolality and catheterise the bladder. Admit to ICU.

a. Give 10–15 ml/kg/h 4% dextrose/0.18% saline for 1–2 hours until there is good urine output. Beware fluid overload.

b. 1 g KCl in each 500 ml bag.

c. Up to 1 mmol NaHCO₃/kg/h to keep urine pH > 7.5.

d. Check blood gases and U & E 2-hourly.

9. With potentially fatal levels, i.e. > 1000 mg/l, or with oliguria or anuria, dialysis is indicated.

LEAD POISONING WITH ENCEPHALOPATHY

Lead encephalopathy may present suddenly with convulsions, signs of raised ICP and coma, or more gradually with drowsiness, ataxia, hyperactivity and retarded development.

Other findings suggestive of lead poisoning include X-rays showing a line of increased metaphyseal density of the long bones, abdominal films showing radio-opaque material in the gut, basophilic stippling of the red cells and iron deficiency anaemia.

Investigations

Obtain blood lead and erythrocyte protoporphyrin. Admit any child with symptoms or if blood lead level exceeds 50 µg/dl. Chelation therapy should be instituted if blood lead levels are > 50 µg/dl (2.4–2.9 µmol/l) or if the patient is symptomatic.

LP is contraindicated.

Treatment

Lead intoxication with encephalopathy should be treated as a medical emergency.

1. In recent substantial ingestion, perform gastric lavage with cuffed ETT leaving activated charcoal in the stomach. Give one dose of cathartic.

2. Consider a cleansing enema if lead is found on AXR.

3. Give maintenance fluids and ensure a good urine flow. Excessive fluids further increase cerebral oedema.

4. Cerebral oedema: may be managed by ventilation and administration of 1.5 g/kg of 20% mannitol over 20 min. Dexamethasone up to 1–2 mg/kg per 24 hours i.v. in divided doses.

5. Seizures: diazepam 0.25–0.4 mg/kg i.v., max. 10 mg/dose. If uncontrolled give phenytoin.

6. Chelation therapy: start dimercaprol (BAL) i.m. in a dose of 3–5 mg/kg/dose every 4 hours for 2 days, then every 5 hours for 2 more days, then every 5–12 hours up to an additional 7 days.

Start Ca – EDTA 50–75 mg/kg per 24 hours deep i.m. injection in 3–5 divided doses for up to 5 days.

It is important to continue chelation therapy because cerebral oedema will not respond to therapy unless the amount of lead in the body has been reduced.

7. Monitor U & E, Ca^{2+}, blood lead, 24-hour urine lead, and EEG if necessary.

NB. It is important to follow children to ensure the source of lead is removed. As follow-up care penicillamine may be given daily until the blood lead level falls below 3 µmol/l.

Lead poisoning without encephalopathy also requires treatment. (Consult a larger text.)

ACID INGESTION

Treatment

1. Do not induce vomiting; do not give HCO_3^- to neutralise. Activated charcoal is of no value.
2. Irrigate all contaminated areas with copious amounts of water.
3. After oral exposure immediately dilute with milk. Use water if milk is not immediately available.
4. Steroid use is controversial.
5. Evaluate for oesophageal and gastric burns; consult surgical colleagues if serious.

Delayed pyloric stricture may occur.

ALKALINE (CORROSIVE) INGESTION

Exposure to alkaline corrosives may result in severe burns.

Treatment

1. Use of diluents is controversial. Residual perioral alkali should be rinsed with milk. Activated charcoal is not indicated. Neutralisation is contraindicated.
2. Emesis or lavage is contraindicated.
3. Keep nil by mouth and acquire surgical opinion. Endoscopy may be indicated.
4. Consider administration of 1 mg/kg prednisolone where deep oesophageal burns are seen.
5. Antibiotics only for specific indications.

Specific antidotes

A few ingested substances have specific antidotes. Some of these are listed below together with their antidote. Before giving the antidote, check thoroughly with the poison centre on the need for it, additional management strategies required and the dose to be given. Some of the antidotes may be toxic themselves.

Carbon monoxide. Give 100% oxygen.

Methaemoglobinaemia. Caused by drugs such as sulphonamides and substances such as nitrates. Give methylene blue (1–2 mg/kg) i.v. as a 1% solution and repeat after 4 hours if required. Vitamin C may also be helpful.

Cholinesterase inhibitors, e.g. in some insecticides. Atropine is used as an antidote.

Antifreeze (ethylene glycol). Ethyl alcohol acts as a competitor, slowing down the metabolism of ethylene glycol to its toxic metabolites.

Warfarin. Give vitamin K 2–5 mg/kg i.m.

16

Ear, nose and throat problems

Beware of the child with signs of mild upper respiratory signs but who has severe constitutional symptoms. Look for alternative diagnoses, e.g. meningitis, pneumonia, etc.

The common cold

Management is symptomatic.
1. Ensure adequate fluid intake in young babies.
2. Paracetamol for fever (approximately 10 mg/kg/6-hourly).
3. If feeding is difficult due to nasal obstruction, advise clearing the nose with a damp cotton wool bud. Instillation of 1–2 drops of vasoconstrictor nasal drops (0.5% ephedrine) may also help. Use only if necessary and for **a maximum of 1–2 days only**.
4. Explain to parents that symptoms may last up to 2 weeks.

Pharyngitis and tonsillitis

Cause: either group A beta-haemolytic streptococci or viral infection. A white tonsillar exudate in teenagers may be due to glandular fever.

DIAGNOSIS

There is no reliable way of distinguishing bacterial from viral infection clinically. In practice we do not usually perform a throat swab or ASO titre to support the diagnosis of bacterial infection. Do a monospot test to exclude glandular fever if indicated.

TREATMENT

1. Oral penicillin V if considered bacterial; must be continued for 10 entire days. Give erythromycin if the child is allergic to penicillin.
2. Paracetamol for pain and fever.

Indications for adenotonsillectomy

There is no uniform agreement as to indications for surgery. Upper airway obstruction, especially if associated with sleep apnoea, a previous episode of quinsy and suspected malignancy (i.e. unilateral enlargement) are indications for surgery. Children with recurrent tonsillitis only rarely warrant surgery.

OBSTRUCTIVE SLEEP APNOEA

Obstructive breathing at night (i.e. prominent snoring) associated with apnoeic episodes. May cause significant FTT.

Diagnosis is often from history alone. Admit to hospital for overnight observation and O_2 saturation study (patients often show episodes of < 90% O_2 saturation).

TREATMENT

Adenotonsillectomy is usually curative.

NB. Adenotonsillectomy performed for obstructive sleep apnoea must be done in a centre with paediatric intensive care facilities as postoperative respiratory arrest may occur.

Post tonsillectomy bleed

TREATMENT

1. Within 24 hours (reactionary): usually requires return to theatre; treat seriously; insert an i.v. line and crossmatch. Close observation of the child is needed. Contact the ENT surgeon.
2. Secondary haemorrhage (after 1 week). This is usually much less serious; however, admit, observe closely and give penicillin. Inform the surgeon.

Cervical adenitis

Marked enlargement of the lymph nodes due to localised or systemic infection. (Minor cervical lymphadenopathy is commonly due to simple viral infection or tonsillitis.)

INVESTIGATIONS

1. Examine the drainage area of the nodes affected.

2. ASO titre, monospot test, FBC (film and differential) and blood cultures.
3. An USS of the neck may help in the detection of an abscess.
4. Rarely, *Mycobacterium tuberculosis* may be the cause. If suspected, a Mantoux test and CXR are indicated. Atypical *M. tuberculosis* may also be causative.

   Malignant disease may occasionally be responsible.

TREATMENT

1. Penicillin and flucloxacillin (or Augmentin) (for 14 days) to cover group A haemolytic streptococci and *Staph. aureus*. Severity of illness determines whether antibiotics are given p.o. or i.v.
2. Surgical drainage or excisional biopsy should be considered for infected nodes that are refractory to antibiotic treatment or are fluctuant (i.e. abscess formation). Material should be cultured for anaerobic and aerobic organisms and *Mycobacterium*.

Peri-tonsillar abscess (quinsy)

Seen in older children. Inspection shows a bulge in the soft palate with deviation of the uvula to the opposite side in association with inflamed tonsils. Stridor may be present. Rupture may cause aspiration pneumonia.

TREATMENT

1. Admit and take blood cultures; give i.v. penicillin (300 mg/kg per 24 hours in six divided doses).
2. Nil by mouth and nurse with head up.
3. Refer immediately to the ENT surgeon for opinion with regards to surgical drainage. Tonsillectomy is indicated when well.

Retropharyngeal abscess

Uncommon after 3 years of age. The diagnosis is made on history and X-ray changes.

CLINICAL FEATURES

The child may have signs of infection, drooling, dysphagia and stridor.

INVESTIGATIONS

As the child's airway may be threatened, investigations should be carried out in ICU.

1. Lateral neck X-ray characteristically shows an increase in the normal distance from vertebral column to air in the pharynx (i.e. greater than the width of a vertebral body). Gas may also be seen in the soft tissues.
2. Direct inspection by the ENT surgeon.

TREATMENT

1. Do not palpate as this may cause rupture.
2. Urgent ENT opinion; surgical drainage may be necessary.
3. Chloramphenicol and penicillin i.v.

Diphtheria

Very rare but consider if unimmunised. Inflamed tonsils and pharynx and signs of infection are seen. There may be a thick grey membrane over the tonsils and removal may cause brisk bleeding. Airway occlusion may occur. Throat swab and blood cultures are needed.

TREATMENT

1. ET intubation may be needed for airway obstruction.
2. Penicillin 300 mg/kg per 24 hours i.v. in six divided doses.
3. Antitoxin: give as soon as possible. Test dose to exclude hypersensitivity.

Acute sinusitis

CLINICAL FEATURES

Include fever, nasal congestion, sensation of fullness or pain, with tenderness over the sinuses.

AETIOLOGY

Viral or bacterial (*Str. pneumoniae, Haem. influenzae*, group A streptococci, *Branhamella catarrhalis*).

INVESTIGATIONS

Plain X-rays of the sinuses are usually unhelpful in the management of sinusitis.

TREATMENT

1. Augmentin or co-trimoxazole for 10 days.
2. Nasal decongestants (ephidrine 0.5%) may be used but only for 1–2 days.

If there is no improvement after 48 hours or if the child's condition deteriorates prior to this, refer to the ENT department. If symptoms have improved but the child has not completely recovered at 10 days, continue antibiotics for a further week. In patients with chronic sinusitis, continue antibiotics for 4 weeks and arrange for ENT follow-up.

COMPLICATIONS

These include extension of the infection into the CNS and orbital infection. In an older child with maxillary sinusitis, consider a dental cause.

Acute otitis media

CLINICAL FEATURES

Earache and fever. A young child often pulls at his ear.

DIAGNOSIS

A bulging eardrum that appears inflamed although the eardrum may initially be indrawn. Perforation with discharge may occur.

AETIOLOGY

Viral or bacterial (*Pneumococcus, Haem. influenzae, Br. catarrhalis*). Consider gram negative organisms and *Staph. aureus* in the neonatal period.

TREATMENT

1. Neonatal:
   a. Admit because of the risk of sepsis.
   b. Consider tympanocentesis (by the ENT surgeon) and a full sepsis screen.
   c. Broad spectrum i.v. antibiotics, e.g. cefotaxime and flucloxacillin.
2. > 3 months:
   a. Amoxicillin (or erythromycin) for at least 5 days. If no improvement is seen within 2–3 days, treat with Augmentin as organisms may be beta-lactamase pro-ducers. Use erythromycin for bullous otitis media

(multiple blisters on tympanic membrane and canal) caused by *Mycoplasma* infection.

b. Paracetamol 4-hourly for fever or pain.

c. Aspiration of the ear (by the ENT surgeon only) should be considered if the patient is seriously ill or for failure of antibiotic treatment, extreme pain, postauricular tenderness and swelling suggesting early mastoiditis, inadequate drainage through spontaneous perforation, and if facial palsy develops or if an unusual organism is suspected (e.g. in an immunocompromised child). Discuss with the ENT surgeon.

NB. Review at 3 weeks to ensure clearance of middle ear fluid. Review at 12 weeks and refer to the ENT department if still present.

Recurrent acute otitis media

Usually due to re-infection.

TREATMENT

1. If ear drums are of normal appearance between infections consider antibiotic prophylaxis (e.g. amoxycillin 20 mg/kg or co-trimoxazole once per 24 hours). Continue for 6–12 weeks then discontinue and observe the child.
2. Myringotomy with insertion of tympanostomy tubes is an option for failure of antibiotic prophylaxis.

Children whose ear drums do not return to a normal appearance between attacks should be referred to the ENT department for consideration of tympanostomy tubes.

Acute mastoiditis

CLINICAL FEATURES

Cellulitis, swelling and/or marked tenderness in the postauricular region following acute otitis media.

MANAGEMENT

1. Urgent admission.
2. Blood cultures.
3. Antibiotics, e.g. i.v. flucloxacillin and cefotaxime in acute mastoiditis. *Pseudomonas* infection should be covered if there has been long-standing ear pathology/infection (e.g. ceftazidime).

4. Immediate referral to the ENT surgeon who will assess the need for tympanostomy tubes and cortical mastoidectomy.
5. Mastoid X-ray is often unhelpful in children; therefore await ENT opinion with regards to further investigations/ management.

Chronic otitis media (glue ear)

CLINICAL FEATURES

Appearance of the ear drum suggesting glue ear includes loss of translucency, change in colour (i.e. to yellow), loss of light reflex and retraction. Definitive signs include presence of fluid level and/or an air bubble. Objective diagnosis is by pneumotoscopy and/or tympanometry.

MANAGEMENT

1. Assess hearing.
2. Medical management consists of 6 weeks of oral antibiotics (e.g. ceclor or co-trimoxazole). No other medical or physical treatment has been shown to be useful.
3. Referral for grommet insertion by the ENT surgeon should be considered if there is a functionally significant hearing loss after 3 months' observation, if effusion fails to clear after medical management or if structural abnormalities are suspected.

COMPLICATIONS

Permanent ear damage and conductive hearing loss.

Removal of ear wax

Wax is a normal secretion and need only be removed if it interferes with a proper view of the ear drum or causes deafness.

TREATMENT

Wax can be softened before syringing of the ear with topical $NaHCO_3$ or olive oil drops (warm to body temperature). Show parents how to use drops.

Otitis externa

This is an eczematous reaction of the meatal skin.

MANAGEMENT

1. Analgesia as required (i.e. paracetamol 10 mg/kg/6-hourly).
2. Avoid wetting the ear.
3. Exclude underlying otitis media and perforation before treatment.
4. Many cases recover after thorough cleansing of the external canal e.g. by gentle use of a cotton wool bud.
5. If infection with inflammation and eczema is present a topical anti-infective agent and a corticosteroid are needed, e.g. Betnesol-N (betamethasone plus neomycin); apply ear drops (3–4 warmed) every 2–3 hours or ear ointment 2–4 times daily.
6. If the ear is closed, not allowing easy insertion of drops, a wick soaked with the above agents should be inserted.
7. i.v. antibiotics are indicated for acute infection causing severe pain, cellulitis of the pinnae and for failed treatment. If a boil is present, treat with oral flucloxacillin or erythromycin.
8. Fungal infections (suggested by blotting paper-like debris) may be treated with clotrimazole solution. Apply 2–3 times daily continuing for at least 14 days after disappearance of the infection.

NB. When otitis externa is treated topically with preparations containing chlorhexadine, aminoglycosides (i.e. neomycin) or polymyxins, in patients with a perforation of the tympanic membrane there is an increased incidence of drug-induced deafness.

A foul-smelling discharge may indicate a gram negative infection (e.g. *Pseudomonas*). A cholesteatoma should be excluded by the ENT surgeon.

Foreign body in the ear

Many foreign bodies can be removed in casualty.

MANAGEMENT

Cooperation is essential. If the object does not completely obscure the canal, use an ear loop to remove the object. For insects, fill the ear with mineral oil and then irrigate.

NB. If the canal is swollen, if there is bleeding or if the foreign body cannot be *easily* removed, refer to the ENT surgeon.

Foreign body in the nose

Presentation includes pain, foul smell from nose, discharge and bleeding.

MANAGEMENT

If the child is cooperative and the foreign body can be seen, it may be removed using a loop, hook or forceps. Topical anaesthesia may help.

If there is doubt about ability to remove the foreign body refer to the ENT surgeon for removal under GA.

NB. Small batteries should be removed immediately as they may cause extensive damage.

Laryngeal and oesophageal foreign bodies

May cause life-threatening stridor. The inhalation may have been witnessed and a history of a coughing or choking episode is obtained. However, one out of eight episodes of foreign body inhalation is not witnessed and presentation may be with a voice change (e.g. hoarseness) and/or breathing difficulty (e.g. stridor).

Immediate referral to the ENT surgeon and continuous supervision of the child are mandatory until the foreign body is removed. The foreign body may cause sudden obstruction and death.

INVESTIGATIONS

1. An AP and lateral neck X-ray may show a radio-opaque foreign body. The X-ray should be performed in ICU and not in the X-ray department.
2. As radiological examination may be normal, laryngoscopy/ endoscopy is necessary as a matter of urgency.

NB. Emergency mechanical efforts (i.e. Heimleich manoeuvre) to dislodge the foreign body should only be performed in the presence of life-threatening obstruction.

Foreign body in the oesophagus

Usually lodge in the upper third of the oesophagus. Pain, coughing, vomiting, choking, stridor and wheeze may occur.

MANAGEMENT

1. Chest and lateral neck X-ray.
2. Oesophageal foreign bodies require prompt removal. Sharp objects usually require endoscopic removal under GA. Refer to the ENT surgeon.

The majority of foreign bodies that pass into the stomach will eventually pass through the GI tract safely.

NB. Batteries must be removed as a matter of urgency.

Allergic rhinitis (hayfever)

Nasal congestion, watery discharge and sneezing. Allergic conjunctivitis may be present.

MANAGEMENT

1. Avoid suspected allergens.
2. Nasal symptoms may be relieved by topical SCG (Rynacrom nasal spray, 1 puff into each nostril 4–6-hourly). If symptoms are not controlled, change to:
3. Topical nasal steroids (e.g. Beconase nasal spray, 100 µg (2 puffs) into each nostril 12-hourly in children >6).
   Both should be used from 2–3 weeks before the hayfever season starts and use should be regular.
4. If symptoms warrant an oral antihistamine (e.g. for children 6–12 years, terfenadine 30 mg 12-hourly) may be given. Prophylactic use of the antihistamine prior to known allergen exposure is best.
5. SCG (Opticrom, administered 2–4 times per 24 hours) as ophthalmic drops may be used for allergic conjunctivitis.

Nose bleed (epistaxis)

Identify the bleeding point if possible. If bleeds are serious and recurrent FBC, clotting and BP should be checked and the child referred to the ENT department.

MANAGEMENT

1. Compression of anterior nasal septum between fingers for at least 10 min without release with the patient upright is usually all that is required.
2. If bleeding persists give topical anaesthesia with Xylocaine spray. Then soak pledgets of cotton wool in 1 : 10 000 adrenaline and apply to the bleeding point for 15–20 min only.
3. If bleeding continues after removal of pledgets refer to the ENT surgeon. Do not attempt to pack the nose without expert instruction.

Nasal trauma

1. An X-ray to diagnose a nasal fracture is unnecessary.
2. Examine for a septal haematoma. This is seen as a bulge from one or both sides of the nasal septum. If present, it requires drainage, packing and prophylactic antibiotics (erythromycin). Discuss with the ENT registrar on call.
3. If a cosmetic deformity is present with minimal swelling this may be reduced. Contact the ENT registrar. If swelling is present, review in 5 days. Reductions should be done within 10 days.

Tracheostomy care

It is unwise to change a tracheostomy tube until a tract has formed 3–4 days post-operatively.

TRACHEOSTOMY TUBE CHANGE

Do not attempt an elective change unless you have previously seen this done. Position the patient flat or with downwards head tilt and aspirate secretions. If difficulty is anticipated, a catheter should always be passed through the old tube before it is removed to act as a guide over which the new tube can be inserted.

OBSTRUCTION OF THE TRACHEOSTOMY TUBE

1. Check the position of the tube.
2. Try to pass a suction catheter and aspirate secretions.
3. If this is not possible, pass another tracheostomy tube.
4. If this is not possible and the child cannot exchange air, intubate with an ETT.

Deafness

Routine hearing screening is carried out at 8–10 months. Ideally infants at risk (family history, previous meningitis, very low birthweight, delayed speech, other developmental handicap) and infants who fail screening should be referred to an audiologist.

MANAGEMENT

Refer to the ENT surgeon who will organise full evaluation.

Hearing screening

A child with: a 20-dB hearing loss can miss a soft whisper; 20–40-dB loss can miss soft speech; 40–60-dB loss ordinary speech missed or not understood; > 80 dB cannot understand a shout.

Screening is determined by age and the presence of other problems (e.g. previous meningitis, developmental delay).

NEONATAL

Auditory response cradle may be used in selected cases, e.g. following meningitis.

1. 0–7 months: watch for age-appropriate response:
   newborn: blinking, startle or cry with loud noise;
   4 months: head turning towards sound is consistent;
   5 months: turns to sound and down if the source is low;
   7 months: direct diagonal movement of head to source of sound below ear level.

2. 7–9 months: distraction test — performed in all children by a health visitor, used up to 18 months. Soft sounds 30–35 dB, high and low frequency. If the child fails, re-test in 1 month. If the child fails a second test, unless the cause is obvious (e.g. upper respiratory tract infection), then refer.

3. 18–30 months: test only if parents are concerned, there is language delay or children at high risk, e.g. post meningitis. This can be a difficult age group to test. Cooperative testing is used, i.e. 'give this to daddy, show me the koala bear'. Exclude visual clues (minimal levels < 40 dB at 1 m).

4. 2.5–5 years: auditory discrimination test, e.g. McCormick toy discrimination test or picture cards. This tests discrimination between similar sounding words and requires response at < 40 dB at 1 m each side.

   Performance test: for this the child is taught to respond in a particular way to hearing a sound.

5. 5–6 years: puretone audiometry.

17

Ophthalmology

Before examining the eyes always assess visual acuity in older children and visual performance in younger children.

VISION SCREENING

High-risk groups for visual impairment include premature babies, those with a family history of squint, amblyopia, and visual handicap. Treat any parental concerns seriously.

Birth. Ophthalmic examination for congenital abnormalities and check for presence of red reflex to help exclude opacities of the cornea, lens (cataract), vitreous and retinal abnormalities. The baby will turn his head towards a source of light.

6 weeks. Repeat the ophthalmic examination. The baby fixates and follows a bright object either side of midline and fixes on face.

4 months. The infant will reach towards object in its view.

6 months. The infant can hold fixation for up to 30 sec. Observe for squint. Light from a distant source (e.g. window) should be reflected symmetrically from the cornea of both eyes (corneal light reflex); if not, a squint is present. Refer to the ophthalmologist if squint is present. The cover test is unreliable at this age.

18 months. Observe for squint and abnormal visual behaviour, check for assymetrical corneal light reflex. The cover test is difficult; an abnormal test warrants referral but failure to manage the test does not merit retesting if squint is not suspected.

2.5–3.5 years. Measure visual acuity using 5 or 7 letter Stycar at 3 m. Many children after the age of 3 will be able to match single letters to the Snellen chart at 6 m. This is more reliable. 6/9 in either eye merits retesting in 6 months. 6/12 should be referred. 80% of 3-year-olds are developmentally able to perform this test. A child who peers or moves his head in an effort to see should have his visual acuity carefully assessed and referred if it is reduced.

5 years (school entry). Test visual acuity using a Snellen chart at 6 m. Test with and without glasses and test near vision if there are visual problems.

10 years. Screen for colour vision. Approximately 5% of boys and 0.4% of girls have some degree of colour vision defect.

Handicapped children should be tested according to their developmental level and nature of handicap. Ophthalmological referral may be necessary.

Periorbital cellulitis

Tenderness, erythema and oedema of the lid and adjacent face.
The most common cause in children < 5 is *Haem. influenzae* type B. If there is evidence of trauma then *Staph. aureus* or group A beta-haemolytic *Streptococcus* is usually the cause.

MANAGEMENT

1. Evaluate to rule out eye involvement, i.e. orbital cellulitis (lid swelling may necessitate the use of an eyelid retractor to examine for proptosis and evaluate eye movements). If there is difficulty in examining the eye or if there is any concern, consult the ophthalmologist on call.
2. Blood cultures and eye swabs.
3. Consider LP in infants or sick children because of the risk of associated meningitis.
4. Admit to hospital.
5. If the cause is unknown commence chloramphenicol i.v. or ceftriaxone and flucloxacillin.
6. If obviously secondary to trauma, e.g. scratch, flucloxacillin and ampicillin i.v. may be given.

If the cellulitis is predominantly over the maxilla, consider dental abscess.

Orbital cellulitis

Infection of tissues behind the orbital septum. Associated with proptosis, chemosis, limitation of eye movement, orbital pain and decreased vision.

MANAGEMENT

1. Admit for urgent antibiotic therapy (as for periorbital cellulitis), following blood culture.
2. Immediate referral to the ophthalmologist and ENT surgeon: sinus evaluation with CT is usually indicated. Consider LP to exclude meningitis.

Red eyes

It is important to distinguish conjunctivitis, the most common cause, from more serious causes (e.g. iritis/keratitis).

CONJUNCTIVITIS

Diffuse redness of the conjunctiva with watery or purulent discharge.

Usually there is no photophobia, mild pain only, normal vision and pupiliary reflexes.

Management depends on age.

A. Neonatal

1. Gonnococcal infection: purulent discharge and conjunctival inflammation in the first few days of life. Gram negative diplococci on microscopy of smear.

Management. Admit for i.v. penicillin, saline eye washes and chloramphenicol eye drops (1 drop to each eye 3 hourly).

Infection is usually acquired from the mother's genital tract; therefore refer parents for treatment.

2. Other bacteria, e.g. *Staph. albus, Staph. aureus*, diphtheroids, streptococci: all can cause an eye discharge.

Management. Neomycin eye drops. If symptoms do not improve, consider *Chlamydia* infection.

3. Chlamydia: 3–30 days of age. A conjunctival swab placed in chlamydial medium is required for diagnosis. Rapid diagnosis by a chlamydial fluorescent antibody test is now available.

Management. Erythromycin 50 mg/kg per 24 hours p.o in 4 divided doses for 10 days.

Infection is acquired from the mother's genital tract; therefore refer parents for treatment. Untreated chlamydial infection may cause maternal infertility.

Outside the neonatal period
Causes include:

1. **Bacterial**. Purulent discharge is usually present. Treat with chloramphenicol eye drops (1 drop into each eye 2–3 hourly during the day) and chloramphenicol eye ointment at night. If persistent, consult an ophthalmologist. Chlamydial infection may cause conjunctivitis outside the neonatal period.

2. **Viral.** Usually presents with a clear discharge and clears spontaneously. If herpes simplex conjunctivitis is suspected

(e.g. eyelid or cheek vesicles) check for corneal ulceration, commence idoxuridine ointment 4-hourly and arrange urgent ophthalmological review. Avoid topical steroids.

3. **Allergic.** Itchy with a watery discharge; often seasonal.
a. Attempt to remove allergen.
b. Stop rubbing of eyes.
c. Try topical antihistamine (antazoline 0.5%).
d. Consider topical SCG for chronic cases.
e. For severe cases discuss the use of prednisolone drops with the ophthalmologist.

Never pad a discharging eye.
If eye drops are used, always show parents how to give them.

BLOCKED NASOLACRIMAL DUCT (DACRYOSTENOSIS)

A persistent purulent discharge in children < 12 months is often due to a blocked tear duct. Usually clears spontaneously. Avoid repeated antibiotics. Massage of the lacrimal sac may hasten resolution. Some cases require probing under GA if not resolving by 9 months.

CORNEAL ULCERATION

Presents with pain, photophobia, blepharospasm and lacrimation. Caused by trauma or herpes simplex (dendritic ulcer). Do not give local steroid drops.

Management
1. Local anaesthetic drops to facilitate examination.
2. Examination with fluorescein stain is needed to determine the extent of the ulceration.
3. If ulceration is traumatic and mild, treat with chloramphenicol eye ointment and eye patch. Review in 24–48 hours (usually healed by then). If ulceration has not healed or if in doubt refer to the ophthalmologist.
4. Refer all cases of herpes infection to the ophthalmologist on call. While awaiting the ophthalmologist, give idoxuridine eye ointment 4-hourly and an eye patch.

IRITIS

Unusual in childhood (chronic iritis is frequently associated with pauciarticular juvenile chronic arthritis). Symptoms are as for corneal ulceration but a corneal defect is absent. The pupil is small and does not react well to light. Vision is often blurred.

Management
1. Immediate ophthalmological referral. If delay occurs, dilate

pupils with homatropine drops 2% and instil prednisolone 0.5% drops 4-hourly.
2. Look for other features of connective tissue disease.

Stye (hordeolum)

Small tender swelling of a sebaceous gland usually due to a *Staph. aureus* infection.

Management
Usually drains spontaneously. Warm moist compress for 10–20 min 6-hourly. Neomycin eye ointment 6-hourly may help resolution.

Chemical burns

Can be devastating, especially if due to an alkaline substance.

Management
1. Profuse irrigation of the eye with tap water at the site of injury.
2. In casualty apply 1–2 drops of a topical local anaesthetic to the eye to facilitate continuous irrigation with normal saline (at least 2 litres).
3. Refer immediately to the ophthalmologist.

Thermal burns

Ocular surface is rarely involved despite extensive lid involvement. Check for corneal ulceration with fluorescein. Give chloramphenicol ointment in cases of corneal ulceration or extensive lid oedema (as lubricant). Discuss management with the on call ophthalmologist.

Foreign bodies

1–2 drops of a topical local anaesthetic may be instilled to facilitate examination. **If local anaesthetic is used the eye must be padded for 24 hours following examination.**

Management
1. Conjunctival: eversion of the lid may be necessary. Most foreign bodies can be removed with a moist cotton wool swab. Refer to the ophthalmologist if any difficulty is encountered.

2. Corneal: if not easily removed with a moist cotton wool swab, refer to the ophthalmologist on duty.
3. Intraocular: signs include perforation site, distorted pupil or small conjunctival haemorrhage. If the history is at all suggestive, arrange an AP and lateral orbit X-ray and refer immediately to the ophthalmologist on duty. Suggestive history includes striking metal on metal, using power tools or lawn mower and explosion of any sort.

Ocular trauma

Every suspected eye injury should be treated with as much respect as if it were known to be a penetrating injury. Perform complete eye and fundal examination including visual acuity in all cases. Specific injuries include:

A. PENETRATING INJURY

1. Test visual acuity.
2. X-ray orbit.
3. Protect the eye with a cone which prevents pressure on the eye (**not** a pad as this will increase pressure on the open damaged eye).
4. Vomiting is common; treat with an antiemetic (e.g. metaclopramide).
5. Urgent referral to the ophthalmic surgeon.

B. HYPHEMA

Blood in the anterior chamber. There is a possibility of secondary haemorrhage and loss of vision, thus patients should be admitted and referred to the ophthalmic surgeon on call.

C. BLOWOUT FRACTURE THROUGH THE ORBITAL WALL

Should be suspected if there is restricted eye movement with double vision, enophthalmos or infraorbital nerve anaesthesia. Refer to the ophthalmologist on call.

Squint

All children with a squint or suspected squint should be referred to the ophthalmology department. Refer any child whose parents suspect a squint even if you cannot detect it on examination. Broad epicanthic folds may give the appearance of a squint but corneal light reflexes are central and there is no movement on cover testing.

If in doubt, refer.

NB. A newly recognised paralytic squint merits urgent neurological referral.

Congenital cataract

White pupil or impairment of the red reflex. Refer urgently to the eye clinic as immediate surgery is now considered advisable. Retinoblastoma also needs to be excluded.

Congenital glaucoma

Early diagnosis is important as surgery offers a high chance of cure.

Presentation is with hazy or enlarged cornea, watery eyes and photophobia. Refer to the ophthalmologist.

Visual impairment

A child is never too young to be referred for an ophthalmological opinion. To assess vision it is important to know the normal visual attainment at various ages (see p. 281). Severe visual impairment interferes with all aspects of development but speech and gross motor are much less retarded than fine motor and social skills.

An obvious cause of visual handicap is often present (e.g. cataracts, optic atrophy, retrolental fibroplasia, etc.); however, significant visual handicap may still be present even if the examination is normal. If in doubt, refer.

18

THE SKIN

Identification of skin lesions is best done by reference to a colour atlas. The commonest skin disorders which junior paediatric staff are required to treat are eczema, skin infections and infestations, including warts and candida, and nappy rash. Particular features or the distribution of a skin lesion may give a clue to the diagnosis:

Gingivitis/stomatitis: most likely diagnoses are:

— Apthous ulcers (common in well children but also following stress or neutropenia; treat with 1% hydrocortisone in glycerine ointment 2-hourly alternating with chlorhexidine mouthwash 2-hourly)
— Dental infection or malocclusion
— Herpes simplex I
— Coxsackie
— Vincent's angina (mixed spirochaetal/anaerobic infection in ill, debilitated children, often with poor dental hygiene. Treat with oral metronidazole 7.5 mg/kg 8-hourly and penicillin 12.5 mg 6-hourly).
— *Candida* (see pp 219, 292, 297).
— Allergic stomatitis (to chemicals in toothpaste, sweets or drugs)
— Angio-oedema (follows exposure to specific allergen and is due to hereditary Cl esterase deficiency. Give parents emergency box containing adrenaline and hydrocortisone and explain i.m. injection)
— Phenytoin gum hypertrophy
— Lead poisoning (blue line on gums)
— Vitamin deficiency
— Some skin diseases involve the mouth (erythema multiforme — Stevens–Johnson syndrome, chicken pox, measles, lichen planus, pemphigus)

Lesions affecting palms or soles: most likely diagnoses are:

— Coxsackie infection
— Kawasaki's disease (fever and four of: bilateral conjunctivitis; oral erythema; erythema, desquamation or oedema of hands or feet; lymphadenopathy; rash)
— Erythema multiforme
— Scabies
— Pompholyx (bullous eczema)

Desquamation:

— Streptococcal infection
— Kawasaki's disease
— Toxic epidermal necrolysis

Photosensitive rashes:

— Suntan!
— Contact with plant psoralens
— Drugs (sulphonamides, thiazide diuretics)
— The others are all very rare (SLE, dermatomyositis, porphyria, phenylketonuria, albinism, vitiligo)

Itchy skin lesions

1. Eczema — usually cheeks, hands and limb flexures.
2. Uritcaria — causes include idiopathic, dietary allergen, insect bite, contact with plant allergen. There is a wheal (raised and white) and flare (red). Treat with terfenadine (non-sedating antihistamine) 1 mg/kg 12-hourly.
3. Insect bites — look for punctum of blood.
4. Fungal infections (tinea capitis — itchy scalp; tinea pedis or athlete's foot — itching between toes; tinea corporis or ringworm — itchy patch on trunk, called tinea versicolor if hypo- or hyperpigmented).
5. Head lice — pediculosis capitis.
6. Scabies — itchy wherever mite burrows, commonly finger webs or buttocks.
7. Psoriasis — erythematous patches with silvery scales and thickened skin (lichenification) over knees and elbows. Scalp and nails involved.
8. Dermatitis herpetiformis — vesicles or itchy papules. Usually affects genitalia, perineum or buttocks and is associated with coeliac disease although age of presentation is later (6–12 years); treat with dapsone.
9. Pityriasis rosea — the herald patch is single, raised and sometimes itchy.
10. Chicken pox.

Conjugated hyperbilirubinaemia and uraemia cause generalised itching, and dermatitis artefacta is a behavioural disorder with repeated itching of the same site, typically the neck.

Blisters and vesicles

NEONATE

Infections

1. Bullous impetigo — 'neonatal pemphigus', a staphylococcal skin infection (see p. 317).

2. Congenital chicken pox — infant is most at risk if the mother's rash first appears within 4 days before or after delivery. May be fatal. If the mother develops chicken pox rash between 4 days before and 4 days after delivery, give 1.25 ml zoster immune globulin i.m. as soon as possible. If the infant develops clinical varicella, give 10 mg/kg acyclovir 8-hourly i.v.

3. Congenital herpes simplex (type II) — infant is most at risk if delivery is vaginal and the mother has active cervical lesions. May be fatal. If the baby has clinical herpes simplex infection, swab the lesions and eyes, mouth and urine for viral culture and take serum for HSV IgM. Consider LP. Treat with acyclovir 10 mg/kg 8-hourly i.v. for 10 days.

Others

1. Inherited bullous disorders (epidermolysis bullosa and incontinentia pigmenti).

CHILD

Infections

1. Chicken pox — macules first, then papules but usually vesicular within hours. Unusual > 10 years (unless immunosuppressed) although second attacks do rarely occur. Axillae are almost always affected.

2. Herpes zoster (shingles) — usually unilateral and confined to a sensory dermatome. A close contact may catch chicken pox from shingles.

3. Herpes simplex (cold sores) — usually type I in childhood (classically affects lips, chin, tongue and buccal mucosa but, confusingly, the first attack may present with genital herpes lesions in either sex). Recurrence at a particular site, usually lips, is common and may be precipitated by viral upper respiratory tract infection or pneumococcal pneumonia. Give regular analgesia and i.v. fluids if oral intake is inadequate. Acyclovir 5% topical cream 4-hourly for 5 days may reduce the duration and severity of the lesions but only if started within 4 days of the first 'cold sore'.

4. Coxsackie A16 virus — blisters on 'hand, foot and mouth' and sometimes maculopapular rash over buttocks.

5. ECHO virus — vesicular rash, often with GI upset.

6. Staphylococcal infections may cause blisters or pustules (see p. 289) and scabies may cause vesicles (see p. 289).

Others

1. Dermatitis herpetiformis (see p. 289).

2. Bullous pemphigoid — usually < 6 years. Face, limbs, genitalia or groins may be affected. Bullae may be bloodstained but are not itchy.

3. Papular urticaria — hypersensitivity reaction, usually to insect bites and usually in the summer.
4. Erythema multiforme — can cause blisters as well as the typical 'target lesions', especially if there is mucosal involvement (Stevens-Johnson syndrome). Follows viral (especially herpes simplex) or mycoplasma infection or sulphonamides.
5. Burns — thermal, solar, chemical.
6. Simple friction — new shoes!
7. Pompholyx — bullous eczema.

Skin infections and infestations

All are potentially infectious. Swab lesions for culture if admission is warranted.

IMPETIGO

Staphylococci or streptococci. May complicate nappy rash, eczema, scabies, pediculosis. Localised area of pustules and crusts and sometimes large blisters.

Clean with saline solution, apply topical 3% chlortetracycline ointment 8-hourly or with nappy change, oral penicillin V and flucloxacillin 6-hourly for 1 week. Avoid contact with other children. If surrounding erythema/swelling suggest cellulitis or erysipelas, admit for parenteral flucloxacillin and penicillin after blood cultures.

SUPERFICIAL INFECTION IN THE NEWBORN

'Whiteheads' on skin, usually staphylococcal. If lesions are few, use Ster-zac powder only. If more extensive or in groins or axillae, apply fusidic acid cream topically. If the infant is febrile or not feeding, take blood cultures and start oral flucloxacillin. Check for conjunctivitis, paronychia and umbilical infection.

TOXIC EPIDERMAL NECROLYSIS

'Scalded skin syndrome' (Lyell's or Ritter's disease). Due to staphylococcal toxin. Presents with erythema and epidermal separation on friction (Nikolsky's sign) and occasionally large, fragile blisters. Admit for parenteral flucloxacillin and to ensure hydration and body temperature are maintained.

SCABIES

Pruritic papules wherever the mite burrows (fingerwebs, wrists, axillae, palms and soles, head and neck, genitalia). Vesicles and bullae may occur as hypersensitivity reaction and secondary bacterial infection is common.

Treatment

1. Bath first.
2. 1% gammabenzene hexachloride (Lindane) lotion to whole body, including genitalia and soles of feet (and including face and scalp in infants), allow to dry and leave applied for 24 hours.
3. Repeat 1. and 2. for another 24 hours.
4. Calamine lotion for residual itching (may persist for 3 months).
5. Treat all 'kissing contacts' twice also, irrespective of symptoms (avoid Lindane in pregnant contacts).
6. All clothing/bed linen must be laundered.

Re-infection common.

PEDICULOSIS CAPITIS

Head lice or nits (the eggs are easier to identify) infect hair including eyebrows/lashes. Usually preschool children. Secondary scalp impetigo occurs.

Treatment

1. 1% malathion cream shampoo, leave application for 12 hours.
2. Wash hair and comb rinsed hair with a fine comb. Repeat this sequence three times at 3-day intervals.
3. Launder all headgear, discourage sharing of combs, encourage frequent hair washing.
4. Treat all family and close contacts irrespective of symptoms.

FUNGAL INFECTIONS (see 'Nappy rash')

1. *Candida* ('thrush' or monilia) is common. Infection at one site should suggest other sites:
   — mouth (white plaques which are difficult to remove)
   — oesophagus
   — nails (paronychia)
   — perineum and genitalia (if there are small, round 'satellite' lesions on the periphery of the main area of erythema, *candida* is probable)

Predisposed to by antibiotics or immunosuppression (including preterms) when candidaemia, endocarditis or meningitis may occur. Treat topical infection with nystatin cream 6-hourly or with every nappy change and continue for 7 days after lesions disappear. Treat oral *Candida* with nystatin suspension

100 000 u/ml, 1 ml 6-hourly after food. Treat systemic *Candida* with i.v. amphotericin and flucytosine combined.

2. Tinea infections of the nails (tinea unguium) and the scalp (tinea capitis — may cause alopecia or a 'kerion', a pustular mass) are treated systemically with griseofulvin 10 mg/kg once per 24 hours for 1 month as this is concentrated in keratin. Treatment may be ineffective until the animal source (cats, dogs, cows) is controlled. Skin dermatophyte infections (tinea pedis, cruris, corporis) respond to topical miconazole 2% 12-hourly until 10 days after lesions heal.

Warts and other viral skin infections

These are infectious and autoinfection by scratching (Koebner phenomenon) is common.

1. WARTS

Papovavirus; usually school age; usually hands, face or feet (genital warts must always arouse suspicion). 2/3 disappear within 2 years and all disappear eventually. A verruca is a plantar wart which grows inwards because of the pressure of the sole.
a. Treat warts and verrucas with Salactol (salicyclic and lactic acids). Paint daily, cover with a plaster, and remove dead skin at intervals with a pumice stone. Minimum trial of therapy is 3 months before referral to a dermatologist for 'freezing' *if the child wishes.*
b. Anogenital warts should be treated with 15% podophyllin paint. Cover the surrounding skin with soft paraffin, apply for 6 hours, then wash off.

2. MOLLUSCUM CONTAGIOSUM

Pox virus; preschool age; multiple on face or trunk. The wart has a central dimple ('umbilicated'), and treatment, if deemed necessary for cosmesis, is by piercing each lesion with a stick dipped in 10% podophyllin. Spontaneous resolution is invariable.

The exanthemas of childhood

Common (Table 18.1) and rarely require admission. Measles and rubella are overdiagnosed and a past history is definitely not a contraindication to immunisation (see Ch. 13).

Table 18.1 Exanthemata and mumps

Disease	Incubation (days)	Duration (days)		Infectious (days)	Site	Complications
Measles	10–14	Prodrome Rash	4 4	2 days prior to prodrome until 5 days after onset of rash	Koplik spots on buccal mucosa during prodrome Rash on face and then whole body	Conjunctivitis/Rhinitis Otitis media Pneumonia Encephalitis (acute or chronic)
Rubella	14–21	Prodrome Rash (25% have no rash)	1–7 4	1 week before rash to 1 week after onset of rash	Post-auricular lymphadenopathy Rash starts on face and trunk	Thrombocytopenia Encephalitis Arthritis
Chickenpox	14–17	No prodrome Rash	10	4 days before rash until all vesicles are crusted	Trunk more than face or limbs	Cerebellar ataxia Purpura fulminans Guillain–Barré syndrome Pneumonia
Roseola infantum (also known as exanthema subitum, 3-day fever or sixth disease) probably due to human herpes virus type 6	10	Prodrome Rash	4 1–2	For the course of the illness	Fine pink truncal rash follows lysis of high fever Cervical and post-auricular lymphadenopathy	Febrile convulsion
Fifth disease (erythema infectiosum due to human parvovirus B19)	7–14	No prodrome Rash	3–7	For the course of the illness	'Slapped cheek' syndrome Reticulate maculopapular rash may then appear on trunk, spreading to limbs a few days later	None

Table 18.1 (Contd)

Disease	Incubation (days)	Duration (days)		Infectious (days)	Site	Complications
Scarlet fever (scarlatina)	2 – 4	Prodrome Rash	2 6	Until penicillin is given	Tonsillitis, pinpoint rash on trunk and neck which blanches on pressure, strawberry tongue, circumoral pallor, desquamation	Glomerulonephritis Rheumatic fever
Mumps	16 – 21	Prodrome Parotid gland swelling	1–3 7	Few days before glands swell until they return to normal	No rash	Pancreatitis Encephalitis

The erythemas

— erythema multiforme (see pp 289, 291)
— erythema nodosum (painful raised swellings on shins associated with streptococcal infections, TB, inflammatory bowel disease, sarcoidosis, sulphonamides)
— erythema annulare = erythema marginatum (rheumatic fever)
— erythema induratum (TB)
— erythema granulare (usually idiopathic)

Atopic eczema

BACKGROUND

5% of children affected, 70% of whom have family history of atopy. Onset is usually > 3 months with remission between 2 and 4 years and in puberty common. There is some evidence that exclusive breast feeding protects.

DIAGNOSIS

Red, itchy rash; usually face or flexures; may be dry or moist; sometimes raised and thickened (lichenified); secondary infection (bacterial — impetigo; herpes simplex — eczema herpeticum or Kaposi's varicelliform eruption) may occur.

MANAGEMENT

Emollients (moisturizers)

Add 'Oilatum' to a cool bath daily. Soaps are contraindicated (as are 'biological' washing powders for clothes); instead, clean the skin by applying 'Unguentum Merck' to wet skin, massage and rinse. Apply aqueous cream (e.g. 'E45') generously and frequently throughout the day and especially last thing at night.

Topical corticosteroids

1% hydrocortisone 6-hourly can be used in all but the very smallest infants, even on the face, long term. Ointment is better for chronic, dry eczema, cream for moist eczema. More potent steroids (Eumovate, Betnovate, Dermovate in ascending strength) require dermatological advice and growth suppression is possible. Nevertheless, under-use is the major reason why hydrocortisone fails; 50 g per week of ointment may be required for a widespread eczema exacerbation.

Antimicrobials

Use 'Terra-Cortil' (1% hydrocortisone and oxytetracycline) for 2 weeks for exacerbations when secondary infection is mild. Impetigo should be swabbed and treated with systemic flucloxacillin and penicillin V for 1 week. Use topical and oral acyclovir for herpes.

Antihistamines

Benefit is related to sedative effect more than antipruritic properties, e.g. trimeprazine 2 mg/kg at night. Avoidance of woollen clothing, trimming of nails and wearing of cotton mits at night, and topical calamine lotion may relieve itching.

Dietary restriction

Controversial. Empirical elimination of egg and cow's milk protein for a 6-week trial is justified, especially in young children provided a soy milk is substituted. Abandon dietary restriction if there is no definite improvement after 6 weeks; if eczema improves, continue for 12 months and then gradually re-introduce. Only a few additional children are helped by more sophisticated diets. (House dust mites, pollen and pets may aggravate eczema but are difficult to avoid.)

SEBORRHOEIC DERMATITIS

Eczema occurring at sites of increased sebaceous activity (face, neck, chest, scalp — 'cradle cap') but there is no abnormality of the sebaceous glands. Not itchy and no treatment (other than baby oil applications before shampooing) is required unless there is secondary *Candida* infection.

Nappy rash

Usually a contact dermatitis, but secondary infection may occur. Risk factors:
— neonatal skin is thin and susceptible to irritants
— poor hygiene and prolonged contact with urine and faeces
— urea-splitting organisms cause ammoniacal dermatitis
— secondary *Candida* infection
— change from breast feeding to formula foods

MANAGEMENT

1. Use disposable nappies and change frequently to keep the area dry and clean.
2. Expose to air whenever feasible and avoid plastic pants.
3. Apply emollient (e.g. E45 cream) after every change.

4. Topical nystatin ointment after every nappy change for *Candida* infection.
5. 1% hydrocortisone 6-hourly for 1 week if the above measures are ineffective.

Once skin has recovered, liberally apply zinc and castor oil barrier cream to prevent recurrence.

19

Neonatology

Resuscitation and asphyxia

High risk deliveries

A paediatrician should be present in cases of:
1. Fetal distress, meconium stained liquor, or antepartum haemorrhage.
2. Forceps, breech or caesarean section.
3. Multiple pregnancy (a doctor for each infant).
4. < 35 weeks' gestation.
5. Concern because of antenatal diagnosis (eg. congenital abnormality, rhesus incompatibility) or maternal disease (e.g. diabetes, myasthenia, severe pre-eclampsia).

A paediatrician should be informed after delivery in cases of:
1. LBW (a rough guide is to admit all infants < 2 kg or < 36 weeks to the NNU).
2. PROM.
3. Any congenital abnormality.
4. Previous abnormal infant or perinatal death.
5. Maternal thyroid or parathyroid disease, thrombocytopenia, infection (genital or systemic), previous hepatitis B infection, family history of TB.

Resuscitation

Immediately following delivery (unless there is meconium stained liquor), dry and wrap the infant, place under a radiant heat source, oropharyngeal suction and aspiration of the nares, face mask O_2.

MECONIUM STAINED LIQUOR

Once the head is delivered, clear the upper airway with a wide-bore suction catheter. Once on resuscitaire, suck the meconium from the oropharynx and insert an ETT ('inspection of the cords' is an unreliable test). If the baby is too vigorous to intubate, he is unlikely to have severe meconium aspiration. Pass suction catheter through ETT and aspirate vigorously. This can be continued for 2 min if the infant is in groups (1) or (2) below, but only for 1 min if in category (3), before IPPV is given via the ETT. Never give mask IPPV. Pneumothorax, hyperinflation and PFC are possible sequelae.

BY 1 MINUTE

Assess the Apgar score (Table 19.1). Further resuscitation is determined by pulse and respiration. There are three groups:
1. Heart rate > 100, regular breathing — the infant should become pink soon with the above measures. If not, see p. 81.
2. Heart rate < 100 but not asystolic or white — give IPPV with 100% O_2 by bag and mask at 40 breaths/min once the airway is clear. If heart rate falls further, or is static after 1 min of mask IPPV, continue as for 3.
3. Asystolic or white — cardiac massage 100/min, laryngoscopy and tracheal suction under direct vision, endotracheal intubation (3.0 mm tube if > 32 weeks, 2.5 mm tube if < 32 weeks), IPPV 40/min with pressure of 30 cmH_2O. If no response is seen, insert a UVC and give 1 mmol/kg NaHCO$_3$ (2 ml/kg 4.2%), 0.25 ml/kg 1 : 10 000 adrenaline and 2 ml/kg 25% dextrose, flushing the drugs through with 2 ml saline. If there is still no response, give 1 ml/kg 10% calcium gluconate and 0.05 ml/kg atropine (0.6 mg/ml solution) via the UVC.

If the infant remains white, or ECG shows complexes but pulses are not palpable, or if there has been antepartum haemorrhage, give 20 ml/kg O negative uncrossmatched blood (or plasma if blood is not available).

If there is respiratory depression, and maternal opiates have been given within 6 hours of delivery, always give neonatal Narcan 0.01 mg/kg i.v. (0.02 mg/ml solution; dose can be repeated 6 times at 3-min intervals and 0.01 mg/kg i.m. (max. 1 ml at one site) as depot.

Table 19.1 Apgar scores

	Score		
	0	1	2
Heart rate	Absent	< 100/min	> 100/min
Respiratory effort	Nil	Gasping or irregular	Regular
Colour of trunk	White	Blue	Pink
Tone	Atonic	Decreased	Normal
Response to suction	None	Decreased	Normal (grimace or cry)

If i.v. access is difficult, give double the above doses of adrenaline, atropine or naloxone via the ETT followed by IPPV.

When not to resuscitate and when to stop
(see Ch. 2 also)

THE VERY IMMATURE INFANT

Different units vary in their enthusiasm to resuscitate infants < 26 weeks' gestation. Therefore, ask about your own unit's policy towards very immature infants AS SOON AS YOU START YOUR JOB. If you are in any doubt about viability, attempt resuscitation. Intensive care can be withdrawn later following assessment by a more senior colleague and discussion with the parents.

'BIRTH ASPHYXIA'

All mature infants who are thought to have been hypoxic during labour should be vigorously resuscitated since fetal monitoring, cord pH and Apgar scores are unreliable predictors of outcome. An infant experiencing acute total asphyxia during labour may be born with no sign of life but recovery is possible. Again, care can be withdrawn later if severe encephalopathy develops and the parents agree.

CONGENITAL ABNORMALITY

The commonest situations are:
1. Cardiopulmonary resuscitation is possible but there is an additional severe anomaly visible (e.g. large myelomeningocele, severe arthrogryphosis). If a management plan has not been agreed beforehand, the infant must be resuscitated.
2. Cardiopulmonary resuscitation is possible but the infant does not breathe spontaneously. Consider maternal drugs, intracerebral bleeding, cerebral malformation, cervical cord injury. Give naloxone 0.01 mg/kg i.v. or i.m. and transfer intubated and ventilated to the NNU for further assessment.
3. Infant is resuscitated and breathes but goes blue on extubation. Consider choanal atresia.
4. Cardiopulmonary resuscitation is ineffective if:
   a. intubation is impossible — tracheal agenesis or stenosis.
   b. no chest wall movement — O_2 supply not connected, ETT is in the oesophagus or there is severe pulmonary hypoplasia (look for typical facies of Potter's syndrome; absence of a history of oligohydramnios does NOT exclude this diagnosis).

    c.   the infant can be ventilated but remains blue — diaphragmatic hernia (pass NGT to decompress) or cyanotic heart disease.

In all these situations, persistent cyanosis is not a reason to stop resuscitation but if the infant is asystolic or bradycardic after 20 min of appropriate resuscitation, resuscitation should be stopped.

Birth asphyxia

BACKGROUND

At increased risk are:

1. Preterm infants
2. SGA infants
3. Abnormal fetal heart rate pattern
4. Meconium stained liquor (rare in preterm labour)
5. Fetal scalp pH < 7.2
6. Abnormal umbilical Doppler velocities

NB. Some infants born asphyxiated do not have these features. In many, a pre-existing abnormality (e.g. neurological abnormality or sepsis) renders the fetus liable to complications of labour and perinatal asphyxia.

ASSESSMENT AT BIRTH

Usually pale, hypotonic and apnoeic but the early Apgar score is a poor predictor of neurological outcome (Apgar score ≤ 5 at 5 min, 95% subsequently normal) and simply determines mode of resuscitation (see p. 300). A low Apgar score at 10 min and beyond is worrying. Umbilical cord pH is also poor predictor.

Table 19.2   Severity and outcome of hypoxic–ischaemic encephalopathy

	Grade		
	I	II	III
Clinical	Hyperalert Staring Irritable Poor suck Tone may be increased or decreased	Require tube feeding Asymmetric tonic neck reflex Difference in tone between upper and lower limbs	Hypertonia Seizures Coma Require ventilation
Outcome	> 95% normal	75% normal	20% normal 50% die in newborn period

Better predictors are clinical severity of subsequent HIE (Table 19.2) and cranial USS at follow-up.

COMPLICATIONS

Cerebral oedema (usually 24–48 hours), cerebral haemorrhage or infarction, seizures, SIADH, ARF, cardiac failure, hypotension, RDS, MAS, DIC, hypoglycaemia, hypocalcaemia, persistent acidosis, NEC.

MANAGEMENT FOLLOWING RESUSCITATION

1. Nil orally. 10% dextrose i.v. at 2/3 maintenance (Table 19.3). There is little evidence that mannitol or steroids prevents cerebral oedema. Increase the dextrose concentration rather than rate to maintain blood glucose > 2.5 mmol/l.
2. Plasma and urine electrolytes and osmolality daily. Anticipate renal failure if haematuria is detected. Urinary catheter if oliguria persists beyond 12 hours and give frusemide 1 mg/kg i.v. provided the infant is normovolaemic and normotensive. If there is no response, start dopamine infusion 5 µg/kg/min i.v.
3. IPPV for lung disease, apnoea or frequent anticonvulsant doses but not prophylactically. Aim for $PaCO_2$ 3.5 kPa to limit cerebral oedema, and pH > 7.25.
4. Insert an arterial line and monitor BP. In the first few days of life, 5th centile for mean BP (mmHg) is the same as gestation (weeks). If hypovolaemia is suspected (mean BP < 5th centile, oliguria, metabolic acidosis or peripheral–core temperature difference of > 2.5°C), give 4% albumin 15 ml/kg i.v. over

Table 19.3   Parenteral fluid requirements (ml/kg bodyweight per 24 hours)

	Fullterm	Preterm
1st 24 hours	40	60
2nd 24 hours	60	90
3rd 24 hours	80	120
4th 24 hours	110	150
5th 24 hours	150	150–180

Notes:
1. Add 20 ml/kg per 24 hours if the infant is receiving phototherapy.
2. Fluid restriction as above may not be appropriate if the reason for admission to NNU is hypoglycaemia.
3. Review feed/fluid intake daily based on electrolytes — in the first week, hypernatraemia is *usually* due to inadequate water intake.
4. Routine fluids as 10% dextrose on day 1, 10% dextrose/0.18% saline thereafter.
5. The above rates assume the infant is in an incubator; if nursed under a radiant warmer, check electrolytes 6-hourly initially as intakes > 250 ml/kg per 24 hours may be required for VLBW infants.

30 min (or FFP — see below). If hypotension persists, infuse dopamine 5–15 µg/kg/min i.v.
5. Anticonvulsants of choice in the newborn, in order, are:
Phenobarbitone 20 mg/kg i.v. over 5 min and 5 mg/kg per 24 hours maintenance.
Clonazepam 0.25 mg i.v. then 0.05 mg i.v. b.i.d.
Paraldehyde 0.3 ml/kg p.r. in equal volume of arachis oil.
Phenytoin 15 mg/kg i.v. over 15 min with ECG monitor; can be repeated 8-hourly.
Diazepam infusion 0.1 mg/kg/h i.v.
6. Vitamin K 1 mg i.m. Give FFP or platelets as lab. results dictate (see Ch. 14).

Outcome

Prognosis is worse if:
1. Apgar score is < 4 at 20 min (2/3 develop major handicap)
2. There is severe HIE (see Table 19.2)
3. HIE persists > 5 days
4. Parenchymal changes are seen on USS
5. There are seizures

Newborn examination

Examine all infants whose delivery you attend immediately after resuscitation.

Healthy infants should be examined within 24 hours of birth. Start at the top and work down, leaving unpleasant tasks until the end. Common queries are:
1. Gynaecomastia and lactation (normal in either sex). Abdomen: check for organomegaly and that there are three vessels in umbilical cord.
2. All infants should pass urine within 24 hours. If not, and the bladder is palpable, exclude urethral valves. If the bladder is impalpable, the cause is either hypovolaemia (usually overtly ill) or renal agenesis (usually pulmonary hypoplasia, abnormal facies and contractures).
3. 95% pass meconium by 24 hours and 98% by 48 hours. If constipated and rectal examination gives 'toothpaste tube' sign of meconium plug, consider Hirschsprung's disease.
4. Vaginal bleeding (normal).

The following should be checked at the end of the examinaton:
Measure OFC.
Femoral pulses.
Hips — dislocated hips will not abduct fully. Dislocatable hips (girls, breeches, family history) can be dislocated and reduced by Barlow's manoeuvre.

Eyes — red reflex to exclude cataract, subconjunctival haemorrhage (common).

Feeding (see Ch. 4 also)

See Table 19.3 for fluid requirements. Once feeding is established, aim for a daily weight gain of 15 g/kg after the first week (initial weight loss of approximately 10% of birthweight, by day 4, is normal).

Vitamins

VITAMIN K

1 mg to all infants (0.5 mg if < 1.5 kg), p.o. with the first feed or i.m. (always i.m. in the NNU) at birth. Haemorrhagic disease of the newborn affects 1 in 50 000 neonates, usually days 3–7 but also (a late form) up to 6 weeks. Most likely if the infant is breast fed, preterm, vitamin K given orally, given antibiotics, or maternal anticonvulsants or warfarin.

VITAMIN D

If < 2.5 kg at birth, 500 iu p.o. once per 24 hours when enteral feeding is established, until discharge (1000 iu if < 1.5 kg).

DSS VITAMIN DROPS (ACD)

If < 2.5 kg at birth, 5 drops p.o. daily when enteral feeding is established, until 6 months beyond EDD.

IRON

If < 2.5 kg at birth, start 0.3 ml Sytron p.o. 12-hourly at 1 month of age, increase to 1.0 ml Sytron p.o. 12-hourly at 3 months, stop at 6 months.

FOLIC ACID

0.25 mg/kg p.o. per 24 hours for documented Coombs' positive haemolytic anaemia, exchange transfusion, or anaemia of prematurity (Hb < 10 g/dl). Stop at 2 months if Hb > 9 g/dl.

Hypoglycaemia

Definition. Whole blood glucose < 2.0 mmol/l for term infants and < 1.5 mmol/l for preterm infants.

Always confirm low 'Reflomat' or test strips by laboratory estimation of plasma glucose. Discrepancies may arise because of old test sticks, wrong Reflomat technique, or blood taken proximal to dextrose infusion. There is increasing evidence that recurrent moderate hypoglycaemia (< 2.6 mmol/l) may also alter neuro-developmental prognosis and that the distinction between symptomatic and asymptomatic hypoglycaemia is erroneous (the symptoms of apnoea, jitteriness, poor feeding occur equally commonly in normoglycaemic infants) unless there are frank convulsions.

Prevention

1. Early milk feeds (see p. 34). *Not* enteral glucose solutions.
2. Immediate blood glucose measurement in all infants who have hypothermia or symptomatic hypoglycaemia.
3. Monitoring at risk infants with regular heel prick blood glucose measurements (lateral margins of heel only): on admission, at 2 hours and 4-hourly thereafter in all at risk infants (Table 19.4) initially.

   In all seriously ill infants, measure blood glucose 6-hourly; hourly during and for 4 hours after an exchange transfusion. If glucose < 2.0 mmol/l is measured, increase frequency of measurements to 2-hourly and if < 1.0 mmol/l, measure hourly. Revert to 4-hourly once glucose is > 2.0 mmol/l.

Management of hypoglycaemia

1. If the infant is well, milk feed hourly by breast or bottle initially. If infant refuses the feed, give a bolus via an NGT. If glucose remains low 1 hour after a feed, proceed as for (2) below.
2. If the infant is ill or too preterm to tolerate bolus NGT feeding, give a bolus of 2 ml/kg 25% dextrose i.v. over 2 min followed *always* by 10% dextrose infusion 3 ml/kg/h initially. Monitor glucose hourly and increase the rate (or increase concentration to 15–20% if hyponatraemia is likely to ensue) accordingly. Only reduce infusion (and simultaneously increase feeding) once blood glucose has been stable for 24 hours.

Table 19.4 Causes of hypoglycaemia

Decreased glucose production	Hyperinsulinism
	Any detectable insulin in the presence of significant hypoglycaemia is suspicious
A. *Usually transient* Preterm or post-mature Birth asphyxia Hypothermia SGA Infection CHD Maternal beta-blockers	A. *Usually transient* Excessive maternal glucose administration during labour Infant of diabetic mother Severe rhesus haemolytic disease Beckwith – Wiedemann syndrome (macroglossia, omphalocele and organomegaly)
B. *Often persistent* Hypopituitarism (micropenis or midline facial defects) Cortisol deficiency (adrenal hyperplasia, hypoplasia or haemorrhage — cortisol and 17-hydroxyprogesterone concentrations) Galactosaemia (reducing substances in urine but no glycosuria) Glycogen storage disease Organic acidaemia (low arterial pH and typical urine chromatogram) or defect of fatty acid oxidation	B. *Often persistent* Pancreatic tumour

Investigations of hypoglycaemia (see Table 19.4)

Only if severe, persistent or recurrent:
1. Dextrose 10% infusion of ≤ 5 ml/kg/h maintains normoglycaemia: the problem is lack of glucose (inadequate intake, absorption or production of glucose, including defective glycogenolysis).
2. Dextrose 10% > 6 ml/kg/h required: problem is excess of insulin. Urine ketones are absent.

Drugs to increase blood glucose include:
hydrocortisone 5 mg/kg i.v. 12-hourly (of little benefit in hyperinsulinism)
glucagon 0.1 mg/kg i.m.

diazoxide 5 mg/kg p.o. 8-hourly (if hyperinsulinism is documented
but hypotension a risk)
chlorthiazide 5 mg/kg p.o. 12-hourly (dehydration a risk)

Jaundice

BACKGROUND

Neonatal unconjugated jaundice is extremely common (50% of term, 80% of
preterm infants), partly because of the relative polycythaemia at birth and the
relative hepatic immaturity. A number of diseases (Table 19.5) can exacerbate
this underlying predisposition and investigation is aimed at identifying these.
Conjugated hyperbilirubinaemia always abnormal.

CLINICAL DIAGNOSIS

Jaundice is detectable when SBR > 85 μmol/l but it is difficult to
'eyeball' the level of jaundice. Artificial light and skin pigmentation add further confusion. *Always* measure SBR in preterm
infants and in term infants if in any doubt.

INVESTIGATION

Only the following groups warrant investigation.

Table 19.5 Conditions associated with neonatal jaundice

Unconjugated hyperbilirubinaemia	Conjugated hyperbilirubinaemia
Haemolysis	A. *Hepatocellular*
Polycythaemia	Idiopathic (i.e. in many preterm or SGA
Excessive bruising	infants, no specific cause is found)
Preterm	Infection (congenital or acquired,
Dehydration	including UTI)
Decreased calorie intake	TPN (cholestasis)
Infection (congenital or acquired)	Inspissated bile plugs (following severe
Meconium retention	rhesus disease)
High GI obstruction (e.g. pyloric	Hypothyroidism
stenosis)	Hypopituitarism
Hypothyroidism	Hypoadrenalism
Galactosaemia	Galactosaemia
Fructosaemia	Fructosaemia
Down's syndrome	Tyrosinaemia
	CF
	Alpha-1-antitrypsin deficiency
	B. *Ductal*
	Abnormal biliary tree (extrahepatic
	biliary atresia, choleductal cyst or
	Alagille's syndrome — biliary hypoplasia
	and peripheral pulmonary artery
	stenosis)

Early onset jaundice (< 24 hours old)

Usually haemolytic (see Ch. 14), of which commonest in the new-born are:

1. Rhesus haemolytic disease
2. ABO incompatibility
3. Congenital spherocytosis (50% present as neonate and 25% have negative family history — autosomal dominant but variable severity)
4. G6PD deficiency (boys only, usually ethnic minorities) and rare enzymopathies
5. Congenital infection (toxoplasmosis is rare in the UK but CMV is common, herpes and parvovirus occur, and rubella is not excluded by immunisation) can cause unconjugated (haemolysis) and/or conjugated (hepatitis) hyperbilirubinaemia.

Check:

1. SBR and conjugated/unconjugated split
2. Hb and blood film: spherocytes are common in normal neonates
3. mother and infant's blood groups and infant's DCT (positive DCT confirms immune aetiology although it may be negative in ABO incompatibility)
4. maternal haemolysis (anti-A or anti-B IgG antibodies) if (3) is suggestive
5. G6PD screen for black, Asian or Mediterranean infants
6. congenital infection screen if there are corroborative signs (hepatosplenomegaly, petechiae, cataracts, SGA).

Jaundice beginning on days 2–5

Usually 'physiological' jaundice. More likely if there is excessive bruising, polycythaemia, or if the infant is breast fed or preterm. Only investigate if SBR > 170 μmol/l to exclude causes which exaggerate unconjugated hyperbilirubinaemia in the neonate.

1. Investigations as above.
2. Infection screen if the baby is ill, including urine culture.
3. Ask about family history (Gilbert's syndrome is the common-est inherited defect of bilirubin metabolism).

If all of the above are negative:

4. Urine for reducing substances (galactosaemia and fructosaemia).
5. Thyroid function tests (hypothyroidism).

For conjugated hyperbilirubinaemia, see below.

Prolonged jaundice (persisting or recurring > 14 days old)

A. If unconjugated and the baby is well, usually 'breast milk' jaundice. Do not stop breast feeding. If not breast fed, inves-tigate as above.
B. If conjugated, investigate as for Table 19.5.
    1. Urinalysis and urine culture. Colour of stools.

2. USS of liver and biliary tree to exclude anatomical problem.
3. Coagulopathy and elevated transaminases suggest 'hepatitis' (may be infection or metabolic).
4. TORCH screen and hepatitis B serology.
5. Thyroid function tests.
6. Alpha-1-antitrypsin phenotype.
7. Sweat test unreliable <6 weeks after EDD. High levels of blood immunoreactive trypsin in CF.

MANAGEMENT (Table 19.6)

Conjugated bilirubin is not neurotoxic. Unconjugated hyperbilirubinaemia is neurotoxic. Total circulating bilirubin is measured but it is free bilirubin (not bound to albumin) which can cross the blood–brain barrier and this is increased by
1. hypoalbuminaemia
2. competitive drugs (all penicillins, some cephalosporins, caffeine, frusemide, digoxin, i.v. diazepam)
3. stressors which increase free fatty acid levels (hypoxia, hypoglycaemia, acidosis, catecholamines, infection)

PREVENTION OF DANGEROUS LEVELS OF UNCONJUGATED HYPERBILIRUBINAEMIA

1. Ensure adequate intake of fluids and calories, especially in breast fed infants.
2. Phototherapy (side-effects are dehydration, loose stools, cataracts): ensure extra 20 ml/kg fluids per 24 hours (see Tables 19.3 and 19.6).
3. Exchange transfusion (see below) for maternofetal blood group incompatibility and if
   a. cord Hb < 10 g/dl, irrespective of cord SBR (if hydrops is

Table 19.6 Management of unconjugated hyperbilirubinaemia

| Gestation (weeks) | Unconjugated bilirubin level (μmol/l) | | | | |
| | To commence phototherapy | | | To perform exchange transfusion | |
	1st 24 h	2nd 24 h	> 48 h	Ill baby	Well baby
<30	70	85	100	150	175
30–31	90	100	135	175	225
32–33	110	135	170	225	275
34–35	120	170	205	275	325
36–37	130	205	240	325	350
>37	140	240	320	350	375

present resuscitate, remove pleural fluid and ascites, and partial exchange, i.e. 90 ml/kg)
b. cord Hb 10–12 g/dl, cord SBR > 80 µmol/l
c. cord SBR < 80 µmol/l but postnatal SBR rises > 20 µmol/hr despite intensive phototherapy

TREATMENT OF DANGEROUS LEVELS OF UNCONJUGATED HYPERBILIRUBINAEMIA — EXCHANGE TRANSFUSION

Monitor

Aspirate the stomach and monitor pulse, temperature and respiration every 15 min and ECG continuously.

Blood

Exchange 180 ml/kg using warmed, fresh, CMV negative, rhesus negative packed cells of same ABO group as the infant. 1 ml 10% calcium gluconate for every 100 ml of citrated donor blood, mixed with the next aliquot.

Route

In/out via a UVC or UAC, or in via a peripheral i.v. cannula and out via a UAC or peripheral arterial cannula.

Establish a 10 ml deficit initially and use aliquots of 10 ml (< 32 weeks) or 20 ml (term), 5 min for each cycle.

Investigations

Initially. SBR, Hb, PCV, glucose, blood gases (if there is a base deficit > 8, half correct with $NaHCO_3$ prior to exchange; see p. 30) and umbilical swab.

At the end of the procedure. SBR, Hb, PCV, glucose, blood gases, blood culture via the catheter and catheter tip. Do not leave the UVC in unless a second exchange is likely within 24 hours.

OUTCOME

1. Mortality < 1% if no hydrops.
2. SBR should be < 50% of pre-exchange level. Start 'double phototherapy' immediately to limit rebound. Check SBR 4-hourly. Restart feeds 1 hour after exchange if umbilical catheters are removed.
3. Measure Hb weekly, discharge on folic acid 0.25 mg/kg per 24 hours until 6 weeks, defer the Guthrie test until 4 days after the last exchange, outpatient hearing test.

Respiratory problems in the newborn

BACKGROUND

Causes:

Usually preterm

1. RDS ('hyaline membrane disease'): due to surfactant deficiency; affects 80% at 28 weeks, 50% at 32 weeks, < 3% at term. Risk is increased by caesarean section, asphyxia, maternal diabetes and decreased with SGA, PROM or maternal steroids. Onset after 8 hours virtually excludes RDS.
2. Apnoea of prematurity: associated with RDS; also see (10) below; accompanied by bradycardia.
3. BPD: chronic CXR changes and O_2 dependency > 28 days as a complication of IPPV.

Usually term

4. TTN: often caesarean section, onset 2–4 hours and resolves by 72 hours.
5. PFC: associated with asphyxia and MAS, often mistaken for cyanotic CHD (see Ch. 7).
6. MAS: see p. 299.

Preterm or term

7. Infection: congenital (group B streptococci, TORCH, *Listeria*) or acquired (*Staph. aureus, E. coli*, late onset group B streptococci after 1 week, *Chlamydia* usually 6 weeks).
8. Air leak: pneumothorax (any infant on IPPV, term infants breathing spontaneously), PIE (preterm on IPPV).
9. Congenital abnormalities: diaphragmatic hernia, tracheo-oesophageal fistula, choanal atresia, pulmonary hypoplasia (± renal agenesis).
10. Neurological problems: asphyxia, haemorrhage, meningitis, seizures (see Ch. 12), sedative drugs (including maternal), myasthenia (infant or maternal).

CLINICAL DIAGNOSIS

Tachypnoea > 60/min, expiratory 'grunting', sternal and intercostal recession, and cyanosis are common to all types of respiratory disease. In contrast, CHD is rarely accompanied by severe respiratory distress.

Initial management is the same in all infants with respiratory distress.

INITIAL MANAGEMENT

1. Resuscitate (see p. 299).
2. Headbox and humidified O_2 or IPPV to keep the infant pink.
3. If FiO$_2$ < 40%, TcPO$_2$ electrode on the right chest and calib-

Table 19.7 Initial ventilator settings

	Infant with respiratory distress	Infant with apnoea (lungs thought to be normal)
PIP (cmH$_2$O)	20	12
PEEP (cmH$_2$O)	4	2
Inspiratory to expiratory ratio	1 : 1	1 : 2
Rate	40	30
FiO$_2$	21–95% to maintain PaO$_2$ 7–10 kPa	Air (21%)

Notes:

1. If the infant was previously in a headbox, start with FiO$_2$ 10% higher. These are the initial settings pending blood gas analysis (see Table 19.8). However, do not wait for blood gas confirmation if the following are observed.
2. If no discernible chest wall movement is seen, increase inspiratory pressure in increments of 4 cmH$_2$O until movement is apparent.
3. If the infant is breathing spontaneously faster than IPPV breaths, increase the rate to 60/min.

rate with arterial gas. If FiO$_2$ > 40%, insert a right radial or umbilical arterial catheter (tip at T4–T8 level; maximum enteral feeding 0.5 ml/h).

4. Adjust FiO$_2$ to maintain PaO$_2$ 7–10 kPa. For initial IPPV settings, see Table 19.7.
5. All infants: ear, umbilical, rectal swab and blood cultures and start penicillin 60 mg/kg i.v. 12-hourly (until culture-negative at 48 hours).
6. If infection is suspected (two of PROM, maternal pyrexia or vaginal discharge, neonatal pyrexia or rash), also perform an LP and SPA and send the gastric aspirate for microscopy; start penicillin 60 mg/kg i.v. 12-hourly and gentamicin 2.5 mg/kg i.v. (daily if ≤ 28 weeks, 18-hourly if 29–35 weeks, 12-hourly if > 35 weeks).
7. FBC (polycythaemia or anaemia exacerbates RDS; WBC is an unreliable guide to infection).
8. 10% dextrose i.v. (see Table 19.3).
9. Defer CXR until 4 hours unless an air leak is suspected or ETT position is uncertain (aim for 2 cm above carina).
10. ECG monitor, apnoea alarm, FiO$_2$ monitor, BP 6-hourly or continuously from arterial catheter (Fig. A. 1), blood glucose 6-hourly (see p. 306).

SUBSEQUENT MANAGEMENT

1. Arterial blood gases 6-hourly (Table 19.8). If pH is low despite normocapnia (PaCO$_2$ 4–6 kPa), there is metabolic acidosis. Commonest causes are:
   a. hypoxia: adjust FiO$_2$ to keep PaO$_2$ 7–10 kPa

Table 19.8 Anticipated effects from changes in ventilator settings

Parameter changed	PaO_2	$PaCO_2$
PIP increased	Increased	Decreased
PEEP increased	Increased	Increased
FiO_2 increased	Increased	Unchanged
Rate increased	Unchanged	Decreased

Notes:
1. Always check arterial gas 20 min after changing IPPV.
2. Max. settings are PIP 40 cmH$_2$O, PEEP 8 cmH$_2$O, FiO_2 95%, rate 100/min.
3. When weaning, reduce PIP first in 2 cmH$_2$O decrements until <20 cmH$_2$O, then FiO_2 in 5% decrements until < 80%, then the rate by 5/min decrements. Extubate into a headbox when 5/min is reached.

    b. hypovolaemia — low BP, poor skin perfusion (core temp — skin temp > 2.5°C or PaO_2 – TcPO_2 > 2.5 kPa), tachycardia > 160/min, bruising or antepartum haemorrhage, > 10 ml/kg blood sampling since birth: transfuse 15 ml/kg whole blood

    c. infection

      If pH is < 7.25 due to metabolic acidosis despite attention to the above, correct with NaHCO$_3$ i.v. over 20 min (mmol = 0.3 × weight × base excess). Give half of this dose initially as 4.2% NaHCO$_3$ (0.5 mmol/ml).

2. Intubate and give IPPV if:
    a. insipient apnoea/collapse
    b. PaO_2 < 7 kPa in FiO_2 of > 90%
    c. $PaCO_2$ > 9 kPa.

3. If still on IPPV at 5 days, start TPN (sooner if VLBW). NG feeding can start once the UAC is out and the respiratory rate ≤ 60/min in a headbox.

4. Daily electrolytes: hyponatraemia in the first week is usually due to excessive i.v. 10% dextrose; after the first week, it is usually due to excessive Na$^+$ losses in urine. Hypernatraemia is usually due to inadequate i.v. 10% dextrose, especially if the infant is under a radiant warmer.

MAJOR COMPLICATIONS

Acute. Air leak, infection PVH, PDA.

    If the baby goes blue on the ventilator:

1. Chest not moving:
    a. the ventilator may be malfunctioning or disconnected from supply, the tubing may be disconnected or kinked — hand ventilate if necessary.
    b. the ETT may be displaced or blocked — re-intubate and aspirate.

2. Chest movement decreased:

a. pneumothorax — insert a 12G chest drain in the midaxillary line.
b. decreased lung compliance — increase the peak inspiratory pressure.
3. Chest movement unchanged:
   a. right-to-left shunting — correct pH < 7.25, consider tolazoline 1 mg/kg i.v. bolus followed by 1 mg/kg i.v. infusion (give 10 ml/kg plasma if hypotension occurs)
   b. large periventricular haemorrhage.

Chronic. BPD (5%), major handicap (approx 20% if VLBW).

OUTCOME

Peak severity is at 3–5 days; 50–75% survival at 26 weeks, 90% survival at 29 weeks, $> 95\%$ survival for > 29 weeks' gestation.

Apnoea in the newborn

BACKGROUND

Causes are legion — hypoxia from any cause but especially RDS and airway obstruction, prematurity and > 3 days old, handling or suction, infection, hypoglycaemia, electrolyte abnormalities, abnormal temperature, anaemia, HIE, seizures, PVH, depressant drugs (including maternal).

CLINICAL DIAGNOSIS

It may be possible to distinguish central apnoea from obstructive apnoea (respiratory efforts continue in the latter) but often it is a combination of the two. Cyanosis (or desaturation on pulse oximetry) and bradycardia rapidly ensue.

MANAGEMENT

A. Immediate treatment

Increase FiO$_2$ to 100% and stimulate the infant by gentle shaking. If the pulse does not increase, bag and mask IPPV and proceed as for resuscitation (p. 3) if no response is seen.

B. Look for the cause

1. Check temperature and BP. Listen for stridor, observe tongue size and pass NGT down both nares. If already on IPPV, aspirate and check ETT placement.
2. Adjust FiO$_2$ to maintain $PaO_2 \approx 10$ kPa.

3. Blood glucose, FBC, U & E, Ca^{2+}, arterial blood gases.
4. Minimal handling.
5. Consider naloxone (see p. 300).

Start preventive measures (see below).

If apnoeas/bradycardias persist:

6. Full infection screen.
7. Cranial USS.

C. Prevention of further apnoeas

1. Aminophylline 5 mg/kg i.v. loading dose over 20 min.
   Maintenance: aminophylline 4.4 mg/kg per 24 hours i.v.
   infusion
   or theophylline 1 mg/kg 8-hourly p.o.

   Adjust doses to maintain random blood levels at 10–14 mg/l. Reduce the dose if vomiting, pulse > 180/min, seizures occur.
2. Connect the ventilator to an apnoea mat to provide regular stimulation.
3. Give CPAP 6 cmH$_2$O via a nasal prong (Vygon ETT advanced via the nares to the nasopharynx).
4. IPPV (see Table 19.7).

Neonatal infections (Table 19.9)

Always take cultures *before* commencing antibiotics.

1. **Sticky eye.** See Ch. 17. (Usually culture-negative but may be *Gonococcus, Staph. aureus, Chlamydia*). Swab both eyes (including chlamydial transport medium and chlamydial scrapings from the inside of the lower lid). Wash both eyes with saline and start chloramphenicol 0.5% drops to both eyes 4-hourly. If *Gonococcus* is confirmed, add penicillin 60 mg/kg 12-hourly i.v. If the infection is chlamydial, change to tetracycline 1% ointment 3-hourly. For periorbital oedema, perform a full infection screen and give i.v. flucloxacillin 50 mg/kg 12-hourly and i.v. gentamicin (see p. 313 for doses).
2. **Umbilical and skin infections** (see Ch. 18).
3. **Paronychia.** If single, swab and clean with spirit swabs and advise cotton mits. If multiple, give flucloxacillin 25 mg/kg p.o. 12-hourly. Do not attempt to cut nails.
4. **Oral and perineal *Candida*** (see Ch. 18).
5. **Pneumonia or RDS** (see p. 311).
6. **NEC.** Penicillin 60 mg/kg i.v. 12-hourly, gentamicin (p. 313) and metronidazole 7.5 mg/kg i.v. 8-hourly (plus 6-hourly decubitus AXR — right side up, nil by mouth and TPN) for 7 days minimum.
7. **Meningitis:** all doses are for the first week of life.

a. Organism unknown: cefotaxime 50 mg/kg i.v. 6-hourly and gentamicin i.v. (p. 313).

b. Group B streptococci: penicillin 60 mg/kg i.v. 6-hourly and gentamicin.

c. *Listeria* ampicillin 75 mg/kg i.v. 12-hourly and gentamicin i.v. (p. 313).

d. *Staph. aureus:* flucloxacillin 75 mg/kg i.v. 12-hourly.

e. *E. coli:* cefotaxime 50 mg/kg i.v. 6-hourly and gentamicin i.v. (p. 313).

f. *Candida:* amphotericin 0.1 mg/kg per 24 hours i.v. infusion, increased to 1.0 mg/kg per 24 hours by day 5, *and* flucytosine 12.5 mg/kg p.o. 6-hourly.

Table 19.9 Features of neonatal infection

'At risk' groups
1. LBW
2. PROM, maternal fever, offensive liquor
3. Indwelling cannulae or catheters and exchange transfusion
4. IPPV
5. Congenital abnormalities of respiratory or GU tract or neural tube defects

Signs of systemic infection (very non-specific)
1. Lethargy, hypotonia, seizures
2. Fever or hypothermia
3. Refusal to feed, abdominal distension or discoloration, vomiting, diarrhoea or bloody stools
4. Apnoeas, bradycardias, cyanotic episodes
5. Late onset or persistent jaundice
6. Petechiae or skin rash
7. 'Sick looking' baby — poor perfusion, mottled skin, low BP, oliguria

Investigations if systemic infection is suspected
1. Hypo- or hyperglycaemia
2. Core–skin temperature difference > 2.5°C; metabolic acidosis on arterial gas.
3. FBC — corrected WBC normal up to 30 000 immediately after birth and then falls during first week; serial increase in polymorphs, absolute neutropenia (< 2000/mm³) and thrombocytopenia all suggest sepsis
4. Cultures (including LP fungi, if present, will grow without special cultures), SPA, blood cultures
5. CXR
6. AXR and 'right side up' decubitus if NEC is suspected
7. Gastric aspirate for microscopy if < 24 hours and not fed
8. Stools for echo and coxsackie viruses if diarrhoea or maternal gastroenteritis
9. TORCH, varicella, HIV (mother or father i.v. drug abuser, or father bisexual or seropositive haemophiliac)

20

Child abuse

Presentation

1. NAI
2. FTT (see Chs 5 and 9)
3. Emotional deprivation (which may contribute to growth failure)
4. Sexual abuse
5. Deliberate poisoning
6. Munchausen syndrome by proxy (e.g. deliberate suffocation, fictitious seizures, nappy stained with parent's blood, etc.)

NON-ACCIDENTAL INJURY

NAI is the commonest form of child abuse and all doctors who deal with children in any capacity must be aware of NAI and have a simple grasp of how to deal with this difficult problem.

Suggestive symptoms and signs

There is rarely one feature of the history or examination which is pathognomonic of NAI; rather, it is the constellation of a number of the following factors which suggests the diagnosis:

1. Many cases are referred to the paediatric service by social workers, GPs, teachers or police who already suspect NAI.
2. Clues from the history:
   a. The parents admit the injury is not accidental.
   b. The child's age. Accidental fractures of any type are extremely rare in children < 18 months. Fractures of the clavicle or humerus from obstetric trauma are exceptions but callus should definitely be present by 2 weeks.
   c. The explanation of how the injury occurred is not consistent with the site(s)/severity of the injuries. Neither 'bruises easily' nor 'brittle bones' are acceptable explanations. In an infant, a fracture of a limb is often ascribed to forcing the infant into a 'baby-grow' — this can never be considered an adequate explanation. There is good evidence that falls from up to 1 m (e.g. off a sofa or out

of bed) even on to a hard surface are only very rarely associated with fractures and never with multiple fractures of the ribs or limbs.

    d. The details of the explanation vary on each repetition.

    e. Delay in presentation of > 48 hours.

3. Clues from the examination:

    a. The distribution of soft tissue injuries — genuinely accidental bruises are very common in normal children on the lower limbs, especially the knees and below, and in toddlers on the forehead. In NAI, bruising to the trunk, lower back and buttocks, and head and neck area are relatively more common. Bruises or burns confined to palms or soles are suspicious.

    b. The distribution of fractures — genuinely accidental fractures are usually simple skull fractures or transverse or greenstick fractures of the limbs, usually distal. Rib fractures are very rare in children as a result of accidents other than road traffic accidents. In contrast, multiple rib fractures are common as a result of NAI, skull fractures may be depressed and limb fractures may be oblique or spiral and involve the humerus or femur. Metaphyseal chip fractures are often the result of NAI.

    c. Multiple injuries, in time and space — if bruises are of very different colours or if some bruises are swollen and tender and others fading, this suggests more than one injury and is therefore not consistent with a single explanatory incident. Seek a radiological opinion on the relative age of callus if fractures are multiple; again these suggest separate injuries.

        Ask yourself whether bruises or fractures of several different anatomical parts can be explained by a single incident. Do previous notes or casualty records suggest previous attendances which, taken together, constitute multiple injuries?

    d. 'Classical' injuries — cigarette burns; torn frenulum; black eye (two black eyes are hardly ever accidental unless involved in road traffic accident); slap or belt marks; head, neck or conjunctival petechiae from strangulation; multiple finger grip marks on the arms, legs, cheeks or thorax (once the grip has been applied several times, the bruises no longer fit the imprint of a hand); bite marks (the jaw of most domestic pets is U-shaped and there will be two canine puncture marks, the human jaw leaves a crescent-shaped bite and the size suggests whether child or adult); injuries to genitalia; subdural haematoma; periosteal reaction on X-ray (the result of twisting of a limb); a scald with glove or stocking distribution.

    e. Other features of 'neglect' — inappropriately dressed for cold weather, dirty clothes, dirty nappy, nappy rash, nits or scabies, poor hygiene.

Immediate management

Never accuse the parents of lying or of being the perpetrators of NAI. If a junior doctor suspects NAI, he should always seek the advice of a senior colleague. Detailed documentation *at the time* is vital, even if hard-pressed in a busy casualty department. Record the names and addresses of all people accompanying the child and the time of arrival.

1. Take a full history, including verbatim records of the parents' explanation.

    When and where did the alleged incident happen, what time, what exactly was the detailed sequence of events, who else witnessed the incident, etc.?

    Obtain a full family and social history and record previous accidents and ingestions by siblings. Ask about family history of bleeding disorders and osteogenesis imperfecta. If a baby, record details of the delivery.

2. Perform a full examination. If the parents refuse permission, do not insist or examine the child alone but inform Social Services.

    The child must be completely undressed and all injuries drawn to scale on a diagram, irrespective of whether or not you consider them to be accidental. Note colours and dimensions of all injuries.

    Don't forget to look in the mouth, under the nappy, the external genitalia, and plot height and weight on a centile chart.

    Blue sclerae and wormian bones on SXR suggest osteogenesis imperfecta. The likelihood of osteogenesis imperfecta in the absence of blue sclerae, progressive deformity and a definite family history is of the order of 1 in 1 000 000.

3. Enquire of the local body (usually the NSPCC or Social Services) who maintain the 'at risk' register whether the child or any sibling (who may have various 'aliases' and addresses if by different fathers) is on the register. However, children on the register still sustain genuine accidents and the parents should not be thought 'guilty until proved innocent'.

4. Inform Social Services immediately of your concern, even if out of 'office hours', as they will wish to interview the family. Social Services may also arrange for siblings who are not present to be examined. It is for the Social Services to decide whether to involve the police and not for the paediatric staff. If the parents attempt to remove their child from the hospital, do not attempt to stop them physically but inform Social Services immediately.

5. Skeletal surveys and clotting studies may be indicated in

NAI to provide corroborative evidence and to exclude a coagulopathy but are by no means routine. In children with suspected NAI attending a casualty department, only 5% of these investigations produced an abnormal result. Coagulopathy or thrombocytopenia should always be considered either if there is a single very large haematoma or if there are very widespread bruises or petechiae. The presence of mucous membrane bleeding or haemarthroses is also suggestive. A family history of bleeding disorder is uncommon (e.g. ITP is not inherited and many of the inherited disorders are not dominant). The overall incidence of inherited bleeding disorders is 1 in 15 000.

Haemorrhagic disease of the newborn can occur up to 8 weeks and is a rare but important cause of intracranial haemorrhage.

6. Obtain all old notes and X-rays.
7. The only indication for hospital admission is that the NAI requires treatment (e.g. traction) or observation (e.g. head injury — see Ch. 12). If Social Services are unhappy for the child to return home with the parents, they should arrange temporary foster care.

    Infectious diseases are rife on medical wards which are therefore not 'a place of safety'. If the child is admitted, you must inform the ward staff of the child's legal guardian and whether the child is currently the subject of a child protection order (this information will be necessary if consent is required for a procedure and in deciding who can be given information).
8. If the child is admitted, clinical photographs should be requested (requires parental consent) and the child's GP informed as soon as possible.

Subsequent action

1. A written report should be sent by the most experienced paediatrician who has seen the injuries to the social worker involved. This should state the explanation(s) offered for the injury, the physical signs, and an opinion as to whether 'on balance of probabilities' the medical evidence suggests that the injuries are non-accidental.

    If legal proceedings ensue, police witness statements may be requested (junior doctors should confine themselves to statements of fact, rather than opinion as to causation, and exclude all hearsay) and the solicitors acting for the local authority may seek written evidence from the most senior paediatrician involved as to likely causation.
2. A case conference is usually convened. The paediatric staff involved should either attend or submit written evidence and photographs as above. The case conference tries to reach a consensus view as to whether NAI has occurred, and hence

whether the child should be placed on the 'at risk' register; to arrange support and monitoring of the family; to decide about care proceedings; to decide whether it is safe for the child o continue in the family home. The police decide whether to press criminal charges.

CHILD SEXUAL ABUSE (CSA)

Ideally, strategies should be in place in all hospitals so that junior paediatric staff are not directly involved in the management of CSA cases, except as observers.

However, CSA and NAI frequently coexist and the diagnosis of CSA may first be considered in the casualty department following presentation with UTI, vaginal discharge or bleeding, or trauma of the genitalia/perineum in either sex.

In girls, the most common types of accidental injury to the external genitalia are caused by straddling, accidental penetration, and tearing of the perineum due to sudden forced abduction of the legs during a fall. The presence of a foreign object may cause vaginal discharge and haematuria may follow self-exploration of the urethral orifice with foreign bodies by either sex.

The recommended course of action follows the sequence for NAI (see above), i.e. take a detailed, verbatim history; perform a full external examination (but leave internal examination of the vagina and rectum to an experienced paediatrician, police surgeon or gynaecologist as appropriate) and document the findings; seek the opinion of the most senior paediatric staff available; if they agree with your suspicion, inform Social Services of your concern. Do not attempt to take forensic samples yourself.

21

Death

WHEN NOT TO RESUSCITATE AND WHEN TO STOP

See Chs 2 and 19, pp 15, 301.

Death on the ward

Hopefully, this is anticipated at least enough to allow you to:
— call both parents
— try to explain the situation to both parents together, not separately
— call the chaplain if the parents wish it
— ask about baptism; in extreme circumstances, a lay person can baptise a child by following the order of service as printed
— nominate a key worker (nurse, doctor or chaplain) who can guarantee uninterrupted time with the parents

If the baby dies before the parents arrive, try to intercept them so that they can be given the news in a private room rather than on the open ward. There is no easy way to tell parents that their child has died but some useful guides are given below.
1. The environment in which the news is given is very important. It should be quiet, private and with sufficient chairs for the whole family.
2. It is reassuring to say that the child did not suffer.
3. The parents should decide when and how other family members should be told. Generally, parents should tell the other children and there is little to be gained by delaying this or using euphemisms. Siblings must grieve as well as parents.

If a decision is taken to electively discontinue treatment, the parents must be asked whether they wish to be present at the time of discontinuation and whether they wish to hold the child afterwards. If so:
— discontinue all infusions
— remove the NG tube, ETT, peripheral arterial and venous cannulae
— do not remove chest drain, central venous or umbilical

catheters, transanastomotic or gastrostomy tubes, urethral or nephrostomy catheters; clamp all such tubes
— dress or swaddle the child and take a photograph for the parents; give the child to the parents and ask whether they wish to be alone or accompanied

Checklist of who to inform of the death:
— GP
— consultant paediatrician (and arrange bereavement counselling in 6 weeks)
— consultant obstetrician, postnatal ward and community midwife in a neonatal death
— health visitor
— pathologist if there will be a post-mortem
— coroner if relevant (see below)
— clinical geneticist if relevant
— hospital administration to avoid further appointments being sent

Post-mortem requests

This should not be broached immediately after death.
1. If for medical interest, explain the reason to the parents. They may be reassured to know that the post-mortem examination is not visible when the child is dressed and does not delay their funeral arrangements. The findings may alter counselling of future pregnancies. Written consent should be obtained.
2. If the case is reported to the coroner (cause of death unknown, no medical practitioner attended the death, death during operation or before recovery from anaesthesia, suspicious circumstances) the parents have no control over the decision regarding post-mortem. Warn the parents that they may be interviewed by the police, that this is routine and does not imply suspicion of the parents.

Death certificates

There are different death certificates for neonatal (< 28 days old) deaths and older children. The body cannot be disposed of until the death certificate has been completed and this should not be deferred pending the outcome of a post-mortem, unless this is a coroner's post-mortem. Cremation forms are separate from death certificates.

Brain death criteria

Two independent, experienced doctors should confirm the findings on two independent occasions. 'It is for the doctors to decide on the interval between tests.' An interval of 24 hours should be the maximum and generally it will be considerably shorter.

PRECONDITIONS

1. Core temperature > 35°C.
2. No drugs that affect consciousness or neuromuscular blockers during the preceding 12 hours. In renal or hepatic failure, wait 24 hours after the last dose of drugs before the first test.
3. No profound abnormality of blood glucose, electrolytes or acid–base balance.
4. No spontaneous breathing and no movement within cranial nerve distribution. Reflex limb movement does not preclude a diagnosis of brain death.

APNOEA TEST

Ensure $PaCO_2 > 6$ kPa, ventilate with 100% O_2 for 15 min, disconnect from ventilator and give 6 l/min O_2 via a tracheal catheter. Observe apnoea for 5 min.

BRAINSTEM REFLEXES

1. Pupils fixed
2. No eye movement when the ear is syringed with ice cold water
3. Absent doll's eye response (see Ch. 12)
4. Absent corneal reflex
5. Absent gag reflex

If the second set of tests confirm brain death, the ventilator is reconnected and the parents told together that their child has died but that the breathing machine is maintaining the heartbeat.

Suitability for organ donation should always be considered. If donation is refused, the ventilator is finally disconnected and most parents will want to hold their child at this time.

Organ donation

Suitable donors can be any age but must be brain dead and in a stable cardiovascular state on a ventilator. Written consent must be obtained for organ donation. Seek permission, in a positive way, to use all potential organs (kidneys, heart, liver, corneas) but parents can exclude specific organs. In cases of accidental death, parents should be told that there will inevitably be a coroner's post-mortem whether or not organ donation is undertaken.

If consent is given, adequate ventilation, BP, renal output and control of infection must be ensured. If the death is due to an accident, the coroner must be asked for permission to remove organs.

Blood grouping, tissue typing and matching a recipient are necessary but organ removal should not be delayed for more than 24 hours after the second brain death tests.

Organs are removed in theatre and the time of death for the death certificate is the time of cessation of the heartbeat in theatre.

The parents cannot be given details of the recipients. Parents may wish to see their child afterwards.

Sudden infant death syndrome

BACKGROUND

1 in 500 infants die suddenly and unexpectedly without an obvious cause of death, usually aged 2–4 months and whilst asleep. SIDS is more common in winter, in ex-preterm babies, in lower social class, in sibs of SIDS babies and in babies who sleep prone.

MANAGEMENT

1. Resuscitation — not if evidence that death is not recent (rigor mortis, cold to touch, fixed staining of skin) but if in any doubt or if any cardiac activity attempt full resuscitation (see Ch. 2).
2. Document the following — how the parents or ambulance team found the infant, the infant's clothing, rectal temperature.
3. Examine for clues to cause of death — nasal discharge, vomitus around mouth, loose stool in nappy, nutritional status, trauma.
4. Counsel the parents — explain 'cot death'. Reassure parents that they are not in any way contributory but that the coroner must be informed and that a post-mortem is mandatory. Forewarn parents that police involvement is routine. Offer the parents the opportunity to hold the baby, arrange a photograph of the baby for the parents, who may also want a lock of hair. Offer them the telephone numbers of local self-help groups. Take a full history.
5. Inform — as for death of an in-patient (p. 324).
6. Arrange for the consultant to counsel the parents at 6 weeks, with post-mortem findings

INVESTIGATIONS

1. FBC, U & E, blood cultures, by cardiac puncture if necessary
2. throat and rectal swabs for virology
3. suprapubic aspiration of urine for culture and metabolic screen
4. CXR
5. skeletal survey if there is external bruising

'Near miss' SIDS

BACKGROUND

Apnoea, cyanosis, limpness or stiffness, choking or gasping. Affected children are younger than SIDS population; there is no seasonal or diurnal variation; can occur when asleep or awake and often during or after feeds.

MANAGEMENT

Full history and examination; always admit to observe breathing pattern and assess feeding difficulties; nurse for 24 hours with an apnoea alarm. Home-monitoring with an apnoea alarm does not alter prognosis but parents may feel reassured. Warn that false alarms common and teach basic resuscitation. Advise parents to place the infant on his back when asleep and to use appropriate number of blankets depending on the season/weather rather than a single, thick quilt.

INVESTIGATION

In all cases:
1. FBC, U & E, glucose, Ca^{2+}, blood cultures
2. nasopharyngeal aspiration (15% of near miss SIDS develop bronchiolitis)
3. stool and urine culture
4. CXR
5. urinary organic acids for fatty acid oxidation disorder
6. save urine for toxicology screen

In selected cases, consider:
1. Barium swallow or oesophageal pH monitoring
2. EEG
3. CSF examination
4. cranial USS
5. skeletal survey
6. continuous monitoring during sleep for obstructive or central apnoea

Follow-up

Bereavement is a long process with several phases and the family require continued support. All parents should be given a 6-week follow-up appointment with a consultant paediatrician, even if the child was 'brought in dead'. At follow-up, the parents' questions can be addressed, any post-mortem conclusions communicated and a check made that 'normal' grieving has and is occurring. The feelings of any siblings should also be discussed.

22

Orthopaedics and trauma

Management of major trauma (See Ch. 2)

Additional points in resuscitation of major trauma cases are:
1. Always X-ray cervical spine, erect chest if possible (pneumo- or haemothorax) and pelvis.
2. Always pass an NGT to empty the stomach and a urinary catheter if there are pelvic injuries.
3. In the small child, there can be significant internal damage without visible skeletal injury; e.g. chest injuries, ruptured viscus etc. Therefore anticipate hypovolaemia and do not wait for a fall in BP before giving colloid or blood; cool peripheries, tachycardia and decreasing GCS precede falling BP.
4. Splint limb fractures. Entonox provides immediate analgesia followed, in the absence of significant head injury and once vital signs are stable and the GCS documented, by pethidine 1 mg/kg i.m. or 0.1 mg/kg i.v. If intermittent analgesia is inadequate, titrate opiate infusion against response (start with diamorphine 0.015 mg/kg/h i.v.) and closely monitor BP and respiration. If there is significant head injury, give codeine phosphate 1 mg/kg i.m.
5. See Ch. 20 if NAI is suspected.
6. See Ch. 21 if resuscitation is unsuccessful.

Management of head injuries (see Ch. 12)

Additional points:
1. SXR if the child is unconscious, vomiting, has retrograde amnesia, if the injury is caused by a sharp object, or if you suspect NAI.
2. Admit if loss of consciousness or memory loss (irrespective of duration of either), vomiting, severe headache, seizures, abnormal neurological signs. If the child is not admitted, advise parents to return if there is vomiting, seizure, drowsiness or altered consciousness or if severe headache

develops after a lucid period (extradural haemorrhage).
3. Small, superficial scalp cuts — clean and use histoacryl glue or hair ties.
4. Deep cuts — suture with 4/0 Vicryl (dissolvable — may take up to 3 weeks; keep hair dry for 1 week)

Burns (see Ch. 23)

Non-accidental injury (see Ch. 20)

Lacerations

BASIC RULES

1. Analgesia.
2. Clean before closing.
   — use local anaesthetic and *allow 5 min to act*
   — remove all foreign material from wound
   — debride all dead tissue
   — explore all penetrating wounds
3. Do not remove penetrating objects (knife, arrow) until expert assistance is present.
4. All jagged wounds require suturing for good cosmetic result.
5. If the wound is of any significant depth, close in layers.
6. See p. 228 regarding tetanus prevention.

METHODS OF WOUND CLOSURE

1. Steristrips: for small lacerations which do not require suturing as Steristrips cause minimal pain and scarring. Cannot be used on a part of the body which is constantly moving (e.g. elbow) or where the Steristrip cannot adhere to the wound edges (e.g. eyebrow, scalp).
2. Histoacryl glue: small scalp lacerations only. Does not require removal.
3. Sutures: scalp   3/0 or 4/0 Vicryl
            hands   4/0 Ethilon or Vicryl
            trunk, legs 4/0 Ethilon
            face   5/0 or 6/0 Ethilon
   Removal: Vicryl dissolvable.
            Ethilon from face at 5 days, other sites at 7 days, from continually moving parts at 10 days. Always use Ethilon rather than Vicryl if a good cosmetic result is essential.

SITES OF WOUND CLOSURE

1. Head injures
See p. 330

2. Facial lacerations

Forehead	Steristrip unless there is a large surrounding haematoma
Eyebrow	do not shave eyebrows
Bridge of nose	suture as haematoma often develops
Cheek	suture usually; if the wound penetrates through to the buccal cavity, seek dental advice
Chin	usually Steristrip but it may not adhere if there is extensive grazing
Lip	suture if the wound extends through vermillion border

3. Lacerations to hands and fingers

Exclude neurovascular damage *before* wound closure. Check flexion and extension of the wrist, thumb and fingers (motor supply and tendon integrity) and sensation over dorsum of the hand, thumb and medial and lateral sides of each finger (digital nerves). Check radial and ulnar pulses and capillary return of finger tips.

Incomplete fingertip injury — Steristrip the fingertip back into position immediately; leave the nail in place if the child is < 5 years, remove the nail if > 5 years; suture nailbed lacerations with 5/0 Vicryl; Steristrip rather than suture volar skin; Paratulle dressing; X-ray for bony injury and start oral erythromycin if fracture is confirmed.

Total amputation of the fingertip — clean wound, paratulle dressing, oral erythromycin.

4. Lacerations over joints
— always require suturing
— splint for 5 days and review; hand or digit must be splinted in semiflexed 'position of use'. Refer to orthopaedic surgeon if you are uncertain.
— if the wound communicates with the joint cavity, admit for expert orthopaedic opinion, exploration and give parenteral flucloxacillin and penicillin.

Soft tissue injuries

Basic rules for contusion, sprain or strain:

1. Regular analgesia.
2. Ice packs for 20 min 6-hourly for 48 hours
3. Rest the injured part for first 24 hours
4. Elevate swollen limbs
5. Start active use/weightbearing as soon as pain allows.
   a. Pulled radius: usually 5 months – 5 years, history of child lifted by that arm, pain in elbow and wrist. No follow-up if reduction is successful; if unsuccessful, collar and cuff sling and review at 48 hours — spontaneous resolution is usual.
   b. Sprained wrist: double Tubigrip bandage for 5 days.
   c. Paronychia:
      (i) no visible pus — oral flucloxacillin, $MgSO_4$ dressing, review in 5 days;
      (ii) pus visible — incision and drainage, paratulle dressing, oral flucloxacillin, review in 5 days.
   d. Partially avulsed nail: remove the distal fragment, under ring block if necessary. Seek orthopaedic opinion if the proximal nail or nail bed is damaged.
   e. Subungual haematoma: insert a heated needle through the nail to relieve; no analgesia is required.
   f. Sprained ankle:
      (i) can weightbear — double Tubigrip bandage for 5 days; no crutches and no follow-up;
      (ii) cannot weightbear — double Tubigrip, crutches, non-weightbearing exercises after 24 hours and review at 5 days, never POP;
      (iii) X-ray if: immediate inability to weightbear, immediate swelling, tenderness of bony prominence, extensive early bruising, joint effusion.
   g. Animal and human bites (see Ch. 13).
   h. Stings:
      (i) bee stings — apply $NaHCO_3$ paste and remove the sting;
      (ii) wasp stings — apply vinegar soaks.

Fractures

Regular analgesia *always*. Use of crutches depends on the child's ability.

1. Nose injuries: unnecessary to X-ray a child's nose as management is unaffected; refer to ENT at 5 days (to allow swelling to subside).
2. Clavicle fractures: broad arm sling and review at 10 days.
3. Supracondylar fracture:
   a. undisplaced — collar and cuff sling inside clothes and refer to the next fracture clinic;

      b. displaced — check distal neurovascular supply (see
         p. 331) and contact the 'on call' orthopaedic surgeon.
4. Greenstick and undisplaced fractures of the distal third of the
  radius or ulna:

    < 5 years   above elbow POP;
    > 5 years   below elbow POP.

  Refer all to the next fracture clinic. 'Backslab' instead of POP
  if soft tissue swelling over a fracture.
5. Fractures of the proximal two-thirds of forearm: long arm
  POP.
6. Metacarpal fractures:
    a. undisplaced — crepe bandage and review at 10 days;
    b. displaced — refer to the 'on call' orthopaedic surgeon.
7. Greenstick and undisplaced fractures of the distal third of the
  tibia or fibula:

    < 5 years   split long leg POP;
    > 5 years   below knee POP ('backslab' if site is swollen).

  Refer all to the next fracture clinic.
8. Fractures of the proximal two-thirds of the tibia and fibula:
  long leg POP.
9. Metatarsal fractures:
    a. can weightbear — companion strap toes, apply metatarsal
      bar for support and review at 10 days;
    b. cannot weightbear — backslab and review at 10 days.
10. Finger and toe fractures:
    a. undisplaced — companion strap and review at 10 days;
    b. thumb/great toe — Elastoplast spica;
    c. extensor avulsion fracture — splint digit in extension and
      review at 7 days.

Acute arthropathy

THE SINGLE PAINFUL JOINT

Background

The first aim is to exclude septic arthritis, which occurs at all ages (including
neonate) and all joints (75% in the lower limbs). Commonest pathogens are
Staph. aureus, streptococci and *Haemophilus* (< 4 years), *Salmonella* in sickle
cell disease, group B *Streptococcus* and *Gonococcus* in the newborn. Osteomyelitis commonly coexists, especially in young children.

Clinical diagnosis

Fever (part of differential of PUO); painful, red, hot, tender,
swollen joint, limp or pseudoparalysis; look for a deformity, assess
the range of movement and function of joint.

Differential diagnosis

Septic arthritis, cellulitis, HSP, rheumatic fever, sickle cell crisis, haemophilia, malignancy (or acute gout in tumour lysis syndrome), monoarticular presentation of JCA.
Fever and malaise are *not* features of a sprain.

Investigation

Joint aspiration for M, C & S (and AFB in 'cold' arthropathy) — increased monocyte count in viral arthritis, increased polymorphs in septic, inflammatory and crystal arthropathy; FBC and baseline ESR or CRP; blood cultures; X-ray the joint and also the bone either side of that joint (changes may not appear for 10 days). Sickle test and ASOT titre if indicated.

Management

Drain pus, start i.v. flucloxacillin and fucidin 6-hourly (ampicillin and flucloxacillin if < 4 years or in known sickle disease) and modify depending on cultures; immobilise the affected limb, give regular analgesia. Continue i.v. antibiotics for 1–3 weeks and orally for another 3 weeks. Monitor response by temperature, symptoms and serial ESR and X-rays.

The treatment of any painful joint involves rest, splintage, regular analgesia and physiotherapy as soon as pain allows.

ACUTE POLYARTHROPATHY

Background

'Reactive' arthritis is the commonest cause (few days after onset of viral illness, especially rubella, mumps, varicella, glandular fever) followed by HSP; rarer causes are meningococcaemia, rheumatic fever, Lyme disease, first presentation of JCA ($\frac{2}{3}$ have < 5 joints affected, $\frac{1}{6}$ have > 5 joints, $\frac{1}{6}$ have systemic presentation) or SLE.

Clinical diagnosis

Look for viral exanthema, purpura, psoriasis; macular rash of JCA; erythema marginatum and subcutaneous nodules of rheumatic fever, examine throat, parotids and lymph nodes (post-auricular lymphadenopathy in rubella); hepatosplenomegaly, lymphadenopathy, iritis and pericardial rub in JCA; pericardial rub or murmurs in rheumatic fever; facial palsy in Lyme disease. Ask about back pain and symptoms of inflammatory bowel disease (see Ch. 9).

Investigations

FBC, ESR, viral titres, Paul Bunnell test, ASOT; ANF is positive in SLE and 70% of pauciarticular JCA; rheumatoid factor is positive in 12% of JCA.

Management

General — regular analgesia (ibuprofen 5 mg/kg 6-hourly); rest the joint and splint in the position of 'maximum function', especially at night, but *all* joints should experience a full range of passive movement each day.

Specific — antibiotics for the bacterial causes of polyarthritis. Diagnosis of JCA requires duration of > 3 months; aspirin 15 mg/kg 4-hourly or indomethacin 0.5 mg/kg 8-hourly are useful starting doses for analgesia, with paracetamol 10 mg/kg 4-hourly in addition.

SUDDEN LIMP

Background

Usually the result of pain, anywhere from sole to spine. (In contrast, neurological weakness develops gradually unless the nerve is damaged traumatically.)

— local soft tissue trauma
— hairline or chip fracture
— reactive viral arthritis (see above)
— bacterial arthritis or osteomyelitis (see above)
— sickle crisis
— JCA
— malignancy (leukaemia, neuroblastoma, osteosarcoma, Ewing's tumour — 'onion skin' X-ray)
— slipped femoral epiphysis

   Conditions more common in boys
— irritable hip (see below)
— Perthe's disease
— Osgood–Schlatter disease

   Conditions more common in girls
— chondromalacia patellae

Clinical diagnosis

Observe the gait; look for local trauma, including between the toes for entry point of infection; a tender, hot, swollen joint suggests effusion; examine for limitation of range of movement of all joints, including hips. If pain-free, check power, reflexes and sensation (including perineal) and palpate the bladder.

Investigations

If trauma is the cause, X-ray the relevant bone or joint, in two views plus contralateral side for comparison. If there is no trauma and problem is not neurological, investigate as for arthropathy above. Acute neurological weakness in the legs is a neurosurgical emergency.

HIP PROBLEMS

See Ch. 19 for CDH. If missed in the newborn, CDH may present with delayed walking or chronic limp.

Background

Pain in the thigh or knee in the skeletally immature is hip pathology until proved otherwise. Commonest are:

— irritable hip (transient synovitis); usually boy < 10 years
— Perthe's disease (avascular aetiology); usually boy 2–10 years; 15% bilateral
— slipped upper femoral epiphysis (adolescent coxa vara); usually adolescent girl, obese or rapid height velocity; 25% bilateral

Clinical diagnosis

A hip problem is suggested by

— hip joint kept in fixed flexion
— limited abduction (unable to stand with legs apart)
— limited internal rotation

Investigations

Exclude septic arthritis (see p. 333) if in any doubt, especially if antibiotics were recently given. FBC and ESR are normal and there is no fever in the three common causes (see Background). X-rays (anteroposterior or frog's legs view and lateral) may show slight joint space widening in irritable hip; increased density of the femoral head in Perthe's disease (although initial X-ray may be normal in up to 30% and the child diagnosed as irritable hip); medially displaced capital epiphysis in slipped femoral epiphysis.

Management

1. Irritable hip is a self-limiting condition and traction is only indicated in the most severe or very young cases. The mainstay of treatment is complete bed rest at home until pain-free with regular analgesia; advise parents to return for re-assessment if there is no improvement after 24 hours; otherwise follow-up at 4 days; avoid sport for 3 weeks. 15% will have a recurrence, usually within a year, and 2% develop Perthe's. Therefore repeat X-ray of hip at 3 months if symptoms persist.
2. Perthe's disease — if good prognosis (< 5 years, boy, < 50% of femoral head affected), may resolve with analgesia and traction. If poor prognosis, surgery usually required.
3. Slipped femoral epiphysis — a surgical emergency as early stabilisation of the less severe type improves outcome.

FOOT DEFORMITIES

Congenital talipes equino varus (club foot)

Occurs in 1/1000 births, fixed deformity, may be bilateral. Associated with spina bifida and arthrogryposis at birth and CP later. Refer urgently to the orthopaedic surgeon as expert treatment (manipulation and strapping) should be started as early as possible. Surgery may be necessary. Follow-up until walking.

Metatarsus varus (intoeing)

Very common but 90% correct spontaneously by 3 years.

Pes cavus (high medial arch often accompanied by clawing of the toes)

Over $\frac{2}{3}$ have a neurological cause (Friederich's ataxia, spinal dysraphism, spina bifida, peripheral neuropathy, Duchenne muscular dystrophy, CP, peroneal muscular dystrophy). Treatment is surgical.

Pes planus (the medial arch is flat when standing)

Very common and, if bilateral, mobile and painless, considered normal in children < 3 years. Rarer causes are CP and peripheral neuropathy. Therefore management of the older child is confined to physiotherapy exercises and heel inserts within the shoe. The unilateral, stiff, painful flat foot may be due to trauma, congenital abnormality, previous infection, JCA or malignancy and needs urgent investigation.

Hallux valgus

Usually bilateral and a cosmetic nuisance in adolescent girls. There may be pain over the metatarsal head from a bunion, in which case advice regarding footwear may suffice. Joint pain must be investigated.

23

Burns and heat related problems

Heat exhaustion

CLINICAL FEATURES

Onset is often gradual. Temperature is normal or mildly elevated, BP may be normal or show signs of hypotension. Skin is moist with perfuse sweating. The child may be dizzy, irritable, disorientated or have a headache. Nausea and vomiting may be present. Serum Na^+ is normal or elevated.

TREATMENT

1. Move to a cool environment. The body may be covered with towels cooled with iced water.
2. Replace fluid losses:
   a. This may be done orally if the child is alert, otherwise,
   b. Intravenous volume resuscitation with close electrolyte monitoring. See Ch. 3.

Heat stroke

CLINICAL FEATURES

The onset is usually acute. Temperature (taken rectally) is $> 41°C$. Skin is dry with no evidence of sweating. Agitation, confusion, seizures, lassitude or coma may be present. Hypotension, vomiting and diarrhoea, oliguria or anuria with ARF may occur. Serum Na^+ may be elevated and LFT may be abnormal. Hypoglycaemia and hypokalaemia may also occur.

INVESTIGATIONS

1. Urinalysis for myoglobin.
2. Blood for U & E, glucose, osmolality, creatinine, LFT, FBC PT and PTT.

TREATMENT

1. Cool the patient by:
   a. removing clothing
   b. placing in an ice water bath and cooling until core temperature is 38.3–38.8°C.
2. Replace fluid and electrolyte losses as required. Initial resuscitation: plasma may be required (10–20 ml/kg for shock).
3. Treat fits with i.v. phenytoin (see p. 359).
4. Monitor fluid balance carefully. Treat renal failure if present (see p. 158).
5. Monitor rectal temperature and ECG trace.
6. We do not use antipyretics or drugs that prevent shivering (e.g. phenothiazines).

Heat stroke should be considered regardless of climate when acute encephalopathy in infants is associated with high fever.

Hypothermia

Definition: a core temperature of < 35°C. Cardiovascular abnormalities are most important. Atrial fibrillation may be noted above 30°C and ventricular fibrillation below 30°C. Asystole occurs at approximately 26°C.

EVALUATION

1. History: duration and type of exposure and treatment since exposure.
2. Temperature must be obtained rectally. Assess for presence of poor perfusion and arrhythmias with ECG. Neurological function decreases with decreasing temperature. Below 30°C children are usually unconscious with diminished respiration and reflexes.

INVESTIGATIONS

These depend on the clinical state and include:
1. Blood gases
2. U & E, creatinine, FBC, LFT and clotting studies
3. Save blood and urine for toxicology
4. CXR to assess for aspiration

TREATMENT

1. Basic cardiac resuscitation must be given if required, but must be accompanied by rewarming. Resuscitation should be continued to allow the patient time to warm. Discuss with the consultant on call. Intravenous medications and defibrillation

are usually ineffective when temperature is $< 30°C$. Avoid giving too much $NaHCO_3$ as alkalosis may precipitate ventricular fibrillation, monitor blood gases.
2. If the patient has an output and normal cardiac rhythm, handle minimally to prevent precipitation of arrhythmia.
3. If temperature is $< 32°C$, core rewarming is suggested. Methods include:
   a. Colonic irrigation with warmed ($38°C$) saline
   b. NG lavage with warmed ($38°C$) saline
   c. Humidifying and warming inspired gases to $44°C$
   d. Heating all parental infusions to $37–40°C$
   In addition, renal dialysis or cardiac bypass have been used.

If the temperature is $> 32°C$ external rewarming may be attempted, taking care to avoid burns and hypotension. Heat to the body surfaces may be applied by warm blankets: wet clothing should have been removed. Peripheral vasodilatation may cause hypovolaemia requiring volume replacement with plasma (e.g. 10 ml/kg).

Burns

Assessment of depth
1. Superficial:
   a. First degree burns: may be caused by sunlight or a minor scald. The skin tends to be dry and erythematous with minor blisters only. The lesion is painful.
   b. Second degree burns: often caused by scald. Skin surface is moist, often whitish. Skin is painful.
   c. Deep second degree burn: again may be caused by scalds or flame contact. Skin may be moist with white slough and may be mottled. Skin may be painless.
2. Deep (i.e. complete loss of skin):
   Third degree: due to severe scalds or contact burn or flame. Skin may be dry, charred, whitish, usually painless.

NB. It is important to realise that in many burns there are varying gradations of burn.

Estimation of area of burns
In children < 12 years burned areas should be plotted on a body chart and areas calculated with the aid of the Lund–Browder chart (Fig. 23.1). Overestimation of the burn is common, often leading to excessive fluid administration.

MINOR BURNS
If burns are superficial and involve $< 8\%$ of the body surface area

NAME .... WARD .... UNIT NUMBER .... DATE ....

AGE ....

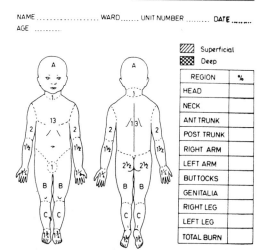

▨	Superficial
▧	Deep

REGION	%
HEAD	
NECK	
ANT TRUNK	
POST TRUNK	
RIGHT ARM	
LEFT ARM	
BUTTOCKS	
GENITALIA	
RIGHT LEG	
LEFT LEG	
TOTAL BURN	

RELATIVE PERCENTAGES AFFECTED BY GROWTH

AREA	AGE 0	1	5	10	15	ADULT
A = ½ OF HEAD	9½	8½	6½	5½	4½	3½
B = ½ OF ONE THIGH	2¾	3¼	4	4½	4½	4¾
C = ½ OF ONE LEG	2½	2½	2¾	3	3¼	3½

Fig. 23.1 Chart for calculating percentage area burned.

they may be managed on an outpatient basis after discussion with a burns registrar. Exceptions to this are burns to the face, neck, hands, feet or perineum, and burns in infants. These should be seen by the burns registrar and are usually admitted.

Treatment

1. Gently cleanse and remove loose skin, leaving blisters intact.
2. Dress the area with tulle gras and an absorbent dressing.
3. If indicated, immobilisation with a firm crepe bandage or sling may be necessary.
4. Leave initial dressing for 5–8 days. If dressing becomes soaked by accident, the lesion may be redressed without the adherent tulle being removed.
5. If you are in any doubt about treatment, contact the burns registrar.

EXTENSIVE BURNS

As a rule children with deep burns or superficial burns > 8% to the body surface area should be admitted. Contact the burns registrar or consultant immediately to discuss transfer of the patient.

Treatment

Following a brief history, which must include the cause of the burn, how and why the patient was exposed, evidence of associated injuries and the possibility of an inhalation burn:

1. Insert an i.v. line. An i.v. line for monitoring CVP in patients with severe burns is very helpful. Burns >12–15%, usually require i.v. therapy.
2. Take blood for FBC, U & E, glucose, creatinine, Ca^{2+}, clotting studies, total protein, LFT, blood group and crossmatch. Urinalysis and CXR are also needed.
3. Weigh the child or estimate the weight.
4. Document the extent and depth of the burn as described earlier.
5. Insert a urethral catheter and monitor urine output in all patients with burns > 15% of surface area.
6. Analgesia and/or sedation should be given as necessary (morphine 0.02–0.04 mg/kg i.v. and/or oral chloral hydrate). Morphine should be used with extreme care (i.e. with anaesthetic supervision) in infants as there is a risk of respiratory arrest.
7. Give tetanus prophylaxis as indicated (see p. 228).
8. Meticulous observation of the patient's condition, including respiration, temperature, BP and fluid balance are essential.
9. Fluid requirements: always discuss with the burns team. Manage on ICU.
   a. **Fluid needed for resuscitation.** Fluid volume required: 3 ml/kg per 1% burned surface area for the first 24 hours. In less severe burns, 2 ml/kg per 1% burned surface area should be sufficient.
      Type of fluid: plasma should make up 25% in burns > 20%, 33% in burns > 30%, 50% in burns > 40% of total fluid requirement depending on the depth and the percent of the burn. The remainder is given as Hartmann's solution in 5% dextrose.

   b. **Maintenance fluid.** For maintenance requirements see p. 18. Use 0.45% saline in 5% dextrose for maintenance fluids.
      Example. Fluid requirements in the first 24 hours:
      First 8 hours: give 50% of the resuscitation fluid plus 33% of the maintenance fluid.
      9–16 hours: give 25% of the resuscitation fluid plus 33% of the maintenance fluid.

16–24 hours: give 25% of the resuscitation fluid plus 33% of the maintenance fluid.

NB. This 24-hour period commences from the time of the burn and not from the time of admission. A urinary flow rate of 0.75 ml/kg/h (in infants > 1 ml/kg/h) is required.

After 24 hours, the maintenance fluid should be given as normal and the replacement fluid is approximately half that given for the first 24 hours. Obviously this will vary between patients and will require biochemical and clinical assessment. Diuresis often occurs 3–5 days following burns.

10. Antibiotics: usually given only for proven infection. On admission, take swabs of the burnt area, nose, throat and rectum. If septicaemia is suspected clinically, take blood cultures and give broad spectrum antibiotics (e.g. gentamicin and flucloxacillin).

11. Vomiting due to gastric dilatation may require a temporary NGT. Most children can tolerate milk 12 hours following a burn.

12. Whole blood is only initially required in severe deep burns. It may be required after the first 24 hours when Hb is falling.

13. Nutrition: a high calorie diet containing adequate protein, vitamins and iron supplements is required. Consult a dietitian.

14. Care of the wound should be supervised by the burns registrar.

15. Escharotomies should be considered if the peripheral circulation to a limb is jeopardised. They may also be required to the trunk if a child has respiratory difficulties. Such children should be in ICU.

ELECTRICAL BURNS

Examine carefully for entrance and exit wounds.

Investigations

In addition to investigations for burns include creatinine, CPK and urine for Hb and myoglobin and perform an ECG.

Management

An electrical burn to the mouth is serious and should be followed by the burns unit because of the possibility of haemorrhage at the site of the burn.

24

Surgical problems

A painful tender scrotum may be due to torsion of the testis and requires urgent surgical attention. Surgical exploration is often required.

Epididymo-orchitis is rare before puberty in the absence of UTI.

Balanitis

Infection under the foreskin.

CLINICAL FEATURES

Erythema, swelling and occasionally a whitish exudate.

MANAGEMENT

1. If the whole penis is red and swollen, hospital admission and i.v. antibiotics are indicated. Discuss with the surgeon on call.
2. For mild erythema and swelling of the foreskin treat immediately with local toilet, antibiotic ointment under the foreskin and oral antibiotics (e.g. erythromycin).

   If in doubt refer to a senior colleague.

Paraphimosis

The foreskin becomes trapped behind the glans which swells, causing acute pain.

MANAGEMENT

Urgent surgical referral if the foreskin cannot be reduced.

Phimosis

Urinary obstruction and ballooning of the foreskin with micturition due to scarring of the preputial opening.

MANAGEMENT

Surgical referral. Circumcision may be required.

Inguinal hernia

Often reported by parents that there is an intermittent swelling in the inguinal region. It is usually painless.

Inguinal hernias always need surgery because of the risk of strangulation of bowel. The younger the child, the greater the risk of strangulation.

MANAGEMENT

Treatment is surgical:
1. Birth–6 weeks: immediate surgical referral to the on call team.
2. 6 weeks–6 months: urgent surgical outpatient opinion; surgery is usually within 2 weeks.
3. > 6 months: surgical opinion within 2 weeks.

Parents and ward staff should be fully briefed concerning signs of strangulation and the need for immediate surgical attention, should they arise.

It is safer to consider a hernia which is even temporarily irreducible as being potentially strangulated. Immediate surgical referral for reduction and operation is required.

Hydrocele

Hydroceles of the scrotum or cord are common.

CLINICAL FEATURES

A painless, brilliantly transilluminable swelling. The upper pole is clearly demonstrable, i.e. the palpating fingers can get above it and there is a narrow cord above the swelling. The swelling does not empty on squeezing.

MANAGEMENT

If the above clinical features are not present, or you are unsure, refer as the swelling may be an irreducible hernia.

If hydroceles persist beyond 2 years, surgery is usually considered.

Central umbilical hernia

This is common in newborns. The majority of umbilical hernias will close spontaneously by the age of 2–3 years. If present beyond this age, a surgical opinion is appropriate.

Para-umbilical hernia

This is a defect in the linea alba, separate but adjacent to the umbilical cicatrix. Most are just above the umbilicus. Spontaneous closure is less likely and surgery is usually performed electively after the first year.

Intussusception

Invagination of a segment of bowel into the adjoining distal bowel.

CLINICAL FEATURES

Age usually 3 months to 3 years, peak incidence 4–6 months. Pain, typically a colic lasting 2–3 min during which the infant screams, draws up his knees, clenches his fists, relaxing as the spasm ceases. Spasms may occur at intervals of 15–20 min. After an hour or more the infant may become exhausted.

Other features may include vomiting, anorexia, persistent unexplained crying. A normal stool is often passed at the onset and a bloody ('red currant jelly') stool may or may not be seen some hours later. An abdominal mass may be felt (66%).

NB. Not all cases are classic; 20% have no colic; vomiting may be absent; rectal blood is absent in 30% and an abdominal mass is not palpable in > 30%.

DIFFERENTIAL DIAGNOSIS

Wind colic — persistent colic for more than 1–2 hours should arouse suspicion that intussusception is present. It is not accompanied by any of the other signs.

Gastroenteritis — when any doubt arises in distinguishing gastroenteritis from an intussusception a diagnostic barium enema should be considered.

MANAGEMENT

1. Erect plain AXR may be of help: fluid levels, dilated small bowel and absent caecal gas shadow may be seen.
2. Urgent surgical opinion. Treatment is either by barium enema which is also diagnostic or by surgical reduction. Peritonitis, significant dehydration or established bowel obstruction are contraindications to a contrast enema.
3. Resuscitation with plasma may be required. Correct fluid and electrolyte loss.

Bile stained vomiting in infancy

Urgent surgical referral is indicated to exclude midgut volvulus.

Pyloric stenosis

Males : females = 5 : 1. Usually occurs from weeks 2 to 6.

CLINICAL FEATURES

Projectile vomiting (not bile stained), FTT, including weight loss, constipation and a hungry baby able to feed again immediately after vomiting.

Signs are visible peristaltic waves and a palpable 'tumour' in the epigastrium or right hypochondrium.

INVESTIGATIONS

Test feed: observe for peristalsis and feel for tumour. Check electrolytes and acid–base. A hypochloraemic alkalosis and hypokalaemia may be seen. Culture urine.

Differential diagnosis includes mismanagement of feeding problem, GOR, intestinal obstruction, intracranial conditions (e.g. meningitis), infections (e.g. renal).

MANAGEMENT

1. Correct dehydration and electrolyte abnormalities, see p. 31.
2. Refer to the surgical team for pyloromyotomy.

Suspected appendicitis

A surgical opinion is essential.

CLINICAL FEATURES

The most common symptom is localised abdominal pain, initially periumbilical then moves to the right iliac fossa. Vomiting is seen in 80%, diarrhoea in 20%. Temperature is only slightly elevated but in about 5% may be $> 39°C$.

Tenderness in the right iliac fossa. Tenderness on rectal examination.

Appendicitis needs to be differentiated from other causes of abdominal pain, such as viral infection, constipation, UTI and from lower lobe chest infection.

NB. Appendicitis in the young child can be difficult to diagnose, and a high index of suspicion is required. Children < 3 and retarded children often present with peritonitis. Delayed diagnosis tends to relate to variable symptomatology in childhood, e.g. there may be few complaints of pain, vomiting may not be present and diarrhoea or dysuria may be predominant features.

TREATMENT

Surgical.

Appendices

Drug doses

NOTES

Adult doses should be used for patients > 40 kg or > 12 years of age unless alterations are detailed below.

Preterm infant drug doses refer to those over 1000 g.

Always consult other references with regard to drug incompatibility and side effects (i.e. BNF or MIMS) or discuss with a pharmacist when prescribing any drug to a child.

Take great care when calculating drug doses; it is good practice to check drug doses with an experienced colleague.

CALCULATION OF DRUG INFUSION RATES

30 µg (0.03 mg)/kg in 50 ml at 1 ml/h = 0.01 µg/kg/min
300 µg (0.3 mg)/kg in 50 ml at 1 ml/h = 0.1 µg/kg/min
3000 µg (3 mg)/kg in 50 ml at 1 ml/h = 1 µg/kg/min
Example: a 10-kg child, 0.1–2 µg/kg/min, infusion 1–20 ml/h: put 0.3 mg/kg (= 3 mg) in 50 ml. Administer via a 50-ml syringe pump.

THERAPEUTIC DRUG MONITORING

Serum drug concentrations may be measured to ensure that therapeutic levels are being achieved and/or to exclude toxicity.
When requesting drug levels always state:
— time blood was taken
— time last dose of drug was given
— route of administration
— other drugs the patient is receiving
Usually samples should only be taken when a steady state has been reached (equivalent to approximately 5 times the drug half-life).

Drugs with a long half-life (e.g. digoxin, phenytoin, carbamazepine and phenobarbitone). Measure levels after at least 5 half-lives and immediately before the next dose.

Drugs with a short half-life (e.g. vancomycin, valproate, gentamicin, tobramycin, chloramphenicol). Take blood for peak level after injection (see individual drugs below for timing) and for trough level (except valproate) just before the **next** dose as well.

CORTICOSTEROIDS

During chronic treatment with corticosteroids maintenance dose should be increased when the child has a significant cause of 'stress', e.g. significant infection or surgical operation. If the total daily dose is < 30 mg prednisolone increase by a factor of 2–3, if > 30 mg double the dose.

Cover for operations

Advised in children on long-term treatment. The aim is to mimic normal response to stress; for example, hydrocortisone 50–100 mg (larger dose, i.e. 100 mg used in children over 8 years) i.m. or i.v. with premedication. Repeat 8-hourly. Dose may be slowly decreased to usual maintenance by 4 days.

If on high dose maintenance steroids, the first day's dose equivalent (see Table A.1) should be the same as on the first day of chronic therapy. Check with the consultant in charge of the patient requiring prolonged steroids.

Table A.1 Relative potencies of corticosteroids

	Glucocorticoid	Mineralocorticoid	Anti-inflammatory
Hydrocortisone	1	1	1
Cortisone	0.8	0.8	1
Prednisolone	4	0.8	4
Methyl prednisolone	5	0.5	6
Dexamethasone	30	0	30

INDIVIDUAL DRUG DOSES

Acetazolamide. *Hydrocephalus:* 7–18 mg/kg p.o. 8–12-hourly. Start at lowest dose, increase as tolerated up to 1–2 weeks. Beware metabolic acidosis and hypokalaemia. *Neonates:* dose as above.

Adenosine. *Supraventricular tachycardia:* 50 µg/kg. Give every 2 min with increments of 50 µg/kg up to a dose of 300 µg/kg until in sinus rhythm. Give as a rapid bolus i.v. (Named patient drug.)

Acetylcysteine. (dose in paracetamol poisoning see p. 261). *Meconium ileus equivalent:* 2.5–5 ml of a 20% solution p.o. 6–8-hourly (should dilute, by a factor of 4, with juice).

ACTH. *Infantile spasms:* 1 u/kg (max. 40 u) i.m. per 24 hours.

Acyclovir. *Varicella zoster and herpes encephalitis:* 10 mg/kg i.v. 8-hourly over 1 hour (concentration of up to 25 mg/ml may be infused if the child is fluid restricted). *Herpes simplex:* 5–10 mg/kg 8-hourly for 5–10 days. Oral dose: < 2 years 100 mg 5-hourly; > 2 years 200–400 mg 5-hourly.

Adrenaline. *Cardiac arrest:* 0.1 ml/kg of 1 in 10 000 i.v. or via ETT (if there is no response, up to 10 times this dose may be required). *Croup:* racaemic adrenaline (2.25%) 0.05 ml/kg or 1 in 1000 (0.1%) 0.5 ml/kg by nebulisation (max. 5 ml). *Anaphylaxis:* 10 µg/kg (i.e. 0.01 ml/kg of 1 in 1000 dilution) s.c. or i.m. injection. May be repeated twice in double dose (max. 100 µg/kg over 3 min).

Alcuronium. Should be administered by an anaesthetist or on ICU. 0.2–0.3 mg/kg i.v.; subsequent dose 0.05 mg/kg.

Allopurinol. 2.5 mg/kg p.o. 6-hourly or 300 mg/m² per 24 hours. Interacts with mercaptopurine and azothioprine.

Aluminium hydroxide. 5–40 mg/kg 8-hourly with food. Gel (64 mg/ml) 0.1 ml/kg 6-hourly p.o.

Amiloride. 0.2 mg/kg p.o. 12-hourly (max. 5 mg/dose).

Aminophylline. *Asthma:* loading dose 5 mg/kg i.v. over 30 min (omit loading dose if taking theophylline) followed by a continuous infusion of 0.75–1 mg/kg/h (e.g. using a 50-ml syringe pump: 40 mg/kg in 50 ml at 1 ml/h = 0.8 mg/kg/h) (therapeutic range 60–110 µmol/l; 10–20 mg/l). *Neonates:* 6 mg/kg i.v. as a loading dose over 30 min. Then 160 µg/kg/h as a continuous infusion (therapeutic range 40–80 µmol/l; 7–14 mg/l).

Amitriptyline. *Enuresis:* 6–10 years 10–20 mg per 24 hours, 11–16 years 25–50 mg per 24 hours p.o. at bedtime.

Amoxycillin. 10–20 mg/kg 8-hourly p.o. in 3 divided doses. *Adult:* 250–500 mg 8-hourly.

Amphotericin B. Test dose 0.1 mg/kg over 2 hours i.v. Increase in increments of 0.2 mg/kg per 24 hours gradually to 1 mg/kg per 24 hours. Infuse over 6 hours. (Hypersensitivity reactions and nephrotoxicity common.)

Ampicillin. 12.5–50 mg/kg p.o. or i.v. 6-hourly. *Neonates:* 30 mg/kg i.v. 12-hourly (day 1–6); 30 mg/kg 8-hourly (7–14 days); 30 mg/kg 6-hourly (14 days plus).

Ascorbic acid. *Scurvy:* 500 mg once and then 100 mg per 24 hours for 1 week; then 25 mg per 24 hours as prophylaxis.

Atenolol. Hypertension: 1–2 mg/kg p.o. 12–24-hourly. *Adult:* 50–200 mg per 24 hours. i.v. 0.05 mg/kg every 5 min until response (max. 4 doses).

Atracurium. 0.5 mg/kg stat i.v. then 5–10 µg/kg/min. By anaesthetist or in ICU only.

Atropine sulphate. *Premedication:* 0.02 mg/kg i.m. (max. 0.6 mg). *Resuscitation:* 20 µg/kg i.v. or via ETT. *Neonatal resuscitation:* 15 µg/kg = 0.025 ml/kg of the 600 µg/ml solution via ETT or i.v. Double the endotracheal dose if response is poor.

Azlocillin. *Neonates:* Preterm 50 mg/kg i.v. 12-hourly, full term 100 mg/kg i.v. 12-hourly. *Infants and children:* 50–75 mg/kg 6–8-hourly. *Very severe infection:* 75 mg/kg 4-hourly. *Adult:* 6–24 g per 24 hours.

Beclomethasone dipropionate. *Asthma:* inhaled via spacer device (MDI 100 µg/puff) 100–400 µg 12-hourly. *Rhinitis:* nasal spray (Beconase) for children > 6 years 100 µg 12-hourly, dose each nostril.

Benztropine. Not recommended < 3 years because of atropine-like side-effects. 0.02 mg/kg stat i.v. or i.m.; may repeat after 15 min. 0.02 mg/kg p.o. 12–24-hourly. *Adult:* 0.5–6 mg per 24 hours.

Bicarbonate. (8.4% = 1 mmol/l) *Under 5 kg:* mmol deficit = base deficit × weight/2 (give half of this only, then review) slowly i.v. *Over 5 kg:* mmol deficit = base deficit × weight/3 (give half of this only, then review) slowly i.v. *Neonates:* use 4.2% (1 ml = 0.5 mmol/l) to correct as burns occur with extravasation. Beware hypernatremia.

Bisacodyl. 2–10 years 5 mg p.o. once daily at night. Rectal (given in the morning): < 1 year 2.5 mg, 1–10 years 5 mg.

Budesonide. Metered dose inhaler via Nebuhaler; 50–200 µg 12-hourly. Also available by Turbohaler (100 µg, 200 µg and 400 µg per dose).

Caffeine. Loading dose 10 mg/kg p.o. or i.v. Maintenance 2.5 mg/kg per 24 hours. Given twice daily.

Calamine. 3–4 times per 24 hours topically.

Calciferol. 600 units per 24 hours (depends on condition).

Calcium gluconate 10% (0.22 mmol/ml Ca^{2+}). *Resuscitation:* 0.5 ml/kg slowly i.v. (max. dose 20 ml). *Hypocalcaemic tetany:* 500 mg/m² over 3 hours. Use a large vein; beware of extravasation. *Neonates:* 0.3 ml/kg i.v. for acute correction under ECG control over 10 min.

Captopril. 0.25 mg/kg p.o. 8-hourly. Increase in steps up to a max. of 1 mg/kg 8-hourly.

Carbamazepine. 2 mg/kg p.o. 8-hourly increasing over 2 weeks (max. 10 mg/kg 8-hourly) (therapeutic level = 20–50 µmol/l; old units = 4.7–11.8 mg/l). Steady state is not achieved for 2–4 weeks; measurement should be delayed until then; sample should be taken immediately before a dose. Phenytoin, phenobarbitone and primidone can lower serum concentration. Cimetidine and erythromycin may increase level.

Carbimazole. 0.25 mg/kg p.o. (max. 10 mg/dose) 8-hourly for 2 weeks, then 0.1 mg/kg 12-hourly.

Cefaclor. 10–15 mg/kg p.o. given 8-hourly (max. 1 g).

Cefotaxime. 30–50 mg/kg 6–8-hourly. *Adult:* 2–12 g per 24 hours. *Neonates:* dose in serious infections; 1–7 days of age 50 mg/kg 8–12-hourly; > 2 weeks 50 mg/kg

6–8-hourly.

Ceftazidime. 30–50 mg/kg i.v. 8-hourly. *Adult:* 1–2 g/dose.

Ceftriaxone. 50–100 mg/kg per 24 hours i.v. in 1 or 2 doses. *Adult:* 1–2 g per 24 hours.

Chloral hydrate. *Hypnotic:* 50 mg/kg stat dose (max. 1 g).

Chloramphenicol. 40 mg/kg stat then 25 mg/kg i.v. or p.o. 6–8-hourly. (max. 1 g/dose) (therapeutic levels 20–30 mg/l peak, trough < 15 mg/l). Take sample after 2–3 days unless toxicity is suspected. Phenobarbitone may lower serum concentration. Phenytoin may increase serum concentration. *Eye:* 1 drop 2–6-hourly for 2–3 days, then increase time between doses.

Chloroquine sulphate. *Prophylaxis:* 5 mg (base)/kg p.o. once a week (300 mg max.). *Treatment:* 10 mg (base)/kg stat p.o. followed by 5 mg (base)/kg in 6-hours then 5 mg (base)/kg per 24 hours for 2 days.

Chlorothiazide. < 6 months up to 17 mg/kg p.o. 12-hourly, > 6 months 5–12 mg/kg 12-hourly. *Adult:* 500–2000 mg per 24 hours.

Chlorpheniramine. 100 µg/kg p.o. *Adult:* 4 mg 8-hourly or 200 µg/kg i.v. single dose.

Chlorpromazine. *Sedation:* 0.5 mg/kg slowly i.v., i.m. or p.o. 4–6-hourly (max. 2 mg/kg per 24 hours). *Neonates:* 500 µg/kg p.o., i.m. or i.v. 8-hourly for alpha blockade and narcotic withdrawal.

Cholestyramine. Resin: 0.05–0.1 g/kg p.o. 8-hourly.

Cimetidine. 5–10 mg/kg p.o. or i.v. 6-hourly over 30 min (max. 200 mg/dose).

Ciprofloxacin. 5–10 mg/kg p.o. 12-hourly. Not licensed for use in children.

Clindamycin. 3–6 mg/kg p.o., i.m. or i.v. 6-hourly. Give over 30 min.

Clonazepam. *Seizures:* Neonates up to 0.25 mg i.v. (DECREASE dose for premature and non-ventilated babies). Children up to 0.5 mg. Adult: 1 mg. *Prophylaxis:* 0.01–0.03 mg/kg per 24 hours p.o. in 2–3 divided doses. Increase by < 0.25–0.5 mg every third day up to 0.05–0.1 mg/kg per 24 hours in 3 divided doses.

Clonidine. *Migraine:* commence with 0.5 µg/kg p.o. 12-hourly.

Clotrimazole. Cream/lotion apply 12-hourly.

Codeine. *Analgesic:* 0.5 mg/kg p.o. 4-hourly.

Cotrimoxazole. 2–5 months 120 mg p.o. or i.v. infusion 12-hourly; 6 months–5 years 240 mg 12-hourly; > 5 years 480 mg 12-hourly.

Desferrioxamine. *Iron poisoning:* see p. 260; *Thalassemia major:* 500 mg/unit of blood i.v.; *s.c. maintenance:* 1–3 g/5 ml over 10 hours, 4–6 nights/week but needs to be tailored to patients' needs (monitor serum iron levels).

Desmopressin (DDAVP). 5–10 µg intranasal every 12–24 hours or 0.3 µg/kg i.v. over 30 min.

Dexamethasone. 100 µg/kg p.o. or i.v. 6-hourly. For treatment of shock 2–6 mg/kg i.v. may be repeated in 2–6 hours if shock persists. *Neonates:* for BPD 0.25 mg/kg i.v. or p.o. 12-hourly for 3 days, then 0.125 mg/kg 12-hourly for 3 days; then reduce by 10% every 3 days until at 0.05 mg/kg 12-hourly when dose goes to every other day. Total initial course = 3 weeks. For extubation 0.5 mg/kg as a single dose prior to extubation, repeat dose 48 hours later for stridor.

Diamorphine. *Neonates:* ventilated patients give 20 µg/kg loading dose i.v. Then 2.5 µg/kg/h as an infusion in 5 or 10% dextrose. Adjust to control pain or to suppress respiration. Respiratory depression occurs in spontaneously breathing babies. ICU monitoring is needed.

Diazepam. 0.2 mg/kg i.v. or 0.2–0.5 mg/kg p.o. 8–12-hourly. Rectal 0.3–0.4 mg/kg. Caution: may cause respiratory depression.

Diazoxide. 2–5 mg/kg i.v.; may repeat in 30 min. *Adult:* 300 mg. May cause severe hypotension. Monitor for arrhythmias and hyperglycaemia.

Dicyclomine. 0.5 mg/kg p.o. 6-hourly (max. 15 mg/dose). *Not* under 6 months.

Digoxin. Digitalisation with loading dose is only needed in the management of arrhythmias or severe acute heart failure. Otherwise start with maintenance dose. Give over at least 5 min; 15 µg/kg stat p.o. or i.v. over 5 min, 5 µg/kg after 6 hours; then 3–5 µg/kg 12-hourly. Therapeutic range — low: < 0.6 nmol/l; borderline low: 0.6–1 nmol/l; therapeutic range: 1–2.5 nmol/l; borderline high: 2.5–3 nmol/l; high: > 3 nmol/l (conversion to old units × 0.7809 = ng/ml). Sample should not be taken for 6 days from starting unless toxicity is suspected. Sample should be taken 6 hours after dose. Absorption may be decreased by antacid, metoclopramide or neomycin. Drugs increasing peristalsis, e.g. tetracycline and propantheline, may increase absorption. Serum concentration may be increased by quinidine and calcium blocking agents and effects of digoxin increased by spironolactone. Renal and hepatic disease and hypothyroidism may cause increased levels.

Dimercaprol. See p. 266.

Dobutamine. 2–20 µg/kg/min i.v. continuous infusion. *Neonates:* 1–2 µg/kg/min initially. Then adjusted between 3 and 10 µg/kg/min for required inotropism.

Dopamine. 2–15 µg/kg/min i.v. continuous infusion (e.g. 3 mg/kg dopamine in 50 ml infused at 5 ml/h = 5 µg/kg/min). *Neonates:* dose as above. 2–5 µg/kg/min for renal vasodilatation, 5–10 µg/kg/min for inotropism,

10–15 µg/kg/min for inotropism, but vasoconstriction may occur at these doses. Give via central vein if possible.

Econazole. 1% topical to skin 2–3 times per 24 hours.

Edrophonium. i.v. test dose of 20 µg/kg, then 100 µg/kg.

Ephedrine. 0.5% nasal drops 1 drop into each nostril 6-hourly (2 days only).

Erythromycin. 10–20 mg/kg i.v. or p.o. 6–8-hourly (15 min before food). *Adult:* 1–4 g per 24 hours. *Neonates:* week 1, 10 mg/kg 12-hourly; weeks 2–4, 10 mg/kg 8-hourly.

Ethosuximide. Commence 125 mg 12-hourly increasing slowly at 4–7-day intervals to 10–20 mg/kg 12-hourly. *Adult:* up to 2 g per 24 hours (therapeutic range 0.3–0.7 mmol/l; conversion to old units × 141.2 = µg/ml).

Ferrous gluconate. (9 mg ferrous gluconate = 1 mg elemental iron). *Prophylaxis:* 2 mg elemental iron/kg per 24 hours. *Treatment:* 6 mg elemental iron/kg per 24 hours. Give in divided doses.

Ferrous sulphate. (200 mg tablets = 60 mg elemental iron). *Prophylaxis:* 2 mg elemental iron/kg per 24 hours. *Treatment:* 6 mg elemental iron/kg per 24 hours. Give in divided doses.

Flecainide. Up to a max. of 2 mg/kg i.v. over 10 min with ECG monitoring. Orally 3–6 mg/kg per 24 hours titrated slowly up to 20 mg/kg per 24 hours in 2–3 divided doses. (Adjust dose according to blood levels.)

Flucloxacillin. 25–50 mg/kg p.o. or i.v. 1–7 days of age 12-hourly; 2–4 weeks, 8-hourly; > 4 weeks, 4–6 hourly.

Flucytosine. 0–4 weeks, 25 mg/kg 6-hourly, > 4 weeks 50 mg/kg 6-hourly i.v. or p.o.

Fludrocortisone. 0.05–0.2 mg per 24 hours.

Folic acid. 250 µg/kg per 24 hours p.o. up to 1 year. 1–4 years, 2.5 mg per 24 hours; 5–12 years, 5 mg per 24 hours.

Folinic acid. 10–15 mg/m² p.o., i.v. or i.m. 6-hourly for rescue after high dose methotrexate (for 48 hours). 100–1000 mg/ m² 6-hourly for methotrexate toxicity. (Dose depends on dose of methotrexate administered and on resulting blood levels of methotrexate; consult the pharmacy.)

Frusemide. 1–2 mg/kg p.o. 12–24-hourly or 0.5–1 mg/kg i.v. 6–12-hourly. May increase to 5 mg/kg in resistant cases.

Fucidic acid. See sodium fusidate.

Ganciclovir. 5 mg/kg i.v. 12-hourly over 1 hour.

Gaviscon. Infants: 1–2 g powder with feed 4-hourly. < 12 years: 5–10 ml liquid or half a sachet of granules after meals.

Gentamicin. 2.5 mg/kg i.v. < 30 weeks' gestation, give daily; 30–35 weeks' gestation, give 18-hourly; term week 1, give 12-hourly; infants and young children, give 8-hourly. (Usual adult dose 80 mg 8-hourly.) (therapeutic range, peak = 5–10 mg/l, trough = < 2 mg/l). In patients with impaired renal function or dehydration it may be necessary to monitor serum levels from the start of treatment. Usually check after 2 days (3 doses). Sample for peak 1 hour after dose and for trough level immediately before **next dose**.

Glucagon. 1 unit = 1 mg. 0.05 u/kg i.m. or s.c. (max. dose 1 unit) or 0.2 µ/kg stat i.v. then 0.005–0.01 u/kg/h for cardiogenic shock.

Glycerin. Rectal: insert appropriate (i.e. infant, child, adult) suppository into the rectum and allow to remain for 15–30 min.

Glyceryl trinitrate. s.l.: 0.01–0.015 mg/kg.

Griseofulvin. 10–15 mg/kg once per 24 hours p.o. with main meal. *Adult:* 500–1000 mg per 24 hours.

Haloperidol. Start 0.5 mg per 24 hours p.o., increase up to 0.025 mg/kg 12-hourly. i.v.: depends on the patient; consult a reference text.

Heparin. Low dose: 75 u/kg stat i.v., then 10–15 u/kg/h. Full dose: 50–200 u/kg stat, then 15–30 u/kg/h. Monitor dose with clotting time or PTT. Antidote: see protamine.

Hydralazine. Oral: initially 0.15–0.5 mg/kg 12-hourly; gradually increase to 2 mg/kg. *Adult:* 25–200 mg per 24 hours. i.v.: 0.25–0.5 mg/kg stat i.v., then 0.1–0.2 mg/kg 4–6-hourly. Max. 3 mg/kg in 24 hours.

Hydrocortisone sodium succinate. 2–4 mg/kg i.v. repeated 3–6-hourly over the first 24 hours, reducing the dose over the next 24 hours. May be changed to oral prednisolone when tolerated.

Ibuprofen. 10–40 mg/kg per 24 hours p.o.; up to a max. of 2.4 g per 24 hours for acute control of disease. Give in 3–4 divided doses.

Idoxuridine. *Eye:* 0.1%; 1 drop hourly while awake; 2-hourly during the night. Continue for 5 days following the disappearance of lesion.

Imipramine. *Enuresis:* 5–6 years give 25 mg p.o. at night; 7–10 years 50 mg; > 10 years 50–75 mg. *Antidepressant:* 5–12 years 10 mg 8-hourly; ≥ 13 years 25 mg 8-hourly.

Indomethacin. *Rheumatoid arthritis, inflammation, pain:* 0.5–1 mg/kg p.o. 8-hourly. *Neonates:* for patent ductus arteriosus: 0.2 mg/kg i.v., give 12-hourly for 3 doses. Check renal function and platelets. Consider concomitant frusemide.

Ipratropium bromide. Nebulised solution (0.025%); 0.4–1 ml diluted to 2 ml with normal saline 4–6-hourly. Metered dose aerosol (20 µg/dose); up to 5 years 1 puff 8-hourly; 6–12 years 1–2 puffs 8-hourly.

Isoniazid (INAH). 10–15 mg/kg per 24 hours in 1 or 2 doses (adults 300 mg per 24 hours).

Isoprenaline. 0.05–0.5 µg/kg/min i.v. by continuous infusion.

Ketoconazole. 3–10 mg/kg once daily at night with a meal. *Adult:* 200 mg per 24 hours.

Ketovite multivitamin. 1–3 tablets plus 5 ml of mixture per 24 hours.

Labetalol. 1–2 mg/kg p.o. every 6–8 hours.

Lactulose. *Laxative:* 0.5 ml/kg 12- or 24-hourly. *Hepatic coma:* 1 ml/kg 6-hourly.

Loperamide. 2–5 years 1 mg p.o. 8-hourly; 6–12 years 2 mg 8-hourly.

Magnesium sulphate. *To treat deficiency:* 50% magnesium sulphate (2 mmol/ml; max. 4 mmol) 0.2 ml/kg 12-hourly i.m. or very slowly i.v.; dilute before giving i.v. (Inj. magnesium sulphate 50% contains 1 g $MgSO_4 7H_2O = 4$ mmol Mg^{2+} in 2 ml.)

Mannitol. 0.25–1 g/kg i.v. (1–4 ml/kg of 25% mannitol) over 20–60 min.

Mebendazole. *Enterobiasis (pin worm):* > 2 years, 100 mg single dose. Repeat in 3 weeks. *Trichuriasis, ascariasis, hookworm:* > 2 years, 100 mg given 12-hourly for 3 days.

Mefenamic acid. *Dysmenorrhoea:* 500 mg 8-hourly with meals.

Methylprednisolone. *Asthma:* 0.5–1 mg/kg 6-hourly for 24 hours then decrease to 12-hourly for 24 hours then 1 mg/kg per 24 hours. Change to oral prednisolone when possible.

Metoclopramide. 0.12 mg/kg i.v., i.m. or p.o. 6–8-hourly (adults 5–10 mg 8-hourly). Antidote for dystonic reaction is benztropine.

Metronidazole. Loading dose 15 mg/kg stat followed by 7.5 mg/kg 12-hourly for neonates (start routine doses 48 hours after loading dose for preterm, 24 hours for term); > 4 weeks 7.5 mg/kg 8-hourly i.v. or p.o.
Rectal: 8-hourly; < 1 year 125 mg/dose; 1–5 years 250 mg/dose; 6–12 years 500 mg/dose; > 12 years 1 g/dose. *Orally for Giardia:* 1–3 years 400 mg/dose; 4–7 years 600 mg/dose; 8–12 years 1 g/dose; > 12 years 2 g/dose 24-hourly for 3 days. *Amoebiasis:* 1–3 years 200 mg 8-hourly; 4–7 years 200 mg 6-hourly; 8–12 years 400 mg 8-hourly; > 12 years 800 mg 8-hourly for 5 days.

Miconazole. 7.5–15 mg/kg 8-hourly i.v. (max. 15 mg/kg/dose).

Micralax enema. < 12 months 1.25 ml; 1–2 years 2.5 ml; > 3 years 5 ml p.r.

Midazolam. *Induction of anaesthesia:* i.v. 200 µg/kg over 5 min then 1–2 µg/kg/min.

Morphine. 0.1–0.2 mg/kg p.o. 3–6-hourly or i.v. infusion 10–40 µg/kg/h. < 1 year, discuss with the consultant. *Neonates:* 0.1 mg/kg single dose i.v. 5 µg/kg/h infusion in dextrose. For ventilated neonates only.

Naladixic acid. > 3 months, 12.5 mg/kg 6-hourly.

Naloxone. 5–10 µg/kg i.v. or i.m. Repeat doses may be needed half-hourly. i.m. dose can be given for prolonged effect if i.v. dose is effective.

Naproxen. 5–7.5 mg/kg p.o. 12-hourly. > 5 years, max. dose 1 g per 24 hours.

Neomycin. 12.5–25 mg/kg p.o. 6-hourly.

Neostigmine. 0.05–0.07 mg/kg i.v. given over 1 min (max. dose 2.5 mg). Antagonise cholinergic effects with atropine 0.025 mg/kg.

Niclosamide. Orally as a single dose for beef, pork and fish tapeworm; < 2 years 500 mg in a single dose; 2–6 years 1 g; > 6 years 2 g.

Nifedipine. 0.25–1 mg/kg 6–12 hourly p.o. or sublingual.

Nitrazepam. *Anticonvulsant:* > 1 year 2.5–5 mg 12-hourly.

Nitrofurantonin. > 1 month. *Treatment:* 1.25–1.75 mg/kg p.o. 6-hourly. *Prophylaxis:* 2–3 mg/kg at night. *Adult:* 200 mg per 24 hours.

Nitroprusside. 0.5–10 µg/kg/min i.v. infusion. Discuss use and length of infusion with the consultant.

Nystatin. *Neonates:* 100 000 units (1 ml) 6-hourly. *Children:* 100 000–500 000 units 6–8-hourly after meals.

Oxandrolone. *Turner syndrome:* 0.1 mg/kg per 24 hours. *Anabolic agent:* 0.1–0.2 mg/kg per 24 hours. Discuss with the endocrinologist.

Omnopon. See papavertum.

Pancuronium. In ICU: 0.1 mg/kg i.v. as required. *Neonates:* as above, give 50 µg/kg for subsequent doses as required. Ventilated patients only.

Papavertum (Omnopon). 20–80 µg/kg/h i.v. infusion. 0.4 mg/kg i.m. Not recommended < 12 months.

Paracetamol. 15 mg/kg p.o. or p.r. 4–6-hourly (max. 60 mg/kg per 24 hours).

Paraldehyde. 0.3 ml/kg diluted 1 in 1 with arachis oil p.r. stat or 0.15–0.2 ml/kg i.m. stat.

Penicillin G (benzyl-). *Serious infection:* 100 000 units (60 mg)/kg i.v.; week 1 of life 12-hourly; 2–4 weeks 6-hourly; > 4 weeks 4-hourly.

Penicillin V. 12.5 mg/kg p.o. 6-hourly. *Prophylaxis:* 12.5 mg/kg 12-hourly.

Pethidine. 0.5–1 mg/kg i.v. or 1–1.5 mg/kg i.m. 100–300 µg/kg/h i.v. infusion. Not recommended < 12 months.

Phenobarbitone. *Neonates:* loading dose 20 mg/kg given as two doses of 10 mg/kg 3–4 hours apart, then maintenance 3–4 mg/kg per 24 hours i.v. or p.o. *Children:* loading dose in emergency 20–30 mg/kg i.m. or i.v. stat; maintenance dose 5 mg/kg per 24 hours p.o., i.m. or i.v. (therapeutic range 80–120 µmol/l (old units = 18–28 mg/ml). Take sample after fixed dosage for 2 weeks. If loading dose is given level may be checked earlier. Serum level may be increased by chloramphenicol, cimetidine, phenytoin and valproate.

Phenoxybenzamine: 0.2 mg/kg per 24 hours p.o. 0.5–1 mg/kg i.v. slow infusion (over at least 1 hour).

Phentolamine. In ICU: 0.1 mg/kg i.v. stat (test for phaeochromocytoma).

Phenytoin. *Emergency:* loading dose 15–20 mg/kg i.v. over 1 hour (max. infusion rate = 1 mg/kg/min). *Maintenance:* neonatal — preterm 2 mg/kg 12-hourly; term 1st week 4 mg/kg 12-hourly; children 4–8 mg/kg per 24 hours in 2 or 3 divided doses (therapeutic level = 40–80 μmol/l; 9.3–18.5 mg/l). When an i.v. loading dose has been given a serum specimen may be taken after 1 hour to determine whether the therapeutic concentration has been reached. Longterm treatment sample after 1–2 weeks and immediately before next dose. Serum concentration may be decreased by antacids, carbamazepine and rifampicin and increased by chloramphenicol, dexamethasone, cimetidine and in liver failure. Level of free phenytoin is increased by salicylate, valproate, hyperbilirubinaemia and uraemia.

Phytomenadione (vitamin K₁). 0.3 mg/kg (max. 10 mg) i.m. or slowly i.v. Prophylaxis in neonates 1 mg.

Piperacillin. 75 mg/kg i.v. 8-hourly.

Piperazine. *Ascaris:* 75 mg/kg p.o. (max. 4 g) per 24 hours for 2 days. *Pinworm:* above dose for 7 days.

Pizotifen: Adult: starting dose 0.5 mg per 24 hours increasing to 1.5 mg per 24 hours in 2 doses. Over 5 years, 500 μg per 24 hours; >10 years, 1 mg per 24 hours.

Platelets. 10–20 ml/kg in a single dose.

Prednisolone. *Acute asthma:* 2 mg/kg per 24 hours p.o. Usual max. dose 60 mg/kg per 24 hours.

Procyclidine. See p. 263.

Promethazine. 0.5 mg/kg p.o., i.v. or i.m. 6–8-hourly.

Propantheline. 0.3 mg/kg p.o. 6-hourly.

Propranolol. 0.01–0.1 mg/kg i.v. stat then 6-hourly. Oral: 0.2–0.5 mg/kg p.o. 6-hourly increasing to 1.25 mg/kg 6-hourly. *Migraine prophylaxis:* commence 10 mg per 24 hours increasing to 2 mg/kg per 24 hours in 2–3 divided doses.

Prostaglandin E₁. *Neonates:* maintenance infusion 0.005 μg/kg/min i.v. (Take 0.5 ml of PGE₁ (0.5 mg/ml) in a 1-ml syringe. Dilute 0.1 ml in 40 ml 5% dextrose in a 50-ml syringe. This solution is 1.25 μg/ml of PGE₁. Give at 0.24 ml/kg/h to achieve 0.005 μg/kg/min.)

Protamine. *Heparin overdosage:* 1 mg/100 units heparin i.v. Subsequent dose 1 mg/kg (half-life 1–2 hours).

Pyrazinamide. 20–30 mg/kg p.o. in 3 divided doses.

Pyridoxine. *Neonatal fitting:* 50 mg i.v.

Quinalbarbitone. *Sedative:* 5 mg/kg.

Quinine. Loading dose of 20 mg/kg i.v. over 4 hours, followed by 7.5 mg/kg 8-hourly (over 2–4 hours). Once the child recovers, give 10 mg/kg p.o. 8-hourly.

Ranitidine. 3 mg/kg p.o. 12-hourly or 1 mg/kg i.v. (over 10 min) 6–8-hourly.

Rifampicin. *Treatment:* 10–20 mg/kg p.o. or i.v. (max. 600 mg/dose). *Prophylaxis:* < 4 weeks 5 mg/kg 12-hourly for 4 doses; > 4 weeks 10 mg/kg (max. dose 600 mg) 12-hourly for 4 doses.

Salbutamol. Severe asthmatic attack, see p. 115. Nebulised: 2–5 mg 4-hourly. Powder inhalation; via Ventedisk or Rotahaler (200 µg) up to 4-hourly. By aerosol inhalation: 100–200 µg (1–2 puffs) up to 4-hourly.

Senna. From 1 year, 0.5 ml/kg p.o. 24-hourly.

Sodium cromoglycate. Nebulised: 20 mg (2 ml) 8-hourly. Powder inhalation of spincaps: 1 capsule 6–8-hourly via Spinhaler. *Eye* (opticrom) 2%: 1 drop each eye 6-hourly.

Sodium nitrite. 3% solution 0.2 ml/kg i.v. over 5 min.

Sodium valporate. Commence 5–7 mg/kg p.o. 8–12-hourly, increasing to max. 50 mg/kg per 24 hours in 2–3 divided doses.

Spironolactone. 1–3 mg/kg per 24 hours p.o. in 2–3 divided doses. *Adult:* 100–400 mg per 24 hours.

Streptomycin. 20 mg/kg 12-hourly i.m. (max. dose 1 g).

Sulphasalazine. Initial dose 12.5–25 mg/kg 6-hourly p.o. Maintenance 10–15 mg/kg.

Suxamethonium. 1 mg/kg i.v. Anaesthetists only.

Terbutaline. Nebulised: ≤ 3 years 2 mg; 3–6 years, 3 mg; 6–8 years 4 mg; > 8 years 5 mg 6–12-hourly. Powder inhalation (Turbohaler) 500 µg (1 inhalation) up to 6-hourly. Metered dose areosol 250–500 µg (1–2 puffs) 4–hourly as required.

Terfenadine. 6–12 years, 30 mg 12-hourly.

THAM 3.6%. *Neonates:* 1 mL equivalent to 0.25 mmol sodium bicarbonate. Used in attempt to avoid sodium and CO_2 accumulation. Apnoea may occur: restrict to ventilated babies.

Theophylline. *Neonatal apnoea:* 6 mg/kg p.o. stat (assuming aminophylline not already given), then 0–1 weeks 2 mg/kg 12-hourly; 1–2 weeks 3 mg/kg 12-hourly; > 2 weeks 4 mg/kg 12-hourly. Sustained release 1–7 years 12 mg/kg (usually 12-hourly), 8–16 years 10 mg/kg (therapeutic level 40–80 µmol/l; 7–15 mg/l). Levels may be checked midway between doses about 3 days after commencing maintenance therapy or sooner if toxicity is suspected. *Asthma:* > 1 year, 5 mg/kg 6-hourly (max. 250 mg/dose) (therapeutic level 60–110 µmol/l; 10–20 mg/l). Taken after stable dosage for at least 48 hours. Slow release, sample 4 hours after dose; other oral forms, sample after 2 hours. Patient with status asthmaticus: samples if needed may be taken 30 min after loading dose or 4 hours after starting constant infusion. Levels may be increased with cimetidine, erythromycin, oral contraceptive, cardiac and liver failure and sustained fever, and lowered by phenytoin, rifampicin or barbiturate therapy or by smoking (conversion of SI to old units × 0.1802 = µg/ml).

Thiabendazole. 25 mg/kg p.o. 12-hourly. Length of treatment depends on condition.

Thiopentone. Given in ICU. 3–5 mg/kg i.v. stat slowly, then 1–2 mg/kg/h.

Thyroxine. *Infant:* initial dose 25 µg per 24 hours p.o., increasing by small increments to keep serum thyroxine in upper half of normal range and serum TSH level suppressed. Dose usually needed is 3–5 µg/kg per 24 hours.

Ticarcillin. Infants and children: 75 mg/kg 6-hourly.

Tobramycin. *Preterm:* 2–2.5 mg/kg i.v. per 24 hours. *Term:* week 1, 2–2.5 mg/kg i.v. 12-hourly, > 1 week 2–2.5 mg/kg 8-hourly (max. 100 mg). Therapeutic range, peak 5–10 mg/l, trough < 2 mg/l. See notes under gentamicin as drugs are similarly affected.

Tolazoline. 1–2 mg/kg i.v. over 1–5 min as test bolus; may cause hypotension: have plasma available. Then 1–2 mg/kg/h maintenance infusion in normal saline. Pediatrics 1986 77: 307

Tranexamic acid. 20 mg/kg 8-hourly to stop bleeding in haemophiliacs.

Trimeprazine. See Vallergan.

Trimethoprim. *Prophylaxis:* 1–5 years 25 mg per 24 hours; 5–12 years 50–75 mg per 24 hours; > 12 years 100 mg per 24 hours. *Treatment:* 6–12 months 25 mg 12-hourly; 1–5 years 50 mg 12-hourly; 6–12 years 100 mg 12-hourly; > 12 years 200 mg 12-hourly.

Vallergan (trimeprazine). *Sedative:* 2–4 mg/kg p.o. *Antipruritic:* 1–12 months 250 µg/kg 8-hourly; 1–4 years 2.5 mg 8-hourly; 5–10 years 5 mg 8-hourly.

Vancomycin. Week 1, 15 mg/kg i.v. 12-hourly; weeks 2–4, 15 mg/kg 8-hourly; > 4 weeks, 10–15 mg/kg 6-hourly (therapeutic range, peak 25–40 mg/l, trough < 10 mg/l). Levels are measured after 2–3 days of therapy. Peak sample 30 min after end of infusion; trough sample immediately before next dose. Impaired renal function will lead to elevated serum concentrations.

Vasopressin. *Bleeding oesophageal varices:* 0.3 u/kg i.v. infusion (max. 20 units) single dose infused over 30 min.

Vigabatrin. Start at 20 mg/kg 12-hourly. This can be increased gradually to 40 to 50 mg/kg 12-hourly. Vigabatrin lowers the concentration of phenytoin.

Vitamin K. (phytomenadione) On NNU: 1 mg i.m. On postnatal ward: 1 mg p.o. For infants < 1.5 kg 0.5 mg i.m. Older children: 300µg/kg/day slowly to max. 10 mg.

Warfarin. 0.1–0.2 mg/kg per 24 hours p.o. Monitor dose with INR.

Normal values

Clinical chemistry

These values are offered as a guide only. Local labs may differ. Check normal values with the lab. you use. For less common tests check with your local lab.

Acid–base:

	pH 7.3–7.45
	PCO_2 4.5–6 KPa (32–45 mmHg)
	PO_2 11–14 KPa (80–100 mmHg)
	Bicarbonate 18–25 mmol/l
	Base excess –4 to +3 mmol/l
Alanine amino transferase (ALT)	Newborn–1 month: up to 70 iu/l; infants and children: 15–55 iu/l
Albumin	Preterm 25–45 g/l; newborn (term) 25–50 g/l; 1–3 months 30–42 g/l; 3–12 months 27–50 g/l; 1–15 years 32–50 g/l
Alkaline phosphatase	Newborn: 150–600 u/l; 6 months–9 years 250–800 u/l
Ammonia	Newborn < 80 µmol/l; infants and children < 50 µmol/l
Amylase	70–300 iu/l
Aspartate aminotrans-ferase (AST)	< 45 iu/l
Base excess	see Acid–base
Bicarbonate	see Acid–base
Bilirubin	Full term: day 1 < 65 µmol/l; day 2 < 115 µmol/l; 3–5 days < 155 µmol/l; > 1 month < 10 µmol/l
Calcium (ionised)	Adult value is 1.19–1.29 mmol/l
Calcium (total)	Preterm 1.5–2.5 mmol/l; infants 2.25–2.75 mmol/l; > 1 year 2.25–2.6 mmol/l; correction for protein binding = measured Ca^{2+} + (40-albumin/40 g/l) mmol/l
Calcium (urine)	Children < 0.1 mmol/kg per 24 hours
Chloride	95–105 mmol/l
Creatinine kinase	Newborn < 600 iu/l; 1 month < 400 iu/l; 1 year < 300 iu/l; children < 190 iu/l (male), < 130 iu/l (female)
Creatinine	0–2 years 20–50 µmol/l; 2–6 years 25–60 µmol/l; 6–12 years 30–80 µmol/l; > 12 years 65–120 µmol/l (male), 50–110 µmol/l (female)
Creatinine clearance	0–3 months 17–50 ml/min/m²; 3–12

	months 26–75 ml/min/m²; 12–18 months 36–95 ml/min/m²; 2 years– adult 50–85 ml/min/m²
Creatinine (calculation of GFR from serum level)	GFR = (49.5 × ht (cm))/plasma creatinine (μmol/l)
C-reactive protein	< 20 mg/l
Gammaglutaryl transferase (GGT)	Neonate ≤ 200 iu/l; 1 month–1 year ≤ 150 iu/l; > 1 year < 30 iu/l
Glucose	Newborn–3 days 2–5 mmol/l; > 1 week 2.5–5 mmol/l
Glycosylated haemoglobin	4.5–7.5%
Lactate	0.7–1.8 mmol/l
Liver function	see Bilirubin, AST, GGT and Protein
Magnesium	Newborn 0.7–1.2 mmol/l; child 0.7–1.0 mmol/l
Osmolality	275–295 mmol/kg
Phosphate	Preterm first month 1.4–3.4 mmol/l; full term newborn 1.2–2.9 mmol/l; 1 year 1.2–2.2 mmol/l; 2–10 years 1.0–1.8 mmol/l; >10 years 0.7–1.6 mmol/l
Potassium	0–2 weeks 3.7–6 mmol/l; 2 weeks–3 months 3.7–5.7 mmol/l; > 3 months 3.5–5 mmol/l
Protein (total)	1 month 50–70 g/l; 1 year 60–80 g/l; 1–9 years 60–81 g/l
Sodium	135–145 mmol/l
Urea	0–1 years 2.5–7.5 mmol/l; 1–7 years 3.3–6.5 mmol/l; 7–16 years 2.6–6.7 mmol/l (male), 2.5–6.0 mmol/l (female)

Haematology

Table A.2   Normal haematological indices for various ages

Age	Hb (g/dl) Mean (range)	MCV (fl) Mean (range)	WBC (× 10⁹/l) Range	Reticulocytes (%) Range
Birth	18.5 (14.5–21.5)	108 (95–116)	5–26	3–7
1 month	14.0 (10.0–16.5)	104 (85–108)	6–15	0–1
6 months	11.0 (8.5–13.5)	88 (80–96)	6–15	0–1
1 year	12.0 (10.5–13.5)	78 (70–86)	6–15	0–1
6 years	12.5 (11.5–14.0)	81 (75–88)	6–15	0–1
12 years	13.5 (11.5–14.5)	86 (77–94)	5–15	0–1

Note: An artefactual high neonatal WBC may be reported because automatic cell counters may wrongly include in the WBC the many normoblasts (red cell precursors) in the neonate.

Blood pressure

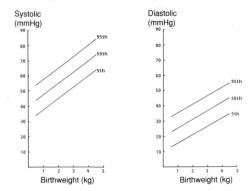

Fig. A.1 Centiles for neonatal systolic and diastolic blood pressure by birthweight (boys and girls).

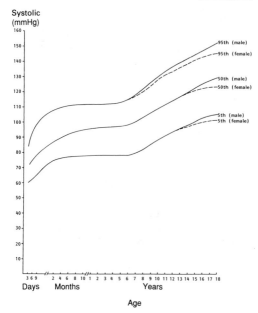

Fig. A.2 Centiles for systolic blood pressure from birth to 18 years (centiles for male and female shown separately only where they differ).

Diastolic
(mmHg)

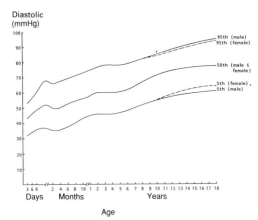

Fig. A.3 Centiles for diastolic blood pressure from birth to 18 years (centiles for male and female shown separately only where they differ).

Calculating the body surface area from height and weight

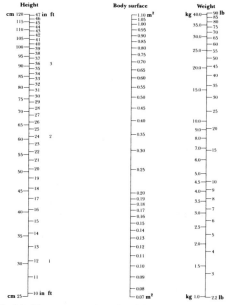

Fig. A.4 This nomogram may be used to calculate the body surface area from the weight and height of the patient. Note the patient's height on the left-hand scale and weight on the right-hand scale, and put a ruler between the two points; the point at which the line intersects the centre scale indicates the patient's body surface area.

Table A.3 Average surface area and weight at six ages

	Weight (kg)	Surface area (m²)
Newborn	3	0.2
1 year	10	0.4
3 years	15	0.6
6 years	20	0.8
10 years	30	1.0
14 years	50	1.5
Adult	70	1.7

Index

Page numbers in *italics* refer to figures and tables.

Abdominal distension, 124
Abdominal migraine, 138
Abdominal obstruction, 137
Abdominal pain, 123
  acute, 137–8
  cystic fibrosis, 114
  recurrent, 138
Abdominal X-ray
  in acute abdominal pain,
    138
  vomiting, 125
ABO incompatibility, 309
N-Acetylcysteine, 114, 262
Acid ingestion, 267
Acid–base balance, 30–1
  problems, *29*
Acidosis
  management in chronic
    renal failure, 164
  metabolic, 19–20, 30
  in metabolic disease, 183,
    184
  in total parenteral
    nutrition, 43
Actinomycin, 251–2
Acute cerebellar ataxia, 70
Acute renal failure, 158–62
  causes, *159*
  investigations, 159–60
  management, 160–2
Acute stridor, 101–6
Acyanotic congenital heart
    disease, 80, 88
Acyclovir, 201, 217, 256,
    297
Addisonian crisis, 181

Addamel, 42
Adenosine, 9–10, 91
Adenotonsillectomy
    indications, 270
Adrenal
  crisis, 180
  disorder and precocious
    puberty, 52, 53
  insufficiency, 16
  tumour, 52, 181, 182
Adrenaline, 106
  endotracheal tube
    administration, 7
Adrenocortical hypofunction,
    180–1
AIDS, 218–19
Air embolus in total
    parenteral nutrition, 44
Airway
  clearance, 2–3
  examination, 106
Alcohol, 264
Alkaline diuresis, forced,
    265, 266
Alkaline ingestion, 267
Alkalosis, metabolic, 30–1
Allergic rhinitis, 278
Allopurinol, 250
Alpha thalassaemia, *239*, 240
Ambubag, 4
Aminophylline, 115, 315–16
Amoebiasis, 220, 221–2
Amoxycillin, 211, 274
Amphotericin B, 220, 256,
    317
Ampicillin, 211, 282

Anabolic steroids, 52
Anaemia, 144, 230–40
  beta thalassaemia, 239–40
  blood transfusion, 240–1
  haemoglobinopathies,
    237–40
  haemolytic, 232–4, 237,
    305
  hypochromic, 230–2
  iron deficiency, 230–2
  macrocytic, 234–6
  management in chronic
    renal failure, 164
  normocytic, 236–7
  of prematurity, 305
Anal fissure, 134
Analgesia, 254
  in acute polyarthropathy,
    335
  for fractures, 332–3
  for wound closure, 330
Anaphylaxis, 5, 224
  cytotoxic drugs, 250
  desferrioxamine, 261
Androgens, 106
  exogenous, 52
Angio-oedema, 105–6
Angioneurotic oedema,
  105–6
Angiotensin converting
  enzyme inhibitors, 99
Ankylostoma duodenale, 223
Anorexia, iron deficiency,
  231
Anorexia nervosa, 39–40
  criteria for hospitalisation,
    40
Anoxia, 13
Antidiuretic hormone
  deficiency, 23
  inappropriate secretion,
    22, 23
Anti-tetanus treatment,
  228–9
Anticholinergic poisoning,
  262
Anticholinesterases, 207
Anticonvulsants, 14, 189,
  190

for newborn, 304
Antidotes, specific, 267–8
Antifreeze poisoning
  antidote, 268
Antihypertensive drugs, oral,
  98, 99
Antipyretic treatment, 185
Antitoxin, diphtheria, 105,
  272
Aortic atresia, 80
  treatment, 88
Apex beat, 81
Apgar score, 300, 302, 304
Apnoea
  acute, 94
  alarm, 13
  in infancy, 121
  in newborn, 315–16
  test, 325
Appendicitis, 137, 347–8
  acute, 114
Arrhythmias, 7, 80, 90–2
  complete heart block, 91
  supraventricular
    tachycardia, 90–1
  in total parenteral
    nutrition, 44
  ventricular
    tachyarrhythmias,
    91–2
Arterial blood gases, 12,
  86–7
Arthritis
  reactive, 334
  septic, 103, 210–11, 333,
    336
Arthropathy, acute, 333–4
Ascaris lumbricoides, 222
Ascites, 142, 143, 145
Ascorbic acid, 37
Asphyxia
  birth, 301, 302–4
  in newborn, 299–305
Aspirin, 216, 247
  Reye's syndrome, 201
Asthma, 22, 103, 115–17
  cystic fibrosis, 114
  inpatient management,
    115–16

Asthma (*contd*)
mild attack, 115, 116
moderate attack, 115
outpatient management, 116–17
pneumomediastinum, 112
pneumothorax, 111
severe, 115–16, 117
wheezy infant, 117, 118
Asystole, 7
following defibrillation, 9
Ataxia, 203, 205
Atracurium, 197
Atrial septal defect, 80
Atrioventricular canal defect, 80
Atropine
anticholinesterase inhibitor antidote, 268
endotracheal tube administration, 7
poisoning, 262
Auditory response cradle, 280
Augmentin, 211, 212, 273
Autoimmune disease, 209
Automatic oscillometry, 97
Azlocilline, 256

Bacterial enteritis, 134
Bacterial tracheitis, 103, 105
Bag urine sample, 152
Balanitis, 164, 344
Barbiturates, 264
Barium swallow, 106, 120, 126
Basilar herniation, 67
BCG, contraindications for immunisation, 226
Beclomethasone dipropionate, 117, 118
Beconase nasal spray, 278
Becotide, 114
Behaviour problems, 71–4
breath holding attacks, 71
odd, *186*
sleep difficulties, 72–3
sleep terrors, 72
sleep walking, 72

teething, 73–4
temper tantrums in toddlers, 71
Bell's palsy, 207
Benzodiazepines, 264
Benztropine mesylate, 264
Benzyl penicillin, 200
Bereavement, 328
Beta thalassaemias, 239–40
Beta-2 agonist, 117
Beta-blockers, *99*
Bilirubin, 310
Biotin, 184
Birth asphyxia, 87, 301, 302–4
Birthweight, milk requirements, 34
Bites
animal, 212
human, 211
Bleeding, abnormal, 243–7
investigation, 245–6
Bleeding varices, 136
Blood examination
in acute abdominal pain, 137
before liver biopsy, 145
for dehydration, 17
following resuscitation, 11
in failure to thrive, *135–6*
in liver failure, *142–3*
in systemic hypertension, 97–8
in vomiting, 125
Blood gas
analysis, 30–1
normal values, 29
Blood pressure, 5, 13, 14
in congenital heart disease, 82
measurement, 97
normal values, *364–6*
systemic hypertension, 95–6, 97, 98
Blood transfusion, 240–2
complications, 241–2
indications, 240–1
rate and volume, 241

Blood transfusion (*contd*)
    see also Exchange
        transfusion
Blue episodes, 187
Body fluid composition, *20*
Body surface area, *367*
Bone
    age, 50, 51
    demineralisation, 43
Bordetella pertussis, 107
Bottle fed infants, gastro-
    oesophageal reflux, 36
Brain death criteria, 325
Brain tumours, 191
Brainstem reflexes, 325
Breast development, 49
    asymmetrical, 49
Breast milk, 32
    contraindications, 35
Breastfeeding
    gastro-oesophageal reflux,
        35
    gastroenteritis, 36
Breath holding attacks, 71,
    187
Breathing, 3–5
Breathlessness, 94
Bricanyl, 116, 117
Bronchial tree, foreign body
    in, 106–7
Bronchiolitis, 109, 110–11
Bronchopulmonary
    dysplasia, 108–10
    management, 109–10
Bronchoscopy, 110
Broviac line, 254–5
Bruising, 243–7
Budesonide, 114, 117
Bulimia, 40
Bullous disorders, inherited,
    290
Bullous impetigo, 289
Bullous pemphigoid, 290
Burns, 291, 340–43
    assessment, 340
    electrical, 343
    extensive, 342–3
    fluid requirements,
        342–3
    minor, 340–1
    tetanus-prone, 228
    to eye, 285

C1 esterase inhibitor, 106
Café-au-lait spots, 207
Calcium, 27–9
Calcium gluconate, 7, 26
    in hypocalcaemia, 28
Calogen-LCT, 37
Caloreen, 37
Calorie nutrition in chronic
    renal failure, 163
Candida infection, 292–3
    nappy rash, 297, 298
    in newborn, 317
Candidiasis, 220
Carbamazepine, 189, *190*
Carbohydrate, 41
Carbon monoxide poisoning,
    antidote, 268
Cardiac anomalies,
    structural, 88
Cardiac arrest, 2
    ventricular tachycardia,
        91–2
Cardiac catheterisation, 87
Cardiac failure, 81
    due to patent ductus,
        89–90
    medical treatment, 88, 89
    see also Heart failure
Cardiac massage, 6
Cardiac output, 6, 15
Carnitine, 184
Carobel, 35, 36, 125
Casein based formula, 32,
    128
Cataract, congenital, 287
Catch-up growth, 38
Cefaclor, 211
Cefotaxime, 198, 199, 200,
    273
    acute mastoiditis, 274
    for meningitis, 317
Central nervous system
    depressant poisoning,
        264
    tumours, 191–2, 247

Central venous catheters, 13, 254–5
Cereals, 34
Cerebellar tumours, 70
Cerebral oedema, 13–14
  lead poisoning, 266
  in neonate, 303
Cerebral palsy, 63–5
  late walking, 69
Cerebrospinal fluid (CSF)
  in meningitis, 198, *199*
  normal, *199*
Cervical adenitis, 270–1
Cervical injury, 193
Cervical spine X-rays, 12
Charcoal
  activated, 260, 265
  slurry, 262, 263
Chelation therapy, 266–7
Chemical burns in eye, 285
Chemotherapy, metabolic
  problems, 249–50
Chest
  auscultation, 10
  disease, 22
  drain, 112
  infection, 80, 94, 113–14
Chest X-ray, 12, 86
  bronchiolitis, 110
  chronic stridor, 106
  foreign body in bronchial
    tree, 107
  pneumonia, 118, 120
  in systemic hypertension,
    97–8
  wheezy infant, 118
Chicken pox, 216–17, 226,
  289, 290, *294*
  congenital, 290
  maternal, 35
Child abuse, 318–22
  sexual, 318, 322
Chlamydia infection, 283
Chloramphenicol, 103, 105,
  210, 211, 272
  eye drops, 283
  eye ointment, 284, 285
  periorbital cellulitis, 282
Chloroquine, 221

Chlorpromazine, 253
Chlorthiazide, 110, 307
Choanal atresia, 301
Cholesteatoma, 276
Cholinesterase inhibitor
  poisoning, antidote,
  268
Chromosomal analysis, 48
Chronic systemic disease,
  delayed puberty, 50
Cimetidine, 136
Circulation, 5–10
  assessment and immediate
    management, 6–10
Circumcision, 164
Cirrhosis, 144
  causes, *144*
  in cystic fibrosis, 115
Cisplatin, 249
Clinical chemistry, normal
  values, 362–3
Clonazepam, 189, *190*
Clotrimazole, 276
Clotting
  abnormalities, 244
  factor abnormalities,
    246–7
Club foot *see* Talipes equino
  varus, congenital
Clumsy child, 70
Co-trimoxazole, 274, 275
Coagulation, 243–7
  tests, *245*
Coagulopathy, 143, 144
Coarctation of aorta, 80
  treatment, 88
Coeliac disease, 129–30
Coma, 192–4
Common cold, 269
Congenital abnormality,
  resuscitation, 301–2
Congenital adrenal
  hyperplasia, 179–80
Congenital adrenocortical
  hyperplasia,
  hyperkalaemia, 26
Congenital heart disease,
  79–94
  apex beat, 81

Congenital heart disease (*contd*)
  arrhythmias, 80, 90–2
  arterial blood gases, 86–7
  blood pressure, 82
  cardiac catheterisation, 87
  cardiac failure, 89–90
  chest X-ray, 86
  clinical diagnosis, 81–2
  cyanosis, 79–80, 81
  detected after first week, 80
  detected within first week, 80
  ECG, 82–5
  echocardiogram, 87
  embolism, 80
  heart sounds, 82
  hypertension, 80
  and immunisation, 94
  infections, 80, 94
  infective endocarditis, 92–4
  investigation, 82–7
  management, 87–8
  medical treatment, 88–94
  murmurs, 81–2
  polycythaemia, 80
  postnatal presentation, 79–80
  pulses, 81
  severe neonatal, 88–9
  signs, 81–2
  stroke, 80
  symptoms, 81
Congenital hip dislocation, 69
Conjunctivitis, 283–4
  bacterial, 283
  viral, 283–4
Connective tissue disease, 209
Consciousness
  level, 10
  loss, *186*
Constipation, 36, 123, 138–40
Constitutionally small child, 133

Continuous positive airway pressure, 109
Convulsions, 28, *186*
  post-traumatic, 195
Copper deficiency, 43
Cor pulmonale, 94–5
Corneal ulceration, 284
Coroner, 324
Cough, 94
  asthma, 116
  paroxysmal, 108
Cow's milk hypersensitivity, 37
Coxsackie A16 virus, 290
^{51}Cr albumin, 136
Cradle cap, 297
Crepitations, inspiratory, 110
Cricothyroid puncture, 102
Croup, 102, 103
Cryptorchidism, 164
CT scan, 13
Cushing's syndrome, 181–2
  obesity, 48
Cyanosis, 79–80, 81, 88, 94
  asthma, 115
  in newborn, 302
  stridor, 104
Cyproterone acetate, 52, 53
Cystic fibrosis (CF), 112–15
  antibiotics, 113
  chest infection exacerbation, 113–14
  diagnosis, 113
  meconium ileus equivalent, 114
  pneumothorax, 111
  respiratory function tests, 113
Cystitis, haemorrhagic, 252
Cytomegalovirus (CMV), 218, 241–2
Cytotoxic drugs, 250–2
  anti-emesis, 252–4
  side effects, 250, *251*

Dacryostenosis *see* Nasolacrimal duct blockage

Daily nutritional
requirements, 33
Danazol, 106
Daunorubicin, 249, 251–2
DC cardioversion, 9, 10, 91
Deafness, 280
drug-induced, 276
Death
brain death criteria, 325
certificates, 324
elective discontinuation of
treatment, 323
follow up, 328
organ donation, 325–6
post-mortem requests, 324
sudden infant death
syndrome, 326–7
on the ward, 323–4
who to inform, 324
Defibrillation, 9
Dehydration, 16–22, 130
assessment, 16
blood investigations, 17
clinical features, 16–17
estimation, 16
fluid administration, 17
hospital admission, 17
hypertonic, 16, 21–2
hypotonic, 18–20
inappropriate ADH
secretion, 22
intravenous therapy,
17–18
isotonic, 20–1
maintenance requirements,
18
management, 17–18
monitoring, 17
Delivery, high risk, 299
Dental infections, 92, 94
Dermatitis
herpetiformes, 289, 290
seborrhoeic, 297
Desamino-D-arginine
vasopressin
in diabetes insipidus, 24
fluid and electrolyte
balance, 25
Desferrioxamine, 261

Desmopressin, 167
Desquamation, 289
Development
assessment, 62–3
behaviour problems,
71–4
cerebral palsy, 63–5
clumsy child, 70
fine motor skills, 76
gross motor skills, 75
language skills, 78
late walking child, 69
mental handicap, 68–9
nervous system
maturation, 63
prematurity, 62
problems, 63–70
reflexes, 63
social skills, 77
speech, 63
spina bifida cystica, 65–7
systemic illness, 63
Dexamethasone, 14, 109–10,
178, 205, 253
Dextrolyte, 18
Dextrose in hypoglycaemia,
307
Di George syndrome, 27
stridor, 105
Diabetes, 168–76
in cystic fibrosis, 114
hypoglycaemia, 174
intercurrent illness, 171–2
surgery, 172–3
vomiting, 171
Diabetes insipidus, 16, 23–5
acute treatment, 24
aetiology, 23
diagnosis, 24
screening test, 25
Diabetic ketoacidosis, 16,
25, 168–70
bicarbonate, 171
fluid management, 169–70
insulin infusion
requirements, 170
plasma sodium, 170–1
potassium requirements,
170

Dialysis, 261
  indications for, 161
Diamorphine, 254
Diarrhoea
  acute, 126–8
  chronic, 128, 129–30
  complications, 128
  dehydration, 16
  diets for chronic, 131
  fluid replacement, 127
  gastrointestinal bleeding,
    127
  hypokalaemia, 25
  hyponatraemia, 23
  infective causes, 127
  isotonic dehydration, 20
  prevention, 127
  specific chemotherapy,
    127
  toddler, 129
  transient lactose
    intolerance, 36
  treatment, 127
  and vomiting, 123–4, 126
Diazepam, 10
  for convulsions, 263
  for newborn, 304
  for seizures, 259, 263,
    264, 266
  solvent withdrawal
    symptoms, 265
  stezolid, 185
Digoxin, 91
  toxicity, 85
Dihydrocodeine, 254
Dihydromorphine, 264
Dimercaprol, 263
Dimethicone, 17, 36, 126
Diphenhydramine, 263
Diphtheria, 105, 272
  adverse immunisation
    reactions, 227
  antitoxin, 105, 272
Disseminated intravascular
    coagulation,
    management, 247
Diuretics, 14, 99
  cause of hypokalaemia,
    25

right-sided heart failure,
  110
Dobutamine, 13
Domperidone, 191, 253
Dopamine, 13, 89
Doppler-assisted
  sphygmomanometry, 97
Down's syndrome, 68
Doxorubicin, 249, 251–2
Drowning, 14–15
  ventricular tachycardia,
    91–2
Duchenne muscular
  dystrophy, 69
Duocal, 37
Duodenal obstruction, 124
Dysmenorrhoea, 50
Dysuria, 148

Ear
  aspiration, 274
  foreign body in, 277
  wax removal, 275
Eating disorders, 39–40
Ebstein's anomaly, 80
Echinococcus granulosus,
  224
ECHO virus, 290
Echocardiogram, 87
Eczema, 289
  atopic, 296–7
Edrophonium chloride, 207
Electrocardiogram (ECG), 7,
  9, 82–5
  axis, 83
  digoxin toxicity, 85
  hypertrophy features, 84
  left atrial hypertrophy, 85
  left axis deviation, 83
  left ventricular
    hypertrophy, 84–5
  monitor, 13
  morphology, 85
  neonatal, 85
  rhythm, 83
  right atrial hypertrophy,
    85
  right axis deviation, 83
  right ventricular

Electrocardiogram (contd)
  hypertrophy, 84
  superior axis, 83
  in systemic hypertension,
    97–8
Electrolyte, requirements, *18*
Electrolytes, 23–9
  calcium, 27–9
  chloride, 26
  potassium, 25–6
  sodium, 23–5
  solutions, 17
Embolism, 80
Emotional deprivation, 318
Encephalitis, 68
  viral, 200–1
Encephalopathy, Reye's
  syndrome, 201
Encopresis, 138–40
Endocardial fibroelastosis,
  80
Endocarditis, 88
Endocrine disorders
  delayed puberty, 50
  short stature, 46, 47
Endotracheal tube (ETT), 3
  atropine adrenaline and
    lignocaine
    administration, 7, *8*
  insertion, 4–5
  for meconium stained
    liquor in newborn,
    299–300
  position, 12
  size, *4*
  for stridor, 104
Enema, 140
Energy supplements, 37
Entamoeba histolytica,
  221–2
Enterobius vermicularis,
  222–3
Entonox, 329
Enuresis, 148, 150, 165–7
  management, 166–7
Ephedrine, 273
Epiglottitis, 102, 103
Epilepsy, 63
  clumsy child, 70

spina bifida cystica, 67
Epistaxis, 278–9
Epstein–Barr virus, 218
Erythema infectiosum, *294*
Erythema multiforme, 291
Erythemas, 144, 296
Erythromycin, 211, 212
  conjunctivitis, 283
  estolate, 108
Escharotomies, 343
Essential fatty acid
  deficiency, 44
Ethosuximide, 189, *190*
Examination of newborn,
  304–5
Exanthemas of childhood,
  293, *294–5*
Exchange transfusion, 27,
  234, 260, 261, 305
  for unconjugated
    hyperbilirubinaemia,
    310, 311
  see also Blood transfusion
Exercise growth hormone
  test, 47–8
Extravasation in total
  parenteral nutrition, 44
Eyes
  chemical burns, 285
  congenital cataract, 287
  congenital glaucoma, 287
  foreign body, 285–6
  iritis, 284–5
  of newborn, 305, 317
  ocular trauma, 286
  pupillary size, 15
  thermal burns, 285
  see also Ophthalmology

Factor VIII, 218, 246
Faecal overflow, 129, 138
Failure to thrive (FTT), 38,
  130–3
  causes, 131, *132*
  child abuse, 318
  constipation, 138
  in coronary heart disease,
    81
  hepatosplenomegaly, 144

Failure to thrive (*contd*)
  inhalation pneumonia, 120
  investigations, *135–6*
  short stature, 46
  trial of feeding, 134, *147*
Fainting, 187
Fallot's cyanotic spells, 88
Fansidar, 221
Fat
  and carbohydrate
    combination, 37
  emulsion, 37
  total parenteral nutrition,
    41
Febrile convulsions, 185–7
Feeding
  bolus for newborn, 306
  of newborn, 32, 34, 305
  parental concern, 36
  problems, 35–7
  see also Eating disorders
Femoral epiphysis, slipped
    upper, 336
Fever
  electrolyte requirements,
    18
  prolonged, 209–10
Fifth disease, *294*
Flecainide, 10, 91
Floppy infant, 206
Flucloxacillin, 105, 210,
    211, 271
  in acute arthropathy, 334
  in acute mastoiditis, 274
  for impetigo, 297
  for meningitis, 317
  in otitis media, 273
  for paronychia, 317
  periorbital cellulitis, 282
Flucytosine, 317
Fludrocortisone, 179, 180,
    181
Fluids, 16–22
  balance in Reye's
    syndrome, 202
5-Fluorocytosine, 220
Folate deficiency, 235
Folic acid for newborn, 305
Folinic acid rescue, 252

Foot deformities, 336–7
Foreign bodies
  aspiration, 3
  ENT, 276–8
  in eye, 285–6
  inhalation, 106–7
  laryngeal, 277
  in nose, 277
Foreskin, 164
Formula milks, 32
Formula S, 37, 128
Fractures, 332–3
  compound, 211
  limb, 10, 329
Fragile X syndrome, 68
Friedreich's ataxia, 70
Frenectomy, 71
Friction on skin, 291
Frusemide, 110
  diuresis, 22
Fucidin, in acute
    arthropathy, 334
Fungal infections, 219–20,
    289, 292–3

G6PD deficiency, *233*, 234,
    237, 309
  precipitants of haemolysis,
    234
Galactomin, 38
Galactosaemia, 35
  soya milks, 37
Gammaglobulin, 215, 216
Gastric lavage, 259–60, 262
  hazards, 264
Gastro-oesophageal reflux
  in bottle fed infants, 36
  in breast fed baby, 35
Gastroenteritis, 126
  in breast fed baby, 36
  transient lactose
    intolerance, 36
Gastroenterology
  abdominal pain, 137–8
  bleeding varices, 136
  constipation, 138–40
  diarrhoea, 126–30
  encopresis, 138–40
  failure to thrive, 130–3

Gastroenterology (*contd*)
  gastrointestinal bleeding,
    133–4, 136
  hepatosplenomegaly,
    140–5
  jaundice, 144, *146*, 147
  liver biopsy, 144, 146
  soiling, 138–9
  vomiting, 122–6
Gastrointestinal bleeding,
  127, 133–4, 136
Gaviscon, 35, 36, 125
Genital development, 49
Genitalia, ambiguous, 178–9
Genitourinary system
  diagnostic imaging, 154
  investigation, 151–4
Gentamicin, 210, 211, 256
German measles *see* Rubella
Giardia lamblia, 222
Giardiasis, 129, 222
Gingivitis, 288
Glandular fever, 269
  see also Epstein–Barr
    virus
Glasgow Coma (GC) Scale,
  10, *11*, 140, 192, 195
Glaucoma, congenital, 287
Glomerulonephritis, 162
Glucagon, 307
Glucose, 26
  blood levels in newborn,
    306
  infusion, 184
  polymers, 37
Glue ear *see* Otitis media,
  chronic
Gluten-sensitive enteropathy
  see Coeliac disease
Glycosuria, 150
Golytely, 114
Gonadal failure, bilateral,
  50
Gonadotrophin-releasing
  hormone test, 55
Gondatrophin secreting
  tumours, precocious
  puberty, 52
Grommets, 275

Growth, 45
  disproportionate, 47
  height, 45–8
  pituitary function tests,
    53–5
  puberty, 48–53
  weight, 48
Growth hormone
  deficiency, 47
  producing tumours, 45–6
  stimulation test, 53
  suppression test, 46
Guedel airway sizes, *3*
Guthrie test, 176
Gynaecomastia, 304
  in boys, 50

Haematemesis, 133, 145
Haematological malignancy,
  248
Haematology, normal
  values, *363*
Haematoma, septal, 279
Haematuria, 149, 150
  in neonate, 303
Haemodialysis, 260
  alcohol intoxication, 264
  salicylate poisoning, 265
Haemoglobinopathies, 232,
  237–40
Haemolysis, massive, 26
Haemolytic anaemia, 232–4,
  237, 305
  classification, *233*
Haemolytic transfusion
  reactions, 241
Haemoperfusion, 260
Haemophilia, 244
Haemophilia A, 247
Haemophilus influenzae,
  210, 211
  type B, 103
Haemoptysis, 94
  in cystic fibrosis, 114
Haemorrhage, acute, blood
  transfusion, 240
Haemorrhagic disease of the
  newborn, 244, 305
Hallux valgus, 337

Hand, foot and mouth
disease, 218, 290
Hayfever *see* Allergic
rhinitis
Head
lice, 289, 292
size, 202–3, *204*
Head circumference
centiles for boys, *56*,
60–1
centiles for girls, *57*, *60–1*
Head injury, 22, 194–5
management, 329–30
Headaches, 190–1
Hearing screen, 280
Heart
atrial enlargement, 86
auscultation, 10
complete block, 91
rate, *5*
shape, 86
situs, 86
size, 86
sounds, 82
toxic effects of
hyperkalaemia, 26
Heart failure, 7, 80
right-sided, 110
see also Cardiac failure
Heart murmur, 80, 81–2
Heat
exhaustion, 338
stroke, 16, 338–9
Height, 45–8, *367*
centiles for boys, *56*, *58*
centiles for girls, *57*, *59*
estimation of mature, 45
short stature, 46–8
tall stature, 45–6
Heimlich manoeuvre, 3, 107,
277
Heinz bodies, 237
Helminth infections, 220,
222–4
Hepatic encephalopathy, 137
Hepatic problems in total
parenteral nutrition, 43
Hepatitis, 145
Hepatitis A, 147

Hepatomegaly
due to cirrhosis, 144
ventricular failure, 82
Hepatosplenomegaly,
140–5
acute liver failure, 140,
142–3, 143
causes, *141*
Herpes simplex, 290
type I (HSE), 200, 201
type II congenital, 290
Herpes zoster, 217, 290
Hickman line, 254–5
Hip
dislocation, 304
irritable, 336
problems, 336
Hirschsprung's disease, 122,
124, 138
Histoacryl glue, 330
HIV
infections, 218–19
screening of donor blood,
241
HIV-positive mother, 35
Homocystinuria, 46
Hook worm, 223
Hordeolum *see* Stye
Hormone replacement, 51
Howell–Jolly bodies, 237
Human immunoglobulin,
246
Hyaluronidase,
administration route,
252
Hydatid, 224
Hydrocele, 345–6
Hydrocephalus, 66, 195
clumsy child, 70
Hydrocortisone, 106, 179,
180, 181
in hypoglycaemia, 307
sodium succinate, 181
topical, 296, 298
Hydronephrosis, 151
Hydroxycobalamin, 184
Hyoscine, 262
Hyperammonaemia in TPN,
43

Hyperbilirubinaemia, *146*, 147
Hyperbilirubinaemia, unconjugated, 310
  exchange transfusion, 311
Hypercalcaemia, 29
  with chemotherapy, 250
Hyperglycaemia
  in diabetes, 171
  glycosuria, *150*
  in total parenteral nutrition, 43
Hyperkalaemia, 26
  with chemotherapy, 249
Hyperlipidaemia in TPN, 43
Hypernatraemia, 23
Hyperphosphataemia with chemotherapy, 249
Hypersplenism, *233*, 234
Hypertension, 80
  acute and chronic, 96
  management in chronic renal failure, 164
Hypertensive crisis, emergency treatment, *100*
Hyperthyroidism, 177–8
  TSH stimulation test, 54
Hypertonic dehydration, 21–2
Hyperuricaemia with chemotherapy, 250
Hyperventilation, 187
Hypoalbuminaemia, 27
  nephrotic syndrome, 157
Hypocalcaemia, 27–8
  stridor, 105
  in total parenteral nutrition, 43
Hypochromic anaemia, 230–2
  causes, *231*
Hypoglycaemia
  assessment, 175–6
  beyond neonatal period, 174–6
  causes, *307*
  in diabetes, 171, 174
  evaluation, *176*

management, 174
  of newborn, 306–7
  in TPN, 43
  treatment, 174–5
Hypokalaemia, 14, 25–6
Hypomagnesaemia, 27
  in total parenteral nutrition, 43
Hyponatraemia, 14, 23
  in cystic fibrosis, 114
  inappropriate ADH secretion, 22
Hypophosphataemia in total parenteral nutrition, 43
Hypoplastic left heart, 80
Hypospadias, 164
Hypotension, 13, 261
Hypothermia, 2, 339–40
  drowning, 14
  electrolyte requirements, 18
  induction, 197
  in poisoning, 264
Hypothyroidism, 176–7
  obesity, 48
  thyroid stimulating hormone stimulation test, 54
Hypotonia, *206*
Hypotonic dehydration, 18–20
  fluid requirements, 19
  management, 19–20
Hypovolaemia, 6, 7, 158, 159
Hypoxia prevention, 109
Hypoxic–ischaemic encephalopathy, *302*, 303

Ibuprofen, 185
Idiopathic hypercalcaemia of infancy, 29
Imipramine, 167
Immunisation, 224–8
  adverse reactions, 227
  anaphylactic shock, 224, 227–8

Immunisation (*contd*)
  contraindications, 225–7
  recommended schedule,
    225
Immunodeficiency, 214–15
Immunoglobulin, 226
Immunological tests, 215
Immunosuppression,
  infection with, 255–6
Impetigo, 291, 297
In–out catheterisation, 152
Indomethacin, 90
Infection, 209
  chest, 80, 113–14
  congenital, 309
  in immunosuppressed
    child, 255–6
  neonatal, *316*, 317
  prevention, 256
  severe, 22
  tinea, 293
  in TPN, 43
  transmission by
    transfusion, 241–2
  treatment, 256
  viral, 216–19
Infectious mononucleosis *see*
  Epstein–Barr virus
Infective endocarditis, 92–4
  diagnosis, 93
  investigation, 93
  prophylaxis, 92–3
  treatment, 93–4
Inflammatory bowel disease,
  129
  laboratory tests, 39
Inguinal hernia, 345
Inherited prolonged QT
  syndrome, 92
Injury, non-accidental,
  318–22
  case conference, 321–2
  head injuries, 329
  management, 320–1
  reporting, 321
  symptoms and signs,
    318–19
Injury, soft tissue, 331–2
Insect bites, 289

Insulin, 26
  formula for calculating
    daily subcutaneous
    requirement, 171
  infusion, 170
  resistance, 171
  tolerance test, 53–4
Intensive care unit (ICU),
  monitoring post-
  resuscitation, 13
Intermittent positive pressure
  ventilation
  pneumothorax, 111
  in severe heart failure, 89
Intestinal obstruction, 114
Intoeing *see* Metatarsus
  varus
Intra-arterial cannula, 13
Intracranial pressure (ICP),
  13, 14
Intracranial pressure (ICP),
  raised, 195–7
  causes, *196*
  large head size, 202
  reduction, 197
  in viral encephalitis, 201
Intralipid, 41
Intravascular volume, 5–6
Intravenous fluids, 17, *18*
Intravenous therapy,
  inadequate as cause of
  hypokalaemia, 25
Intubation IPPV, 4–5
Intussusception, 346–7
Ipecacuanha, 261, 262, 263
  hazards, 264
  paediatric syrup, 259, 261,
    265
Ipratropium, 109
  bromide, 118, 262
Iritis, 284–5
Iron
  deficiency, 43, 243
  for newborn, 305
  normal indices, *231*
  poisoning, 260–1
Iron deficiency anaemia,
  230–2
  normocytic, 236

Isomil, 37
Isoniazid, 213
Isotonic dehydration, 20–1

Jaundice, 144, 147
  beginning on days 2–5, 309
  causes, *146*
  early onset, 308–9
  hepatocellular, *146*
  management of neonatal, 310
  neonatal, 308–11
  neonatal haemolytic, 240
  obstructive, *146*
  physiological, 309
  prolonged, 309–10
Jejunal biopsy, 129–30
  examination in failure to thrive, *136*
Jerks, *186*
Joint pain, hallux valgus, 337
Juvenile pernicious anaemia, 235

Kawasaki's disease, 215–16
  thrombocytosis, 247
Kayser–Fleischer ring, 144
Klinefelter syndrome, 46
  delayed puberty, 50
Kyphoscoliosis, 67

Lacerations, 330–1
Lactation
  in newborn, 304
  see also Breastfeeding
Lactic acidosis with chemotherapy, 250
Lactose intolerance
  diarrhoea, 128
  soya milks, 37, 38
  transient, 36
Lactulose, 114, 139
  with diamorphine, 254
Laerdal mask sizes, *4*
Language
  development, 63

  regression, 63
  skills development, *78*
Laryngeal foreign bodies, 277
Laryngoscopy, 105
Late walking child, 69
Laurence Moon Biedl syndrome, obesity, 48
Laxatives in cystic fibrosis, 114
Lead poisoning and encephalopathy, 266–7
Left ventricular outflow obstruction, 80
Leukaemias, 29, 247, 248
  infection with, 255
Lignocaine, 92
  ETT administration, 7
Limb fractures, 10, 329
Limp, sudden, 335
Liquigen-MCT, 37
Liver biopsy, *143*, 145–6
Liver disease
  chronic, 39
  drugs used with caution, *145*
Liver failure
  acute, 140, *142–3*, 143
  chronic, 144–5
  investigation, *142–3*
  in Reye's syndrome, 201, 202
Lumbar puncture (LP), 12, 198, 201
Lung
  breath sounds, 107
  cyst and pneumothorax, 111
  disease, 87
  function tests, 117
  needle aspiration, 112
Lymphomas, 247
  infection with, 255

McCune–Albright syndrome, 52
Macrocephaly, *203*

Macrocytic anaemia, 234–6
  causes, *235*
Magill's forceps, 3
Malabsorption in CF, 115
Malaria, 221, *233*
Malathion shampoo, 292
Malignant disease, 209
Mallory–Weiss tear, 127,
  135
Mannitol, 14, 144
Mantoux test, 212–13, 271
Marfan syndrome, 46
Mask ventilation, 3–4
Mastoidectomy, cortical,
  275
Mastoiditis, acute, 274–5
Maxijul, 37
Measles, 216, 226, *294*
  adverse immunisation
    reactions, 227
  contraindications for
    immunisation, 226
Mebendazole, 222, 223, 224
Meconium, 304
  ileus, 114
  stained liquor, 299–300,
    302
Medication, maternal, 35
Medium chain triglyceride
  (MCT), 38
Melaena, 133, 134, 145
Menarche, 50
Meningism, 193, 198
Meningitis, 22, 68, 185,
  197–200
  hearing screen, 280
  in newborn, 317
Mental handicap, 68–9
  late walking, 69
  mild, 68
  profoundly retarded
    children, 69
  severe, 68
Mesna, 252
Metabolic acidosis, 19–20,
  30
Metabolic alkalosis, 30–1
Metabolic disease, 182–4
  vitamin-responsive

disorders, 184
Metabolic disorders, short
  stature, 46
Metacarpal fracture, 333
Metatarsal fracture, 333
Metatarsus varus, 337
Methaemoglobinaemia, 87
  poisoning antidote, 268
Methotrexate, 249
  folinic acid rescue, 252
  intrathecal, 252
Metoclopramide, 191, 253
Microcephaly, 203, *204*
Midazolam, 197
Midstream urine (MSU)
  specimen, 152
Migraine, 187, 190, 191
Migraleve, 191
Milks, 32
  in diarrhoea, 128
  quantity, 34
Mist tents, 104
MMR vaccine, 219
Molluscum contagiosum,
  293
Morphine, 197, 264
Motor skills development,
  75, *76*
Mouth-to-mouth breathing,
  3
Multicystic dysplastic
  kidney, 151
Mumps, 216, *295*
  adverse immunisation
    reactions, 227
Munchausen syndrome by
  proxy, 318
Muscle tone, 10
Myasthenia gravis, 207
Mycobacterium tuberculosis,
  212, 271
Myringotomy, 274

Nabilone, 253
Nappy rash, 297–8
Narcan, 300
Narcotics, 264
Nasal decongestants, 273
Nasal polyps, 114

Nasal trauma, 279
Nasogastric aspiration, 13
Nasolacrimal duct blockage, 284
Nausea, cytotoxic drugs, 252–4
Necator americanus, 223
Needle aspiration, 112
Neocate, 38
Neomycin, eye ointment, 285
Neonatology
    apnoea in newborn, 315–16
    examination of newborn, 304–5
    feeding, 305
    hypoglycaemia, 306–7
    infection, *316*, 317
    jaundice, 308–11
    respiratory problems, 311–15
    resuscitation and asphyxia, 299–305
Neostigmine, 207
Nephritic syndrome, 159
Nephrotic syndrome, 157–8, 159
    complications, 158
Neuroblastoma, 154, 247
    clumsy child, 70
Neurofibromatosis, 207
    precocious puberty, 52
Neurology, seizures, 185–90
Neurosurgery, 22
Neutropenia, 255
Niclosamide, 224
Night terrors, 71–2
Normocytic anaemia, 236–7
Nose
    bleed, 278–9
    foreign body in, 277
    injuries, 332
Nutramigen, 38
Nutrition
    in chronic renal failure, 163
    daily requirements, *33*

eating disorders, 39–40
in failure to thrive child, 38
feeding newborn infants, 32, 34
feeding problems, 35–7
special dietary products, 37–8
total parenteral, 40–4
weaning, 34–5
see also Total parenteral nutrition
Nutritional disorders, short stature, 46
Nutritional status, laboratory monitoring, 39
Nystatin, 256, 292

Obesity, 48
Obstruction, abdominal, 136
Ocular trauma, 286
Oedema
    nephrotic syndrome, 157
    see also Cerebral oedema
Oesophageal foreign bodies, 277–8
Oesophageal varices, 133
Oestrogen, 51
    exogenous, 52
Oilatum, 296
Oliguria, 26
Oncology, 247–57
    central venous catheters, 254–5
    pain relief, 253–4
    thrombocytopenia, 257
Ondansitron, 253
Ophthalmology
    blocked nasolacrimal duct, 284
    chemical burns, 285
    congenital cataract, 287
    congenital glaucoma, 287
    conjunctivitis, 283–4
    corneal ulceration, 284
    foreign bodies, 285–6
    iritis, 284–5
    ocular trauma, 286

Ophthalmology (*contd*)
orbital cellulitis, 282
periorbital cellulitis, 282
red eyes, 283–5
squint, 286–7
stye, 285
thermal burns, 285
vision screening, 281–2
visual impairment, 287
see also Eyes
Opticrom, 278
Oral complexion, 261
Oral fluids, 17
Orbital cellulitis, 282
Orchidometer, 47, 50
Organ donation, 325–6
Oropharyngeal airway, 3
Orthopaedics
acute arthropathy, 333–4
acute polyarthropathy, 334–5
foot deformities, 336–7
hip problems, 336
sudden limp, 335
Osteogenesis imperfecta, 320
Osteomyelitis, 210
Ostersoy, 37
Otitis externa, 276
Otitis media, 185
acute, 273–4
chronic, 275
recurrent acute, 274
Ovarian tumours, 52
Oxandrolone, 51
Oxygen
by mask, 3, 4, 10
dependency, 108–9

$PaCO_2$, 86, 87, 110
Paediatric paddles, 9
Pain relief, 253–4
Palmar erythema, 143
Pancrease, 115
PaO_2, 86, 87
Papovirus, 293
Paracetamol, 185, 187, 216, 217, 254, 256
in ENT problems, 269

in otitis externa, 276
in otitis media, 274
poisoning, 261–2
Paraldehyde, 259, 304
Paraphimosis, 344
Parasitic infections, 220–4
protozoan, 221–2
Parathyroid disease, 27, 29
Parenteral fluid requirements
of newborn, *303*
Paronychia, 317
Partial thromboplastin time, 246
Parvolex, 262
Patent ductus arteriosus, 80
cardiac failure, 89–90
Pedel, 42
Pediculosis capitis, 292
Pelvic fracture, 10
Penicillamine, 267
Penicillin, 105, 157, 271
in acute polyarthropathy, 335
conjunctivitis, 283
in diphtheria, 272
for meningitis, 317
in retropharyngeal
abscess, 272
Penicillin V, 269, 297
Pepdite/Prejomin, 38
Peri-tonsillar abscess, 271
Pericardial tamponade, 7
Periodic syndrome, 138
Periorbital cellulitis, 282
Peritoneal dialysis, 22
Peritonism, 137
Peritonitis, 348
Pernicious anaemia, 235, 236
Perthe's disease, 336
Pertussis
adverse immunisation
reactions, 227
contraindications for
immunisation, 226
Pes cavus, 337
Pes planus, 337
Petechial rash, 193

PGE infusion, 88, 89
pH monitoring, oesophageal, 126
Pharyngitis, 269
Phenobarbitone, 189, *190*, 304
Phenothiazine poisoning, 263–4
Phenytoin, 263, 264
  for fits, 339
  for newborn, 304
Phimosis, 164, 345
Photosensitive rash, 289
Phototherapy, 234, 310
Pin worm, 222–3
Piperazine, 223
Pituitary disorder
  delayed puberty, 50, 51
  precocious puberty, 52
Pituitary function tests, 53–5
  combined anterior and posterior function, 55
Pituitary tumour, 181, 182
Pityriasis rosea, 289
Plasmodium spp, 221
Platelets, 243–7
  transfusion, 246, 257
Platinum, 249
Pneumocystis pneumonia, 218, 219
  prophylaxis against, 256
Pneumomediastinum, 112
Pneumonia, 15, 103, 118–20
  antibiotics, 119, 120
  aspiration, 120
  bacterial, 118
  viral, 118
Pneumopericardium, 7, 112
Pneumothorax, 7, 10, 111–12
  asthma, 116
  PO₂, 87
Poison
  centres, 259
  removal, 259–60
Poisoning
  acid ingestion, 267

alkaline ingestion, 267
anticholinergic, 262
central nervous system depressants, 264
deliberate, 318
improvement of excretion, 260
iron, 260–1
lead, 266–7
management, 258–9
paracetamol, 261–2
phenothiazines, 263–4
salicylate, 265–6
solvent inhalation and abuse, 264–5
specific antidotes, 267–8
tricyclic antidepressants, 262
Polio
  adverse immunisation reactions, 227
  contraindications for immunisation, 226
Polyarthropathy, acute, 334–5
Polycal, 37
Polycythaemia, 80, 242–3
Polyuria, 148, 150
Pompholyx, 291
Portal hypertension, 133, 136
  due to cirrhosis, 144
Post tonsillectomy bleed, 270
Post-mortem requests, 324
Post-renal failure, 161–2
Potassium, 25–6
  canrenoate, 143
  total parenteral nutrition, 42
Prader–Willi syndrome, 48
Pre-renal failure, 160
Precocious puberty, 51–3, 179
  false, 181
Prednisolone, 114, 115, 157, 246
Pregestimil, 38, 128

Premature infants, apnoea, 121
Prochlorperazine, 253
Proctoscopy, 136
Procyclidine, 129, 263
Propylthiouracil, 178
Prosobee, 37
Protein
  intolerance, 128
  nutrition in chronic renal failure, 163
  total parenteral nutrition, 41
Proteinuria, 150
  nephrotic syndrome, 157
Prothrombin time, 246
Protozoan infections, 221–2
Pseudohermaphrodite, 178
Pseudohypoparathyroidism, 48
Pseudoseizures, hysterical, 187
Psoriasis, 289
Puberty, 47, 48–53
  delayed, 50–1
  precocious, 51–3, 179
  problems, 49–50
  stages, 49
Pubic hair, 49
Pulmonary atresia
  total, 79
  treatment, 88
Pulmonary hypertension, 94–5
  right-sided heart failure, 110
Pulmonary stenosis, 80
Pulmonary vasculature, 86
Pulmonary venous drainage, total anomalous, 80
Pulse
  in congenital heart disease, 81
  in newborn, 300
  palpation, 6
Pupillary size, 15
Purpura, 144

Pyloric stenosis, 31, 125, 347
Pyloric tumour, 125
Pyrazinamide, 213
Pyrexia of unknown origin, 208–10
Pyrimethamine, 222
Pyroxidine, 213

Quinine, 221
Quinsy see Peri–tonsillar abscess

Radiology
  examination in liver failure, 143
  in failure to thrive, 136
Radiotherapy, 250
Rebreathing into paper bag, 31
Rectal examination, 124
Rectum, empty, 139
Red blood cells
  destruction, 234
  haemolysis, 14
  rare abnormalities, 237
Red eyes, 283–5
Reflexes, 10
Reflomat, 306
Rehydration in diabetic ketoacidosis, 169–70
Renal biopsy, 154
Renal compromise, 27
Renal disease
  common presentations, 148–51
  drugs requiring caution, 165
  dysuria, 148
  glycosuria, 150
  haematuria, 149, 150
  polyuria, 148
  proteinuria, 150
  renal mass, 150–1
Renal failure, 14
  acute, 158–62
  chronic, 162–4
  hyperkalaemia, 26
  laboratory tests, 39
  in neonate, 303
  short stature, 46

Renal impairment and drug prescribing, 165
Renal mass, 150–1
    causes, 151
    investigation of solid, 154
Renal obstruction, urinary tract infection, 156
Renal osteodystrophy, management, 163
Renal replacement therapy, 164
Renal tubular defects, hypokalaemia, 25
Renal vein thrombosis, 151
Resonium, 26
Respiration in newborn, 300
Respiratory acidosis, 31
Respiratory alkalosis, 31
Respiratory arrest, 2
Respiratory distress, 111
Respiratory function tests, 113
Respiratory medicine
    acute stridor, 101–6
    apnoea in infancy, 121
    bronchiolitis, 110–11
    bronchopulmonary dysplasia, 108–10
    chronic stridor, 106
    foreign body inhalation, 106–7
    pneumonia, 118–20
    pneumothorax, 111–12
    wheezy infant, 117–18
    whooping cough, 107–8
Respiratory problems, in newborn, 311–15
Respiratory synctial virus bronchiolitis, 94
Resuscitation, 2–15
    airway, 2–3
    and asphyxia in newborn, 299–305
    baseline assessment, 10–11
    birth asphyxia, 301
    blood investigations, 11
    breathing, 3–5

    cardiopulmonary in newborn, 301
    cerebral oedema, 13–14
    circulation, 5–10
    congenital abnormality, 301–2
    drowning, 14–15
    emergency drug doses, 8
    for extensive burns, 342
    gastrointestinal bleeding, 135
    hypotension, 13
    in hypothermia, 339
    hypotonic dehydration, 19
    initial assessment and management, 2–10
    initial investigations, 11–12
    intubation intermittent positive pressure ventilation, 4–5
    management following, 303–4
    monitoring post-resuscitation, 13
    post-resuscitation care, 12
    respiratory problems of newborn, 312
    seizures, 14
    stopping, 15
    subsequent management, 10–13
    supportive management, 13–14
    transfer of child, 12–13
    trauma, 329
    very immature infant, 301
Reticulocytosis, 237
Retropharyngeal abscess, 271–2
Rewarming, 15, 339, 340
Reye's syndrome, 201–2
Rhesus haemolytic disease, 308
Rickets, 27, 28
    biochemical, 144
Rifampicin, 200, 213

Roseola infantum, *294*
Round worms, 222
Rubella, 217, *294*
  adverse immunisation
    reactions, 227
  contraindications for
    immunisation, 226
Rynacrom nasal spray,
    278

Salbutamol, 115, 116, 117
Salicylate poisoning, 265–6
Salt
  acute severe poisoning, 22
  and water balance in
    chronic renal failure,
    163–4
Salt-free infusions, 23
Sandoglobulin, 246
Sarcoid, 29
Saturation monitor, 13
Scabies, 289, 291–2
Scalded skin syndrome *see*
    Toxic epidermal
    necrolysis
Scarlet fever, *295*
Scrotal pain, 344
Scurvy, 36
Sedative poisoning, 264
Seizures, 14
  afebrile, 187–90
  control in poisoning, 259
  febrile convulsions,
    185–7
  reflex-anoxic, 187
  in Reye's syndrome, 202
Selenium deficiency, 43
Sengstaken Blakemore tube,
    136
Senokot, 139
Septic arthritis, 103, 210–11,
    333, 336
Septicaemia, 5
Sexual identity, designation,
    180
Sexual precocity, 46
  see also Precocious
    puberty
Shingles *see* Herpes zoster

Shock, 5, 6–7
  dehydration, 21
Short bowel syndrome, 39
Short stature, 46–8
  investigations, 47–8
Sickle
  disease, 238
  gene, 239
  trait, 238
Sickle cell disease, 237–9
Silastic catheter breakage,
    44
Sinus bradycardia, 7
Sinusitis, acute, 272–3
Skeletal development,
    accelerated, 52
Skeletal dysplasia, 46
Skin
  blisters and vesicles,
    289–91
  childhood infections, 290
  erythemas, 296
  exanthemas of childhood,
    293, *294–5*
  haemangioma, 136
  identification of lesions,
    288–9
  infections and infestations,
    291–3
  itchy lesions, 289
  neonatal infections,
    289–90
  palms and soles, 288–9
  viral infections, 293
  warts, 293
Skull fracture, basal, 193
Skull X-ray, 194
  for short stature, 48
Sleep
  difficulties, 71–3
  terrors, 71–2
  walking, 72
Sleep apnoea, obstructive,
    270
Smoke inhalation, 105
Social Services, 320, 321
Social skills development,
    77
Sodium, 23–5

Sodium (*contd*)
  total parenteral nutrition, 41
  valproate, 189, *190*
Sodium chromoglycate, 278
Soft tissue injuries, 331–2
Soiling, 138–9
Solvent inhalation and abuse, 264–5
Solvito N, 41
Soto's syndrome, 46
Soya milks, 37–8, 128
  in eczema, *297*
Spasms, *186*
Special formulas, 37–8
Speech
  development, 63
  therapy, 63
Spherocytosis, congenital, 309
Sphygmomanometer, 97
Spider naevi, 144
Spina bifida cystica, 65–7
  renal problems, 66–7
  shunt problems, 66
Spinal cord
  compression, 205, 207
  tumours, 191–2
Spironolactone, 110, 143, 157
Splenomegaly, 232
Squint, 286–7
Staphylococcal infections, 290
Staphylococcus aureus, 210, 211
Starvation, hypokalaemia, 25
Status epilepticus, *188*
Steatorrhoea, 123
Stenosis, severe, 79, 80
Steristrips, 330, 331
Sticky eye, 317
Stokes–Adams attack, 91, 187
Stomatitis, 288
Stools
  examination, 124, 125

frequency, 36
in failure to thrive, *134*
Stridor
  assessment, 103–4
  causes, *101*
  chronic, 106
  expiratory, 101, 104
  inspiratory, 101, 104
  intubation, 102, 103, 104, 106
  tracheostomy, 106
  and wheezing, 118
Stroke, 80
Strongyloides stercoralis, 223
Stye, 285
Sudden infant death syndrome (SIDS), 15, 326–7
  apnoea in infancy, 121
  bronchopulmonary dysplasia, 109
  near miss, 94, 327
Superficial infection in the newborn, 291
Supracondylar fracture, 332
Suprapubic aspiration, 152
Supraventricular tachycardia (SVT), 9, 90–1
Surface area and weight, 6, *367*
Surgery, 344–8
  appendicitis, 347–8
  balanitis, 344
  bile stained vomiting in infancy, 347
  diabetic patients, 172–3
  hydrocele, 345–6
  inguinal hernia, 345
  intussesception, 346–7
  paraphimosis, 344
  phimosis, 345
  pyloric stenosis, 347
  scrotal pain, 344
  umbilical hernia, 346
Sutures, 330, 331
Sweat
  examination in failure to thrive, *134*

Sweat (contd)
  examination in liver
    failure, *143*
  test, 113
Synacthen test
  prolonged, 181
  short, 180
Syringomyelia, 67
Systemic hypertension,
    95–8
  diagnosis, 97
  investigations, 97–8
  management, 98
Sytron, 232, 305

Tachypnoea, 94
Talipes equino varus,
    congenital, 336–7
Tall stature, 45–6
Tape worm, 224
Target cells, 237
Teething, 73–4
Temper tantrums in toddlers,
    71
Terbutaline *see* Bricanyl
Terfenadine, 278
Terra–Cortil, 297
Testes, 164
Testicular tumours, 52
Testicular volume, 47
  measurement, 47, 50
Testis torsion, 344
Testosterone, 51
Tetanus
  adverse immunisation
    reactions, 227
  contraindications for
    immunisation, 226
  status, 211, 212
Tetanus-prone wounds,
    228–9
Tetany, 28
Tethered cord, 67
Tetralogy of Fallot, 80, 81
  treatment, 88
Thalassaemia major, *239*,
    240
Theophylline, 117, 316
Thermal burns to eye, 285

Thiabendazole, 223, 224
Thoracotomy,
    pneumothorax, 111
Thread worm, 222–3
Thrombin time, 246
Thrombocytopenia, 243,
    244, 246
  in child with cancer,
    257
  management, 246
Thrombocytosis, 247
Thrombosis, 158
Thyroid disorder
  delayed puberty, 50
  precocious puberty, 52
Thyroid stimulating
    hormone (TSH) test,
    54–5
L–Thyroxine, 177
Tinea infections, 293
Tissue necrosis
  hyperkalaemia, 26
  in in total parenteral
    nutrition, 44
Tongue tie, 74
Tonsilitis, 185, 269
Tonsillectomy, 270, 271
Total parenteral nutrition,
    40–4
  carbohydrate, 41
  complications, 43–4
  fat, 41
  incompatibilities, 42
  laboratory monitoring,
    42–3
  minerals, 42
  potassium, 42
  protein, 41
  sodium, 41
  technical complications,
    44
  vitamins, 41
Toxacara canis, 223
Toxacara catis, 223
Toxacariasis, 223
Toxic epidermal necrolysis,
    291
Toxoplasmosis, 220
Trace elements, 42

Tracheostomy, 3, 106
  apnoea in infancy, 121
  care, 279
  obstruction of tube, 279
  tube change, 279
Trances, *186*
Transitional circulation, 79
Transposition of great
    arteries, 79
Trauma
  bruising and bleeding,
      243
  fractures, 332–3
  head injuries, 329–30
  lacerations, 330–1
  management, 329
  soft tissue injuries, 331–2
  sudden limp, 335
Tribavirin aerosol, 109
Trichinella spiralis, 223–4
Trichinosis, 223–4
Tricuspid atresia, 79
  treatment, 88
Tricyclic antidepressant
    poisoning, 262
Triglycyl lysine vasopressin,
    137
Trimeprazine, 297
Tuberculosis, 212–14
  contacts, 213
  steroids, 213–14
Tuberosclerosis, 52
Tumour/lysis syndrome,
    249–50
Turner syndrome, 46
  delayed puberty, 50, 51
  obesity, 48
Tympanocentesis, 273
Tympanostomy tubes, 274

Ultrasound scan (USS)
  antenatal diagnosis, 151
  renal mass investigation,
      151
Umbilical hernia, 346
Unsteady child, 203–4
Urinalysis, 151, 152–3
Urinary tract infection,
    155–6, 185

diagnosis, 155
investigations, 155–6
treatment, 155, 156
viral, 185
Urine
  colour, 152–3
  concentration, 153
  in diabetes insipidus, 24
  examination in failure to
      thrive, *134*
  examination in liver
      failure, *142*
  examination in vomiting,
      123–4, 125
  investigations, 12
  investigations in acute
      abdominal pain, 138
  investigations in acute
      renal failure, 159
  microscopy, 153–4
  of newborn, 304
  output, 13
  pH, 153
  sample collection, 152
  testing for poisons, 258
  tests in systemic
      hypertension, 97
Urticaria, 105–6, 289
  papular, 291

Vamin 9 glucose, 41, 42
Varicella zoster
    immunoglobulin, 217
Vascular volume, decreased,
    17
Vasculitis, 247
Vasodilators, 99
Vasopressin, 137
Venous access, 6–7
Venous thrombosis in TPN,
    44
Ventilation
  bronchiolitis, 111
  bronchopulmonary
      dysplasia, 109
Ventilator, 314, 316
  settings, *313*, *314*
Ventricular arrhythmia, 263
Ventricular fibrillation, 7, 9

Ventricular septal defect, 80
Ventricular
   tachyarrhythmias,
   91–2
Ventricular tachycardia, 9
Verapamil, 91
Verrucas, 293
Vertigo, *186*
Vesicoureteric reflux, 156
Vincristine, 251–2
Viral infections, 216–19
Viral laryngotracheo-
   bronchitis, 103
Virilisation, 52
   of females, 179, 181
Vision screening, 281–2
Visual acuity, 47
Visual fields, 47
Visual impairment, 287
Vital signs, 10
Vitalipid N, 41
Vitamin A toxicity, 29
Vitamin B$_{12}$ deficiency, 235
Vitamin C deficiency, 36–7
Vitamin D
   deficiency, 37
   for newborn, 305
   toxicity, 29
Vitamin K
   deficiency, 133, 244, 246
   for newborn, 304, 305
   warfarin antidote, 268
Vitamins
   drops, 35
   supplements in chronic
      renal failure, 163
   total parenteral nutrition,
      41
Vomiting, 122–6
   appendicitis, 348
   assessment, 123–5
   bile stained in infancy,
      347
   causes, 122–3
   chronic in baby, 125
   cystic fibrosis, 114
   cytotoxic drugs, 252–4
   dehydration, 16
   diabetic child, 171

   examination of child,
      123–5
   gastrointestinal, 122
   green, *124*
   hypokalaemia, 25
   infective causes, *127*
   investigations, 125
   management, 125–6
   systemic, 122–3
   whooping cough, 108
Von Willebrand's disease,
   246

Warfarin poisoning, antidote,
   268
Warts, 293
   anogenital, 293
Water
   deficit, 21–2
   deprivation test, 25
   intoxication, 23
Weakness, 204–7
   Bell's palsy, 207
   causes, *206*
   myasthenia gravis, 207
   spinal cord compression,
      205, 207
Weaning, 34–5
Weight, 48
   centiles for boys, *56, 58*
   centiles for girls, *57, 59*
   gain, 130
   and surface area, *6,
      367*
Wheezing, 106, 107
   asthma, 115, 116
   bronchiolitis, 110, 111
   bronchopulmonary
      dysplasia, 109–10
Wheezy infant, 117–18
Whey based formula, 32
Whip worm, 223
White cell count
   abnormalities, *248*
Whooping cough, 107–8
   immunisation, 108
   vomiting, 122
Wilms' tumour, 151, 154,
   247

Wilson's disease, 145
  clumsy child, 70
Wounds
  closure, 330–1
  tetanus-prone, 228–9
Wysoy, 37, 128

X-ray
  abdominal, 125, 138
  chest *see* Chest X-ray
  skull, 48, 194
Xylocaine, 279
Xylose absorption test in
    failure to thrive, *136*

Yankauer catheter, 2

Zinc deficiency, 43